TELe-Health

Series Editors

Fabio Capello, North Cumbria University Hospitals, Cumberland Infirmary, Carlisle, UK

Giovanni Rinaldi, Ospedali Riuniti Marche Nord, Pesaro, Italy

Giovanna Gatti, European Institute of Oncology (IEO), Milan, Italy

Recent advances in technology and medicine are rapidly changing the face of health care. A revolution is occurring in diagnosis and treatment thanks to the implementation of instrumentation and techniques deriving from engineering and research. In addition, a cultural conversion is taking place in which geographical and social boundaries are about to be overcome, resulting in enhanced availability and quality of care. Telemedicine has been considered a possible means of improving health care worldwide that is likely to change the way in which doctors deal with patients and diseases. While various restraints continue to limit the application of telemedicine in different settings and different areas of health, the innovations emerging from eHealth and telecare could stimulate a great leap forward for medicine, provided that some basic rules are taken into consideration and followed. In this series, diverse aspects of tele-health – preventive, promotive, and curative – will be covered by leading experts in the field with the aim of realizing the full potential of the new and exciting technological solutions at our disposal.

Michele Nichelatti

Mathematical Tools for Telemedicine

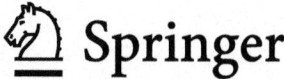 Springer

Michele Nichelatti
Division of Clinical Research
and Innovation
Niguarda Hospital
Milan, Italy

ISSN 2198-6037   ISSN 2198-6045   (electronic)
TELe-Health
ISBN 978-3-031-81708-3   ISBN 978-3-031-81709-0   (eBook)
https://doi.org/10.1007/978-3-031-81709-0

Figures by Andrea Albanese

This Springer imprint is published by the registered company Springer Nature Switzerland AG
The registered company address is: Gewerbestrasse 11, 6330 Cham, Switzerland

If disposing of this product, please recycle the paper.

To Roberta

Foreword

Telemedicine means "the ability to treat at a distance," without the need for physical contact between doctor and patient, that is, without the doctor and patient having to be in the same place at the same time. It is a very composite and multifaceted discipline, ranging from simple teleconsultation to the most sophisticated telesurgery techniques, and therefore its use is not only intended for situations in which the elderly patient is uncomfortable traveling to the nearest hospital, or to the one best equipped for the necessary therapy.

Telemedicine intervenes at the highest levels, in all situations where a patient cannot move and not only when a patient is elderly. Think of oil rig workers, merchant or military navy personnel, when moving a patient by helicopter is not feasible due to distance problems and think of the needs that arise when there are natural disasters such as earthquakes, floods, tidal waves, when local health resources and capacities are severely reduced or when they are completely eliminated.

Telemedicine is evolving rapidly, and this evolution is in turn based on the evolution of neural networks, deep learning, artificial intelligence, and the high-level mathematics that allows this series of improvements in our knowledge of basic disciplines, and that allows us to reach goals that were once unthinkable, but which are getting closer and within reach of healthcare facilities, doctors, and patients. This will improve diagnostic tools, surgical techniques, and the treatment of chronic diseases, and we can hope that the whole thing will benefit all of humanity, in every country in the world.

In this way, the innovative resources of telemedicine, already available today to most doctors in the most technologically advanced countries, will hopefully become commonplace for all doctors all over the world, and then we will be able to say that telemedicine will have contributed to making our planet a fairer place.

As already mentioned, telemedicine is largely based on the growth of knowledge about artificial intelligence, deep learning, and neural networks, and these depend on mathematical techniques, so a textbook that presents these techniques from an elementary point of view could be an interesting resource for those who have to approach telemedicine: this textbook is not a book dedicated to telemedicine, but it contains a series of essential tools for working with telemedicine.

After a very concise overview of the various aspects and issues that need to be understood in order to deal with telemedicine, which will need to be explored in greater depth in texts that deal with individual topics, the book presents the mathematical techniques that may be useful for those who want to deal with telemedicine in order to understand its fundamental basis.

The book presents the various topics, from calculus with one or more variables, to vector and matrix algebra, with its applications to statistics and epidemiology, and then moves on to more advanced topics such as differential equations and an introduction to fractional calculus.

Whenever possible, the applications of the theory to telemedicine are presented during the course of the topics, and this makes the book an interesting reference to keep on the shelf together with other books that deal with the fundamentals to be studied in depth when you are dedicated to telemedicine or when you intend to start studying it and delve deeper into it.

President of the Italian Society of   Professor Antonio Vittorino Gaddi
Telemedicine, Italy

Preface

The available literature on telemedicine is vast and tends to grow rapidly. Particularly relevant are textbooks that discuss the foundations on which telemedicine rests, from neural networks, to deep learning, to artificial intelligence, but these textbooks often have a simplified approach in the theoretical part, while other texts instead aim to present the topics of telemedicine, deep learning, neural networks, and other connected topics from an advanced mathematical approach.

Those approaching the topics of telemedicine may therefore find themselves in an uncomfortable situation if they lack all or part of the mathematical foundation necessary to understand the many excellent advanced texts offered by current publishing production.

This text aims to try to bridge this gap by presenting a quick (and obviously incomplete) exploration of the various topics in telemedicine and then offering a presentation of the mathematical foundations needed to address the same issues, so that the reader will have in front of him or her examples of applications that will hopefully be able to explain and perhaps even encourage further study of the more advanced texts.

The text has been prepared with the utmost care, but despite this, it will be possible to find any errors or omissions in it that should be blamed solely on the writer.

Milan, Italy
March 2025

Michele Nichelatti

Contents

Part I

General Introduction

A Preamble: What Is and What Telemedicine Is For

Telemedicine means assisting and treating patients at a distance, without the need for in-person contact between patient and doctor or patient and nurse, instead offering medical and nursing advice through video or radio communication systems or, otherwise, through computer-managed connections.

Telemedicine, through the remote care and monitoring of patients, offers the appropriate healthcare response to the needs of a population that is experiencing severe aging and an increase in chronic diseases (unable to move freely), but also to isolated populations in rural areas or in the mountains [1].

It is also suitable for the care of sea workers (ships, oil rigs), military personnel on missions abroad, and for many other applications where effectiveness and savings in time and resources can be combined [1, 2].

Telemedicine is one of the systems that can be applied in the redesign, restructuring, and rationalization of the healthcare system, using a number of advanced technologies and a number of innovative organizational models for home care.

To have a clear reference, we consider the definition of telemedicine given by the World Health Organization (WHO):

> "The delivery of health care services, where distance is a critical factor, by all health care professionals using information and communication technologies for the exchange of valid information for diagnosis, treatment and prevention of disease and injuries, research and evaluation, and for the continuing education of health care providers, all in the interests of advancing the health of individuals and their communities"[1]

The definition is certainly interesting, since it comes from a very authoritative source, but it should be noted that perhaps distance is not the main problem to be solved by telemedicine: probably, the critical factor is the possibility of connection between the patient and the healthcare provider.

---

[1] See *WHO. A health telematics policy in support of WHO's Health-For-All strategy for global health development: report of the WHO group consultation on health telematics, 11–16 December, Geneva, 1997. Geneva, World Health Organization, 1998.*

M. Nichelatti, *Mathematical Tools for Telemedicine*, TELe-Health, https://doi.org/10.1007/978-3-031-81709-0_1

This possibility of connection is related to many factors: the availability of fast communication lines, the availability to the patient of hardware systems, if not constantly updated, at least capable of handling the dialog at a distance. Not least, the ability of the patient and relatives, to use the hardware and software appropriately.

In some countries, there was an attitude of mistrust toward telemedicine, because there were fears that medical errors would be realized through doctor–patient conversations without the presence of both of them in a suitable clinic for examination and diagnosis, so this non-positive attitude occurred. However, it was the practice of telemedicine that dispelled these doubts, when it was put to the test, and under conditions that were certainly not easy, at the beginning of the COVID pandemic, and throughout its duration, so doubts about its effectiveness were put aside.

Many health-related computing applications are now available for ordinary smartphones, just as the evolution of telemedicine has also been supported by artificial intelligence and machine learning, with which one can converse naturally and discursively, such as chatbots, which have now become commonplace tools not only in the medical field.

1.1   Telemedicine at a Glance

The word telemedicine refers to all health and care, nursing, psychological, and other services in which using standard and innovative technologies, such that it is no longer necessary for the patient and the health professional to be in the same place (and sometimes not even at the same time).

Telemedicine makes it possible to:

- assist patients and make follow-up visits
- remotely monitor patients' vital parameters
- have health professionals talk to each other for consultations related to particular clinical situations
- send and receive health documents, diagnoses, and reports
- efficiently send images, X-rays, CT scans, MRIs, PET scans, and more

Telemedicine is especially indispensable for those people with chronic or degenerative conditions who require continuous care. For these patients, constant monitoring of clinical conditions and vital parameters (all or only some particulars) may be necessary in order to reduce the risk of compplications and to follow clinical progress [2–4].

In this case, it is then possible to provide better service to the patient, through a quick distribution of information about the subject's health among healthcare professionals, allowing the involvement of specialists who acting outside their local area can help medical and nursing care managers to work at their best, in normal conditions but also in urgent conditions, improving the quality of services for patients and increasing the timeliness of responses to its contingent needs.

The constant evolution of communication and data transmission technologies makes it possible to count on both increasing efficiency and security in the areas of telemedicine and increasing protection of confidentiality and sensitive patient data, remembering that health data are at the top of the list of sensitive data.

Telemedicine represents one of the main areas of development in public and private health care, offering all, or (at present) almost all, of the potential needed to:

- improve equity in access to health and care services
- carry out much of the healthcare activities that are needed in areas that are distant from major hospitals, in sparsely populated and isolated areas, whether for geographical reasons or for reasons caused by environmental disasters such as floods, earthquakes, tornadoes, tidal waves, and more
- improve home care both qualitatively and quantitatively
- decentralize service delivery
- distribute human (in terms of professional expertise) and instrumental resources equitably, among different healthcare managers
- facilitate access to health care for those who are frail, or elderly, or who otherwise lack the financial resources to travel to hospitals

1.2   A Closer Look

It is not widely known that NASA (North American Space Agency) was one of the first companies to get involved and invest in telemedicine back in the 1960s, when it had to take care of the health monitoring of astronauts on the Mercury, Gemini, and Apollo missions (specifically, with regard to the Apollo 13 mission) to record the data and send it back to Earth to mission control at Cape Canaveral.[2] Actually, although almost sensational, this is a very good example of how telemedicine can work.[3]

Only later did the technology used for telemedicine spread to rural areas, to territories lacking efficient and modern healthcare facilities. But probably the best innovation for telemedicine is thanks to the birth of teleconferencing technology, a method widely used today in various fields of everyday work. With video conferencing, information is exchanged in real time between interlocutors, allowing not only communication between doctors where information could be transmitted in real time from one interlocutor to another and vice versa but also enabling communication between doctors, for example, for a consultation.

---

[2] See https://hbr.org/2017/07/how-nasa-uses-telemedicine-to-care-for-astronauts-in-space.

[3] See   https://www.nasa.gov/humans-in-space/innovative-3d-telemedicine-to-help-keep-astronauts-healthy/.

So telemedicine is not only diagnosis and therapy done remotely, but it is a real integration of biomedical knowledge with the most advanced technology that can be used in data transmission, so that the latency time between need and treatment is increasingly reduced. This will mean faster and more reliable care and therefore greater trust between healthcare staff and patient.

The use of information technology in the medical field is part of the natural evolution of medicine, which first passed through knowledge derived from biochemistry and genetics, and then made available to innovations derived from computer science and telecommunications engineering, and applied to biomedical instrumentation starting from measurement methods to sensors that exploit nanotechnologies and which are used for the translation and transfer of information.

Technology, although expensive in terms of investment, is able to yield much more than what is invested, in terms of safety and environmental protection. It is enough to verify how a televisit constitutes a significant saving of time (no time has to be spent on the travel of the doctor or patient) and resources, because the expenses for travel are no longer necessary, and the production of combustion gases from engines (airplanes, ships, cars, trains) or power plants (gas, diesel, coal, other combustible material) that produce electricity is reduced.

Then, it is known that technology advances at an unthinkable speed, and therefore, the use of technologies promotes research on increasingly advanced technologies.

We have already mentioned how engineering progress is driving the development of telemedicine: the ability of engineering to evolve depends on the evolution of mathematical modeling, and this is a consequence of the availability of increasingly advanced software, capable of carrying out very complex mathematical operations in very short times. It will be easy to verify how these software advances also depend on the development of highly advanced computer techniques, based on artificial intelligence. Artificial intelligence, which is a large part of telemedicine, will create a real ecosystem in the future where pure and applied mathematics will find a development that is probably still unthinkable today.

At the same time, the ever-increasing computer capabilities, the new types of chips for calculation (it is likely that quantum computers will soon arrive on the consumer market), and the space available for servers, as well as the data transmission technique and their storage, will allow us to improve patient services while respecting their discretion and privacy.

The availability of big data and data mining techniques will allow us to discard redundant or useless information, to clean it from background noise and parasitic signals, so as to make the most of the analytical capabilities to make predictions about the future of patients and to find hidden correlations between the variables, which these techniques reveal and bring to light. In this way, the quality of information improves and at the same time both the health needs of patients and the needs for efficiency and resource management of public and private healthcare companies are satisfied.

According to a well-known rule that some statisticians call "garbage in, garbage out," you have to work with reliable and clean data. Patient data must be collected free (or at least almost completely free) of errors, must then be translated into error-free signals, and must be transmitted to the recipient equally free of errors, so that the recipient can interpret them correctly and then transform them into a diagnosis. The errors that occur in the collection of information are called "bias" and are real distortions that are almost impossible to remedy. If a sensor is calibrated to work with the units of measurement of the imperial system (feet, yards, ounces, gallons, etc.), the transmitted data will be completely distorted if read by a detector that uses the units of measurement of the international system (meters, kilograms, liters, etc.). The error that occurs during data collection will be transmitted throughout all the processing phases, up to the final result, so that an impeccable processing will be possible and without calculation errors, but with errors in the result. Just like a project for the construction of a skyscraper: the project will be exact in every detail, the calculations for the stability of the structures will be perfect, but if mud is used instead of concrete, the building will collapse.

So the data must be collected accurately, and all efforts must be made and all methods must be performed to exclude errors, just as the data must be checked even after being collected, immediately before their processing. But also the algorithms used for processing must be transparent, crystal-clear, and checked. Only in this way will the results be reliable and usable correctly.

So it seems clear that medicine is constituted starting from a strategic project that has health as its objective, and therefore, telemedicine cannot be seen as the collection of different and incoherent parts, adjusted and assembled as needed: this is not telemedicine. Telemedicine is analysis of needs, identification of problems and search for solutions, which must be obtained from economic, financial, and legal analyses, and from the constant search for an ethical service, which protects the privacy and dignity of patients who are people, and not the numbers of beds where they are hospitalized.

So telemedicine is also protection of the most fragile, it is confidentiality, it is protection of privacy, and all this starts from the protection of data and information collected.

Telemedicine therefore also means interdisciplinary medicine in which all the experiences gathered in the field must be integrated to create something that is not an alternative to traditional medicine in presence, as some might have understood. Telemedicine and medicine in presence must be integrated, just as rescue by ambulance is integrated with that by air ambulance: in some cases, the first option is preferable, in others the second. Telemedicine arrives quickly where traditional medicine would arrive slowly, or telemedicine is able to act in emergency conditions (we all remember what happened with the recent pandemic) so the purpose of telemedicine is not the elimination of medicine in presence, but the replacement of situations in which telemedicine could give a better or faster response than that which medicine in presence would give.

Telemedicine therefore means treating patients remotely, using all the technologies available to be able to do so quickly and economically.

1.3   e-Health

E-Health (or simply eHealth) is often used as an alternative name for telemedicine and perhaps rightly so, because the difference, if you like, is very nuanced and subtle. e-Health is a set of health services that manifest themselves as practical technological applications.

Thus, e-Health would refer to systems used to help doctors formulate a diagnosis, based on the cataloging of symptoms, e-Health contains the electronic prescription and the electronic medical record, as well as all the digital and technical aids to help doctors and nurses, as well as telesurgery systems to operate remotely and data collection systems through wearable biosensors. The difference between e-Health and telemedicine is therefore not perfectly delineated, and it is understandable that in some cases these two terms are used as synonyms.

1.4   Some Definitions in Telemedicine

Within the scope of practical activities and general competencies of telemedicine, we can define the following ones [1–4].

- **Televisit**. The physician interacts remotely and in real time with the patient, in the case even through an assistant. But the televisit cannot be the first medical examination, which must be carried out in the doctor's office, nor can it replace an outpatient visit when one is necessary: the decision on this is up to the treating physician, who must judge according to the patient's best interest. During the televised visit, the physician may use all available telemedicine tools to acquire the clinical data he or she needs. Tele-transmission is, of course, subject to the availability at the patient's home of adequate hardware and software facilities for receiving and transmitting data.
- **Telereferral**. Basically, it is the situation that occurs when a physician, usually a specialist, issues a report not in the presence, but with the patient remote: the report is the medical act that defines a telediagnosis. It is therefore based on the digital communication of documents, which are sent to physicians who have requested them (e.g., the family doctor). It obviously requires the availability of the patient and possibly a caregiver to interface between doctor and patient, if necessary, or if there is some tool to be used to collect some data needed to make the report. Given the importance of telereferral, it is necessary that the tools for communication and transmission of data and files be properly verified.
- **Teleconsultation**. It can take place between physicians or between healthcare personnel with different skills In the first case, a physician interacts with other physicians located remotely to get a consultation, therapeutic direction, or diagnostic opinion, which is then requested from physicians with specific clinical experience in the pathology from which the patient suffers, with whom the physician shares the available information (vital signs, images, electrocardio-

graphic tracings, etc.) in digital format, and thus transmissible in real time or even asynchronously if the patient's condition allows it and if the patient himself does not participate. In the second case, it is a type of advice given by a healthcare provider instructing other staff on a given procedure, whether in the presence of the patient or not. These are situations that help healthcare staff make a position or decision on a given clinical or care problem.

- **Teleassistance**. This is a situation in which healthcare personnel, not necessarily physicians, may contact the remote patient to get or request information about treatment, satisfaction, or other topics, such as administering a questionnaire to obtain a score that quantifies (downward or upward) the severity of the illness, or identifies the patient's "nonmedical" needs. Contacts are generally repeated at a set frequency to monitor the condition of the patient.

References

1. Gogia SB (ed.) Fundamentals of telemedicine and telehealth. New York: Academic Press; 2019.
2. Khandpur RS. Telemedicine: technology and applications (mHealth, TeleHealth and eHealth). Dehli: PHI Learning; 2017.
3. McGrath B. Telemedcine and telehealth. New York: Hayle Medical; 2019.
4. Sorkin C. Field guide to telehealth and telemedicine for nurse practitioners and other healthcare providers. New York: Springer Publishing; 2021.

How the Brain Works

The brain is an organ weighting about 1.4 kg, with a volume of 1.3 l, and a total surface area of about 2,500 cm^2 (e.g., 0.25 m^2, which are equivalent to four A4 paper sheets). The brain is part of the central nervous system (CNS) together with the medulla oblongata, the cerebellum, and the spinal cord (note that in the brain, the gray matter is external and the white matter is internal, while in the spinal cord, the gray matter is internal and the white matter is external). The peripheral nervous system (PNS) consists mainly of the nerves that leave the spinal cord and go to the various organs and districts of the body. Functionally, there is also the autonomic nervous system, which we will not deal with, however.

2.1 Neurons and Synapses

The brain is essentially formed by some hundreds of billions of cells, which in most cases have tasks of processing and transmitting communications by means of electrical signals (the neurons, or nerve cells, which are about 10^{11} in the brain), and in many other cases instead dedicated to other tasks, such as those of structural, mechanical, and metabolic support. A schematic design of a neuron is given in Fig. 2.1, where the most relevant anatomic features are also shown. Each nerve cell connects to an average of 10 thousand other nerve cells by means of a series of cellular structures: the axon for outgoing communication, i.e., going from the neuron to other neurons (the axon coming out of the neuron is unique, although along its path the axon may branch), and the dendrites for direct communication to the neuron coming from other neurons [1]. Neurons are cells endowed with certain anatomo-physiological features that enable them to send electrical signals determined by depolarization of the cytoplasmic membrane that is self-transported along a thin tube (the axon) lined with an insulating sheath of myelin, as shown in Fig. 2.2, just as every electrical wire is lined with an insulating sheath of plastic.

© The Author(s), under exclusive license to Springer Nature Switzerland AG 2025　　11
M. Nichelatti, *Mathematical Tools for Telemedicine*, TELe-Health,
https://doi.org/10.1007/978-3-031-81709-0_2

Fig. 2.1 Neuron

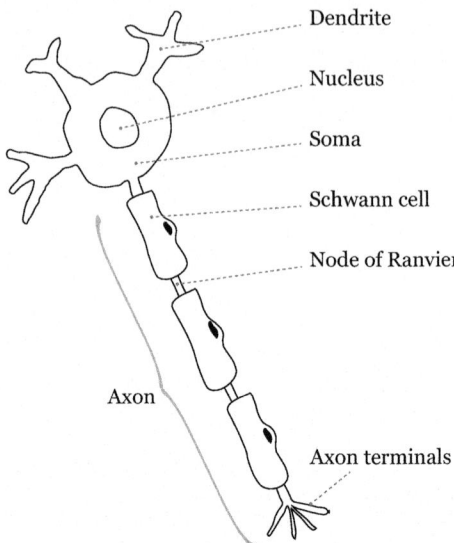

Dendrite

Nucleus

Soma

Schwann cell

Node of Ranvier

Axon

Axon terminals

Fig. 2.2 Myelin Sheath

Axon

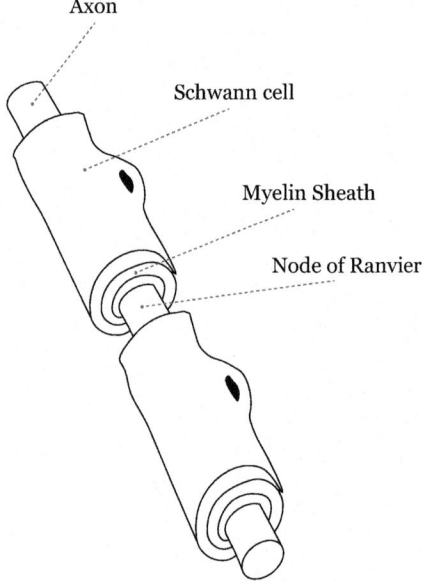

Schwann cell

Myelin Sheath

Node of Ranvier

Generally, the axon (one per neuron, but it can be branched) starts from the nervous cell body and reaches other neurons by transmitting depolarization to them as well, which will then send the signal again to other neurons, until the signal (transmitted along a nerve consisting of a bundle of axons) reaches an effector (a muscle, a gland, and so on) that will respond to the nerve signal by producing a

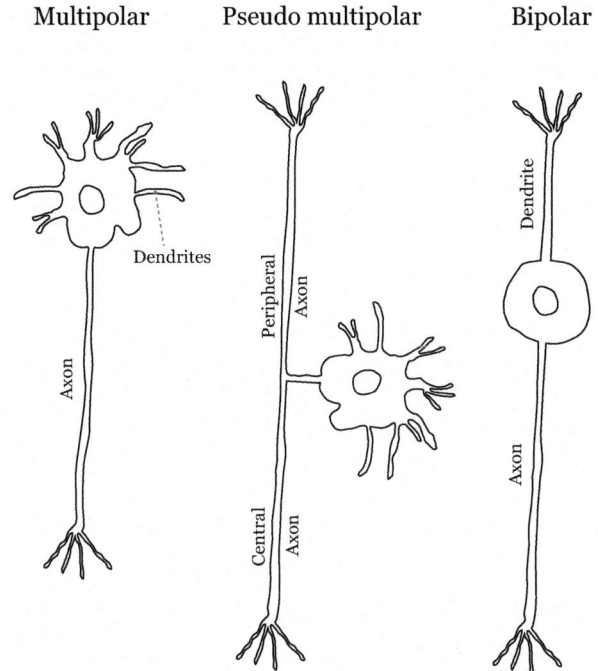

Fig. 2.3 Types of neurons

response (e.g., contraction of a muscle). Some examples of neurons with specific axon structures are presented in Fig. 2.3.

The connection between neurons is allowed by some micoscopic structures called synapses [1].

Synapses are not physical connections between neurons: from an axon carrying the message of the first neuron to the dendrites of the second neuron, there is in fact no real contact, but a small gap. Here, the incoming electrical signal is converted into a chemical signal by the release of certain neurotransmitters, substances that are captured by receptors in the cell membrane of the second neuron. Here the reverse process takes place, and the chemical signal becomes an electrical signal that will be propagated along the axon. It should be pointed out that walking along the axon, the electrical signal propagates in jumps along the nodes of Ranvier, which are the points that the myelin sheath leaves uncovered. It is as if along a normal electrical cable there are breaks in the insulating sheath. Thanks to this jumping pathway, the electrical signal in the brain can reach the speed of 430 km/h.

Nerve cells cannot reproduce or regenerate, so when they die, they are not replaced. The mortality of nerve cells is unsuspectedly high, and reaches after the age of 30 years to about 100 thousand per day, that is, about 4,200 per hour, and 1.2 per second (and to summarize, this corresponds to the loss of about 3.7×10^7 neurons each year); however, the high mortality of neurons does not turn into a decline in cognitive and learning abilities, in fact the reduction of neurons is compensated by the formation of new connections between surviving neurons. This ability to build new synapses and improve communication between neurons and to find new pathways for nerve signal transit is called brain plasticity. Brain plasticity is also responsible for the brain's ability to allow recovery of many functions after localized injury, even if quite severe.

The neurons are among the cells forming the brain, but they form also the nerves that run throughout our bodies, carrying electrical signals from the periphery to the center (by transmitting, for example, the perception of a mosquito bite on an arm) and then from the center to the periphery (causing the movement of a hand chasing the mosquito away from our arm). The reaction can be voluntary or even (partially) involuntary: think, for example, of it happening at night while we sleep.

When a neuron sends a signal to another neuron or cell, the signal can be excitatory, inhibitory, or modulating. Transmission from one cell to another occurs through the mediation of certain molecules that are located in the space between the transmitting and receiving neuron: the incoming signal ruptures certain vesicles that release molecules capable of activating depolarization in the receiving cell. Neurons are connected in real networks that determine pathways and circuits for the passage of signals.

Along with neurons, the nervous system is equipped with other cells that function to perform the task of mechanical scaffolding and metabolic support: these are the glial cells (or simply *glia*). Glial cells are not actively involved in nerve signal transmission, although we will see that one type of glia cells forms the insulating sheath that covers the axon cord. It may be surprising to learn that glia cells are much more numerous than neurons (up to ten times as many, so about the 90% of brain cells are used to maintain and to sustain the remaining 10%), but this, on reflection, was actually to be expected given the tasks they have to perform. Glial cells retain the ability to replicate, which is lost by neurons.

Among glial cells, we recognize the astrocytes (protoplasmic, found in the gray matter of the CNS, and fibrous, found in the white matter), the oligodendrocytes, and the ependymal cells; of great importance are Schwann cells, which line the single axons of neurons with the myelin sheath, isolating the axon cord from surrounding tissues and allowing efficient transmission of the nerve signal. Schwann cells roll up on themselves and wrap around axons with multiple turns, coating them with the myelin sheath, which is formed by their cell membrane. Given their coiling shape, they have a very flattened structure with a reduced capacity for energy production.

Each individual Schwann cell envelops only one tract of axon, so each axon has a myelin sheath formed by multiple Schwann cells; between one Schwann cell and another, the myelin sheath is interrupted for a short distance, so the axon is not covered: these unmyelinated tracts of the axon are called nodes of Ranvier. Between one node of ranvier and another, there is only one Schwann cell wrapping around the axon.

Important among the gray matter cells are the interfascicular oligodendrocytes, which are responsible for the formation and maintenance of the myelin sheath. Their task is similar to that of Schwann cells, except that the latter wrap only one axon, whereas fascicular oligodendrocytes wrap multiple axons.

The brain, whose mass is about 2% of our body, has very strong energy demands, so much so that it consumes more than 20% of the daily energy that comes in through food. Neurons feed on glucose and are unable instead to use for energy purposes proteins or lipids, nor to derive sugars from them. From a structural and functional point of view, this represents an advantage: if neurons during fasting perides could break down lipids for energy purposes in order to obtain the necessary glucose, the myelin sheath (which is very rich in lipids) would be the first target at which neurons would aim (as is the case in multiple sclerosis), and this would prevent the normal functioning of the neuron itself, but also the functioning of the whole brain.

Instead, when one is in the stages of prolonged fasting, the brain obtains sugar by activating a controlled breakdown of muscle proteins, as happens in the glucose–alanine cycle during intensive physical exercise. In simple terms, amino acids (stripped of their amino group) are used to produce energy in the muscles (particularly branched-chain amino acids); instead, the amino group is used together with pyruvic acid to release alanine (an amino acid), which is captured by the liver. Here, the alanine is converted back into pyruvic acid with which the liver produces glucose, which is put into the bloodstream to make it available to the brain at a constant level. Of course, during prolonged fasting, while the brain consumes muscle protein, the rest of the body consumes fat.

2.2   The Central Nervous System (CNS)

Our brain is capable of performing about 1.0×10^{15} processing operations per second (for the most part, without us being aware of it), and holds about 4.7 bits of information per single synapse.

Despite this obvious processing capacity, the amount of information reaching the brain that comes from external (visual, olfactory, tactile, auditory, gustatory) and internal (hormonal, functional, etc.) stimuli is indeed a lot and must be constantly classified and interpreted. To cope with this continuous demand, the brain is aided by the central nervous system (CNS), which, in addition to the brain itself, is composed of the cerebellum (which is responsible for static and dynamic body balance and movement), the medulla oblongata (responsible for, among other things, the various control systems for example, hearing, respiration, and blood pressure), the pons (which is a kind of coordination system for the various sensory and motor transmissions), the midbrain (which is responsible for processing the interconnections between the various motor systems), and the spinal cord (a nerve bundle about 50 cm long—but the length depends on individual height—and protected by the spine that connects nerves from the various districts, in both directions, to the brain).

2.3   How the Brain Stores Information and Learns

Assume that we repeatedly have the same sensory experience, such as smelling a rose (olfactory experience), reading aloud a poem (visual and auditory experience), or listening to a song (another dual experience, made up of music and words).

Depending on personal skills, we should be able to memorize the smell of the rose (not necessarily remembering it, but at least recognizing it among other floral aromas), and in the long run, we should be able to memorize the poem and the song (probably first the music and then the lyrics). In some cases, this memory is permanent (indelible), to the point where we can recite even at 60 years old poems learned when we were children, and to the point where we can sing "Across the universe" by the Fab Four, without getting a single word wrong.

Similarly, we will be able to remember the plot of a movie, recognize a person's face and associate it with a name, evoke a pleasant or unpleasant event that happened many years ago. So we can be sure: our brains process experiences and turn them into memories: in some cases. these are permanent or almost permanent memories, while in other cases, they are short-term memories, which is why, for example, we need a diary where we can mark phone numbers, and always for this reason, even if we recite from memory a poem from 60 years ago, we forget where we left the phone we were holding 5 min ago.

Consequently, we are certain that stored information resides inside the brain, but it is extremely more interesting to understand how it enters our brain. If we look several times at the face of our new colleague at work, the information traveling along the optic nerve will arrive in the area of the brain devoted to handling visual information by passing along an unspecified but very large number of synapses.

As the same signal passes through the same neuronal pathway again, it becomes a kind of highway, where passage is facilitated by "route knowledge." This is what happens when a motorist travels along a road: the first few times his route will be cautious, while after a few times, the motorist will have learned to know the road, will know where there are critical points, where one can speed up, and where one must slow down, and thus, the road will be traveled with increasing efficiency. Thus, signals will also travel along the axon sequence to the brain, with a delineated path, helping memorization [2, 3].

Although the situation is quite clear, our information storage is not a single package that contains everything. So by memorizing a face or a song, or a text, or a tasty dish just eaten in a restaurant, the memory will be fragmented and dispersed in the various districts of the brain dedicated to memorizing the various components of the information, such as words, musical notes, taste, and smell, and when the time comes to recall the memory (the taste of an ice cream), the brain will be able to reassemble the fragments that make it up (the creaminess, the texture, the scent, and more), allowing us to reconstruct the feeling we experienced when we tasted that ice cream. It's easy enough to believe that anyone, without needing to concentrate very hard, is able to remember the smell of an apple pie fresh out of the oven.

Storage of information is due not only to the facilitated transmission along the sequence of neurons, and the unpacking of the overall information that is transformed into its qualitative and quantitative components, but also to the brain's ability to remodel its synapses, to destroy old synapses, and build new synapses. The terminal synapses of an axon can be superstressed onto a new dendrite in order to make possible new connections with other neurons that were previously unreachable. Consequently, the good function of our brain is largely due to its plasticity and its adaptation to new working conditions. For these purposes, the brain must be adequately nourished and have the availability of certain proteins, which serve as adjuvants of synaptic transduction and as drivers of structural shifts and the rearrangement of axons and dendrites in two adjacent neurons.

Studying a new language, or applying ourselves in the study of mathematics or physics, or other scientific disciplines, or learning to draw, are all activities by which we can help brain renewal, or by which we can take advantage of its plasticity.

The study of learning in the brain is possible thanks to certain neuroimaging techniques, it is possible to discover the "physical" path taken by information as they make evident the brain areas that are activated upon receiving a stimulus or producing a response, as an effect of the stimulus [1–3].

Learning takes advantage of the brain plasticity we have just mentioned, based on the a rule of "confidence" in traveling a neuronal pathway and based on the need to frequently and regularly stimulate the synapses of interest. So to learn well the rule of derivation of a given function, one must practice performing the calculation over and over again, until one has understood the method and made it one's own ("to understand" means to make an idea one's own, to carry it within oneself). Thus, as we have seen in our experiences as students, to learn a concept it is necessary to study it over and over again, so that the synapses in the neuronal pathway are stimulated and activated constantly. But the stimulus must be active: we must not only memorize, we must learn to communicate what we have learned, and this is done when we discuss the topic with others, when we listen to them, and when we transmit our knowledge to others, forcing the neurons to remain active. This is what happens during a classroom question or during a learning test.

Our organism listens to us and rewards us: when we learn adequately, when we perform positively a math exercise on the blackboard, or when we manage to tell a piece of the history of the Roman empire correctly, we feel satisfied because we are rewarded by activating reward methods with the production of dopamine, a chemical substance linked to satisfaction with the achievement of a goal, and which stimulates us to continue along the same path, and to continue with the same method. Exactly as it happens to those who, undergoing a food diet and a gymnastic exercise program, feel satisfied and gratified reading on the scale that they have lost the first kilograms of their fitness plan and are driven to continue.

2.4   Intelligence

It is not at all easy to give a definition of intelligence, mainly because there is no unambiguously accepted definition of it. On the contrary, according to psychologist Howard Gardner (b. 1943), there would exist eight different types of intelligence, namely: (1) linguistic intelligence, as the ability to use words correctly in a given context; (2) mathematical and logical intelligence, which enables one to perform even very complex logical and mathematical calculations, using the deductive method; (3) kinesthetic intelligence, which governs the mastery of the body and the coordination of its movements; (4) spatial and visual intelligence, which enables one to process and store information about one's surroundings outdoors and indoors; (5) musical intelligence, which has to do with understanding and processing notes and harmonies and melodies and with talent in the study of the same; (6) interpersonal intelligence, which enables one to understand one's neighbor, to understand his or her point of view, and to empathize with him or her; (7) intrapersonal intelligence, which enables one to understand aspects of one's personality, and which would be a mirror aspect of intrapersonal intelligence; (8) naturalistic intelligence, which is the ability to recognize and classify natural objects such as animal, plants, water, and stones [3, 4].

Other possible kinds of intelligence are sometimes cited: they are the theoretical intelligence, which would correspond to the ability to reason about existential and universal problems, consciousness, or the sistence of God, and so on, and the teaching intelligente, which would correspond to the ability to teach concepts to someone else, and therefore would not belong to the domain of interpersonal intelligence, or logical-mathematical intelligence. Actually, the ability to abstract logical-mathematical concepts may well be associated with a limited ability to transmit them to students: that is, being good thinkers (in any field of knowledge) does not mean being good teachers as well.

Thus, we could define intelligence in a first approximation as being endowed with certain talents and the ability to perform certain activities associated with these same talents.

With these conceptual nuances for the definition of intelligence, possibly, the intelligence quotient(IQ) is mainly to be attributed to an estimate of logical-mathematical intelligence alone.

In practical terms, however, we might consider intelligence as the ability to solve problems never previously faced, that is, to cope with unexpected and new situations.

More generally, we may instead consider intellligence to be a set of mental faculties that enable, through the ability to learn from experience, the meaning of events that occur, adjusting one's attitude and behavior in order to achieve a specific purpose, having perceived and interpreted the information coming from the environment, adapting to it, and retaining memory of it for the future.

Intelligence is not only man's heritage, since animals are endowed with their own individual intelligence (going so far in the case of chimpanzees as to produce tools to be used to obtain food), which enables them to practice hunting, to build even very elaborate dens (such as those of beavers or prairie dogs), and to move with such a sense of direction that they can find their nests after a flight of thousands of kilometers (such as swallows). In addition to individual intelligence, mention should also be made of the possible collective intelligence (which could be attributable to a kind of "collective brain") typical of some insects living in colonies, such as bees and ants.

Not to be forgotten is the new, and in some respects controversial, discipline called plant neurobiology, which deals with the possibility that higher plants are able to receive information and stimuli from the external environment and from other plants and are able to respond to these stimuli. Plants are not endowed with cells resembling animal nerve cells that can propagate stimuli internally, but in spite of this, plant neurobiology is also a very interesting discipline because of its possible future prospects, and still worthy of attention. Recall that plants do work that is indispensable to life all over the planet, creating living tissue from the water and the carbon dioxide in the air, capturing energy to do this work from sunlight. Studying them better and trying to understand the nature of their response to stimuli (a sunflower flower that moves following the apparent movement of the sun, a daisy that opens in the morning and closes in the evening), is certainly an extraordinarily interesting activity.

Intelligence is not only individual: one can very well speak of collective intelligence when an entire population behaves as if it were governed by a single brain. This is the case with bees and especially with ants.

Bees concur to collect pollen from flowers and transport it to the hive. The larvae are grown in perfectly hexagonal cells, which are kept at a constant temperature by the beating of the worker bees' wings [2].

For ants, the concept of a collective brain is even more evident. The search for food occurs along pathways signaled by pheromones and by the exchange of information between two individuals through antennae contact. Some species exhibit even more pronounced behaviors, as in the case of legion ants (*Eciton burchellii*), which do not build nests but live in constant movement. Legionary ants may adapt to do unusual work: for example, they may cling to each other to form bridges to cross small streams.

Other behaviors that can be attributed to a form of collective intelligence is that of flocks of birds and schools of fish, which appear to move in unison: while the movements here are more likely to be dictated by the movements of neighboring individuals, it is nonetheless undeniable that collective movements have to do with a kind of organization that is superior to individual one.

References

1. Bear MF, Connors BW, Paradiso MA. Neuroscience: exploring the brain, 4th edn. Burlington: Jones and Bartlett Learning; 2020.
2. Davis K, Christodoulou J, Seider S, Gardner H. The theory of multiple intelligences. In: Sternberg RJ, Kaufman B, (eds.). The Cambridge handbook of intelligence. Cambridge: Cambridge University Press; 2011. p. 485–503.
3. Demetriou A, Mouyi A, Spanoudis G. The development of mental processing. In: Overton WF, (ed.) The handbook of life-span development: cognition, biology and methods. New York: John Wiley & Sons; 2010. p. 36–55.
4. Herrnstein R, Murray C. The bell curve: intelligence and class structure in American life. New York: The Free Press; 1994.

Some Examples of Logic Reasoning in Humans 3

The word "logic" comes from the Greek word λόγος, which has various meanings, including "verb," "idea," "reason," and identifies the study of the relations between propositions, that is, between statements that can be true or false. Among logic goals there is the study of reasoning, its arguments, and the laws that govern it. Thus, logic is concerned with the study of the methods of proving a statement, how it is derived from prior concepts, and so in a sense, logic is a part of mathematics (and philosophy) that deals with the search for truth.

To a first approximation, it is possible to define logic as a set of rules used to obtain true propositions from a finite number of other propositions, which we call axioms, and which we define as true a priori. Logic may closely resemble arithmetic: in fact, arithmetic is a set of rules for producing data in number form, from other data in number form: to be even clearer, we could say that logic alone should enable us to know the rules of arithmetic; in turn, arithmetic can be classified as a universal algorithm, and consequently, arithmetic is able to transform the propositions of logic into numbers and functions [1–3].

Further, we will look at some very incomplete examples of how logical reasoning can be produced, without any claim to completeness, but just to make it clear how logical reasoning can unravel.

3.1   Modus Ponens

To become familiar with some basic aspects of logic, we need to know some of the symbols that are used. If we must say "if it's raining, then I leave home with an umbrella," then putting $a =$"$it's\ raining$", and $b = $"$I\ leave\ home\ with\ an\ umbrella$" we can write $a \to b$ (or also $a \Rightarrow b$), to mean "if a, then b." We may also write $a \vdash b$ to say that b can be proved by a. Again, one writes $\neg a$ to negate a, thus in our example, $\neg a = $"$it's\ not\ raining$."

© The Author(s), under exclusive license to Springer Nature Switzerland AG 2025   21
M. Nichelatti, *Mathematical Tools for Telemedicine*, TELe-Health,
https://doi.org/10.1007/978-3-031-81709-0_3

The aforementioned example is the first part of a logical reasoning called *modus ponens*, which is composed by three parts: (1) if *a*, then *b*; (2) *a* is true; (3) then *b* follows.

It is represented as

$$a \to b; \; a \vdash b$$

so that, it can be exemplified as *if it's raining (a), then I leave home with an umbrella (b); today it's raining (a), so I leave with an umbrella ($\vdash b$).*

3.2   Modus Tollens

In the *modus tollens*, we use the same division in three parts, but the second and third parts are different: (1) if *a*, then *b*; (2) *b* is false; (3) then not *a* follows

$$a \to b; \; \neg b \vdash \neg a$$

that can also be exemplified by *if it's raining (a), I leave home with an umbrella (b); today I'm not leaving home with an umbrella (¬b), so it's not raining ($\vdash \neg a$).*

Note that a modus tollens can be easily transformed into a modus ponens, and vice versa.

3.3   Syllogisms

The syllogism is a form of deductive reasoning mainly due to *Aristotles* (384–322 B.C.), in which the conclusion is obtained by means of some pre-established truths, whereas the inductive reasoning is given by a conclusion obtained from a series of repeated observations of the facts.

The syllogism also had very important developments after Aristotles, during the Middle Ages and up to modern times, when Boolean syllogism began to develop. We are not interested here in the latter developments, because we are interested just in looking at the syllogism as a method of reasoning [1–3].

All men are mortal; Socrates is a man; therefore, Socrates is mortal. Probably each of us has read or heard this phrase. This sentence is something that looks quite like a syllogism (from the Greek $\sigma\upsilon\lambda\lambda o\gamma\iota\sigma\mu\acute{o}\sigma$, which means "conclusion"), but it is not the best way to present the syllogisms, since it is not exactly a syllogism.

More precisely, a sentence representing one of the possible Aristotelian syllogisms can be written as follows: *all animals are mortal; all men are animals; therefore, all men are mortal.*

There are three sub-sentences in this syllogism (and in all other syllogisms): (1) all animals are mortal; (2) men are animals; (3) therefore, mens are mortal. Thus, we may distinguish

a major premise → *all animals are mortal*

a minor premise → *all men are animals*

a conclusion → *therefore all men are mortal*

where—for the conclusion to be true—we must assume that the major premise and the minor premise are also true. Already from the information in the major premise, minor premise, and conclusion, we can write the relationship "men" $\subset$ "animals" $\subset$ "mortals" to point out that the category "men" is contained in the category "animals," which in turn is contained in the category "mortals."

Note that here, the major premise contains *animals* (a subject) and *mortal* (a predicate), that the second premise contains *men* (a subject) and *animals* (a predicate), and that the conclusion contains *men* (a subject) and *mortal* (a predicate).

Now, if we define "mortal" $= A$, "men" $= Z$, and "animals" $= M$, we may write the major premise as $M \subset A$ (which reads "A contains M"), the minor premise as $Z \subset M$ ("M contains Z"), and the conclusion as $Z \subset A$ ("A contains Z"). Indeed, it's understood that if A contains M, and M contains Z, then A must contain also Z, which can be summarized writing $Z \subset M \subset A$. Given major and minor premises, M is called the *medium*. The syllogism we have just analyzed is called *Barbara* (look at the next lines of text).

The syllogisms are not limited to what above; among 64 potential sysllogisms, 19 are virtually possible (in the sense that they could be theoretically valid), but on a stricly mathematical approach (representable with the Venn diagrams), they are 15. These 15 syllogisms are divided into four *figures* according to the position of the *medium M* in the major and minor premises.

More precisely, in the first figure, we distinguish the following four syllogisms, where M comes first in the major premise and last in the minor premise; these first four syllogisms are given in Fig. 3.1a:

- *Barbara*: any M is A, any Z is M, then any Z is A
- *Celarent*: no M is A, any Z is M, then no Z is A
- *Darii*: any M is A, some Z is M, then some Z is A
- *Ferion*: no M is A, some Z is M, then some Z is not A

In the second figure, we distinguish the following four syllogisms, where M comes last in the major premise and last in the minor premise, as shown in Fig. 3.1b

- *Cesare*: no A is M, any Z is M, then no Z is A
- *Camestres*: any A is M, no Z is M, then no Z is A
- *Festino*: no A is M, some Z is M, then some Z is not A
- *Baroco*: any A is M, some Z is not M, then some Z is not A

Fig. 3.1 List of the
syllogisms represented by
Venn diagrams

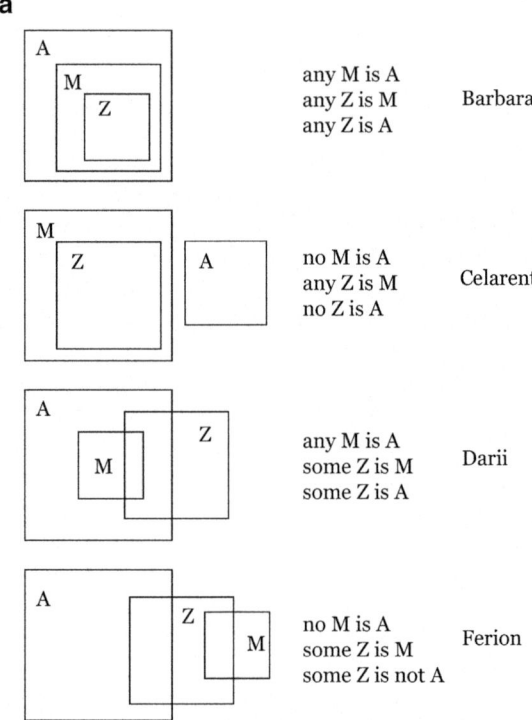

a

any M is A
any Z is M   Barbara
any Z is A

no M is A
any Z is M   Celarent
no Z is A

any M is A
some Z is M   Darii
some Z is A

no M is A
some Z is M   Ferion
some Z is not A

In the third figure, we distinguish the following four syllogisms, where M comes first in the major premise and first in the minor premise; these syllogisms represented in Fig. 3.1c:

- *Disamis*: some M is A, any M is Z, then some Z is A
- *Datisi*: any M is A, some M is Z, then some Z is A
- *Bocardo*: some M is not A, any M is Z, then some Z is not A
- *Ferison*: no M is A, some M is Z, then some Z is not A

Finally, in the fourth figure (which is due to *Galen of Pergamon*, 129–216 a.d.) we distinguish the following three syllogisms, where M comes last in the major premise and first in the minor premise; these syllogisms are presented in Fig. 3.1d:

- *Calemes*: any A is M, no M is Z, then no Z is A
- *Dimatis*: some A is M, any M is Z, then some Z is A
- *Fresison*: no A is M, some M is Z, then some Z is not A

In all the aforementioned definitions, M represents the medium: note that the medium appears only in the major and minor premises, but not in the conclusions. In Fig. 3.1a–d, syllogisms are represented as Venn diagrams.

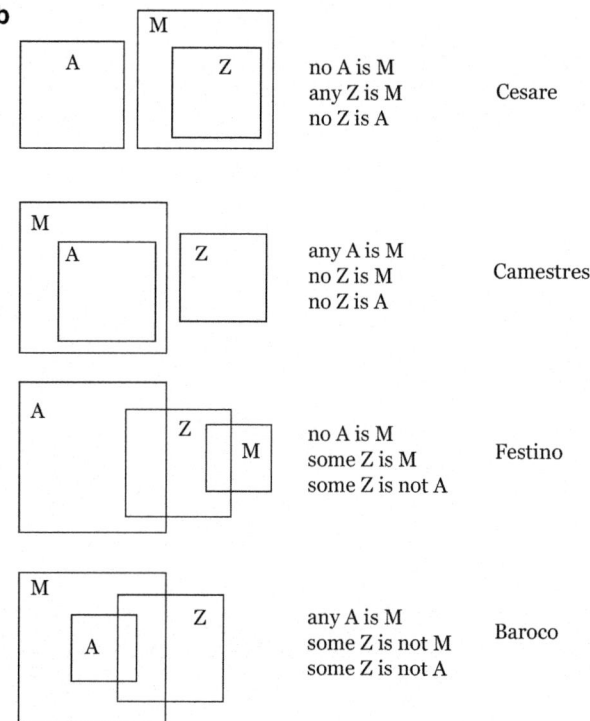

Fig. 3.1 (continued)

The apparently strange names of the syllogisms have a memnomic purpose, on the basis of their major and minor premises and conclusions: in few words, vowels are chosen to remind us of the nature of major premises, minor premises, and conlusions, according to the following table

$$\mathbf{A} \rightarrow \mathbf{A}\text{ffirmo}$$

$$\mathbf{I} \rightarrow \text{aff}\mathbf{I}\text{rmo}$$

$$\mathbf{E} \rightarrow \text{n}\mathbf{E}\text{go}$$

$$\mathbf{O} \rightarrow \text{neg}\mathbf{O}$$

thus, for example, the Barbara syllogism contains three universal affirmative assertions (in the major premise, in the minor premise, and in the conclusion), while the Celarent syllogism contains a universal negative (in the major premise) followed by a universal affirmative (in the minor premise) and another universal negative (in the conlusion).

Note that vowel **A** is used when the affirmative assertion is universal (e.g., absolute, like "any X is Y"), while vowel **I** is used when assertion is particular,

Fig. 3.1 (continued)

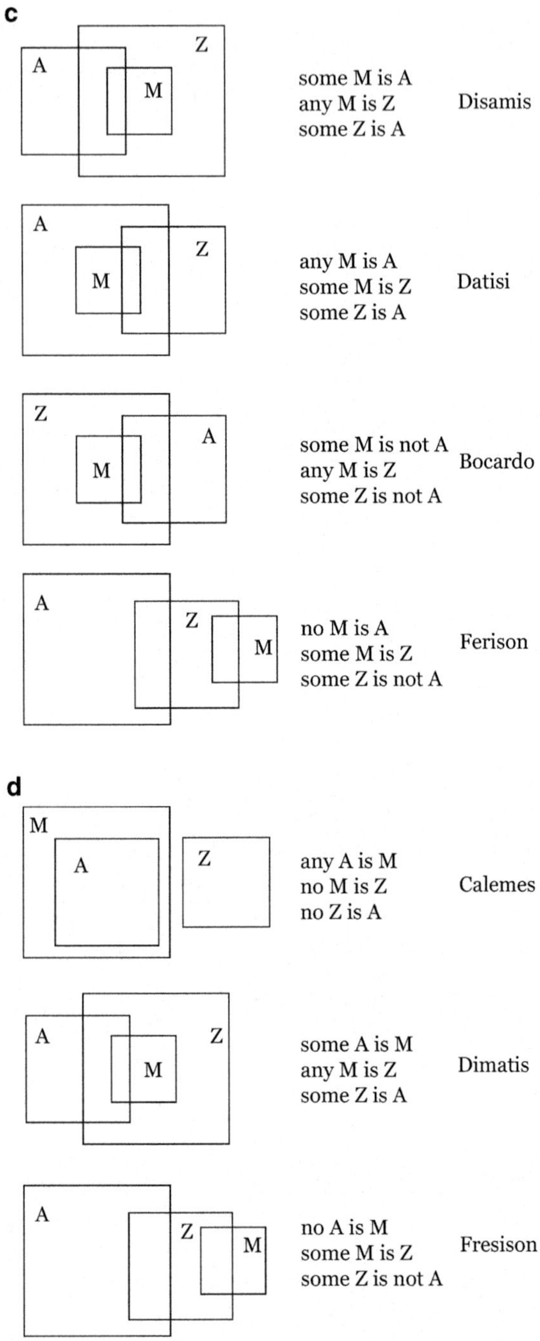

c

some M is A
any M is Z   Disamis
some Z is A

any M is A
some M is Z   Datisi
some Z is A

some M is not A
any M is Z   Bocardo
some Z is not A

no M is A
some M is Z   Ferison
some Z is not A

d

any A is M
no M is Z   Calemes
no Z is A

some A is M
any M is Z   Dimatis
some Z is A

no A is M
some M is Z   Fresison
some Z is not A

e.g., not absolute, and the word "some" is involved (like "some X is Y"): see for example the Datisi syllogism. We see the same for negations: vowel **E** is used for a universal negation (like "no X is Y"), while vowel **O** is used for particular, not absolute negation (like "some X is not Y"): see, for example, the Ferison syllogism.

Let us add a further curiosity, to say that the definition of Baroque art takes its name from the Baroco syllogism: any A is M (universal affirmative), some Z is not M (particular negative); therefore, some Z is not A (particular negative): we could then write the syllogism, for example, in the form *all philosophers are wise, some animals are not wise, so some animals are not philosophers*. All right, no contradiction, but someone may argue that this reasoning can be a bit bizarre, almost twisted in on itself, like the Bernini's altar columns of the Papal Basilica of Saint Peter in the Vatican.

3.4 Probabilistic Reasoning

Assume that one remembers perfectly that the surface area of a circle is $A_c = \pi r^2$ (being r the radius), but does not remember the value of π: however, it is clear that if $r = 1$, then $A_c = \pi$, and so there is at least a probabilistic method to retrieve the π value.

Placing the center of the circle of radius $r = 1$ at the origin O of two Cartesian axes, we immediately realize that the area of the circumscribed square in the circle of unit radius is $A_s = 4$, so that we may apply the Pythagora's theorem by randomly choosing some values along the x axis and a value along the y axis, such that $-1 \leq x \leq 1$ and $-1 \leq y \leq 1$. The hypotenuse of any of these right triangles will be $h = \sqrt{x^2 + y^2}$, thus h is the length of the segment $\overline{OP}$ from the origin of the Cartesian axes to the point P of coordinates (x, y), and if $\overline{OP} = h \leq 1$, then the point P belongs to the circle, whereas, when $\overline{OP} = h > 1$, then P is external to the circle. Thus, one may associate the value 1 to the event $\overline{OP} = h \leq 1$ and the value 0 to the event $\overline{OP} = h > 1$, so that, in the long run, the sum of all 1 values will approximate π: for example, after having evaluated P for $4n$ times (with n great enough), then these belonging to the circle will be πn, so that, at least an approximate value of π can be obtained. The geometric asset of this reasoning is presented in Fig. 3.2.

3.5 Truth Tables

Truth tables are used in logic to connect propositions that can be true or false. A proposition can be denoted by a capital letter, for example, P, while Q will be a second proposition. We may define the negation of P and Q by $\neg P$ and $\neg Q$ respectively (or by $\bar{P}$ and $\bar{Q}$). The proposition composed of P and Q will be referred to as $P \& Q$, or $P \wedge Q$, while the proposition composed as P or Q will be referred to as $P \vee Q$. In this case, $\vee$ corresponds to the Latin word "vel," or a nonexclusive "or": if I say that I drink wine or beer non-exclusively ("wine vel beer"), I mean

Fig. 3.2 Calculating π using probability

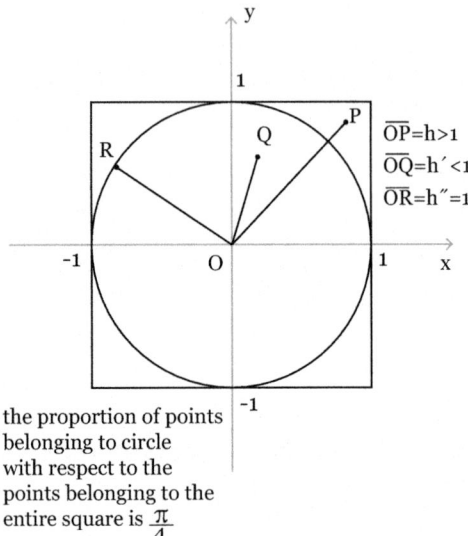

$\overline{OP}=h>1$

$\overline{OQ}=h'<1$

$\overline{OR}=h''=1$

the proportion of points belonging to circle with respect to the points belonging to the entire square is $\frac{\pi}{4}$

that I can drink wine or beer, indifferently, and the choice of one does not affect the choice of the other drink. That is, I can drink both if I feel like it.

On the other hand, if one intends to use an exclusive "or," one uses the symbol $P \veebar Q$, which takes the sense of the Latin word "aut": if I say that I drink wine "or" beer exclusively ("wine aut beer"), it means that tonight I will drink only one beverage between wine and beer, and therefore, by drinking beer, I exclude drinking wine, and vice versa.

We immediately realize that, if P is true, then $\neg P$ is false, and obviously that, if $\neg P$ is true, then P is false. We will write $P = 1$ to say that P is true (and that $\neg P$ is false), and $P = 0$ to say that P is false (and that $\neg P$ is true).

We also use $P \implies Q$ to say "if P, then Q," and $P \iff Q$ to say "P if, and only if, Q."

A very simple truth table may be constructed using these elementary properties, by writing, for example

P	Q	$P\&Q$
1	1	1
1	0	0
0	1	0
0	0	0

or

P	Q	$P \vee Q$
1	1	1
1	0	1
0	1	1
0	0	0

or a still more complete table like

P	Q	$\neg P$	$\neg Q$	$P \& Q$	$P \vee Q$	$P \underline{\vee} Q$	$P \Longrightarrow Q$
1	1	0	0	1	1	1	1
1	0	0	1	0	1	0	0
0	1	1	0	0	1	0	1
0	0	1	1	0	0	1	1

from which one may deduce some other properties: for example, if $P = 1$ and $Q = 1$, then $P \& \neg Q = 0$, $P \vee \neg Q = 1$, $P \underline{\vee} \neg Q = 0$, $P \Longrightarrow \neg Q = 0$, and so on.

3.6   Modern Logic Reasoning

In the modern era, logic got a very strong impetus after the possibility of using mathematical language to study inferences was obtained by Friedrich Ludwig Gottlob Frege (1848–1925), and it was to the study of inferences alone that logic was brought back. Key contributions include, among others, those of Bertrand Russell (1872–1970): famous is his antinomy showing how logical reasoning can lead to contradictions.

In particular, because of its importance in scientific disciplines, it is important to mention fuzzy logic, in which there are not necessarily absolute certainties one way or the other. With classical logic (Aristotelian logic, that of syllogisms) every proposition is either true (i.e., has truth value 1) or false (i.e., has truth value 0), and therefore cannot be both true and false, and especially cannot be something like "60% true." With fuzzy logic, on the other hand, it is permissible to have propositions that are 60% true, or 20% true, or 99% true, thus propositions that are only partially true. If we write "young people dream of their future," who do we mean young people to be? At what age does one stop being young? Is it a quantum leap or is it instead gradual, and starts at the same age for everyone, or does the leap (whether quantum or gradual) from young to old start at various ages, different for each person? Then we might as well turn the sentence around and write "those who can dream about their future are young." More generally, we will define membership functions that assign specific truth values for each possible quantity of the variable we are studying. Thus, the membership function related to how young a person is will be a curve monotonically decreasing from value 1 (at birth) to value zero (at the instant of death); the links between fuzzy logic and some probability concepts are straightforward.

By overcoming Aristotelian logic, it was possible to solve some problems that generated contradictions, such as statements like "all generalizations are wrong, including this one," or "this sentence is false." An in-depth study of this topic is beyond the scope of this book.

References

1. Angell RB. Truth-functional conditionals and modern vs. traditional syllogistic logic. Mind. 1986;95:210–23.
2. Sgarbi M, Cosci M. The aftermath of syllogism: Aristotelian logical argument from Avicenna to Hegel. New York: Bloomsbury USA Academic; 2018.
3. Thompson BER. An introduction to the syllogism and the logic of proportional quantifiers. New York: Peter Lang Publishing, Inc.; 1992.

Working with Data

4

Data are the raw material of all analysis: they can be structured or unstructured, depending on how they are presented. Structured data are tables, such as normal spreadsheets, in which any row is an istance and any column is a variable (actually, there are two main systems to represent structured data in a spreadsheet: the *wide format* and the *long format*, but this is a topic we will not go into here: it is enough for us to know that many software for statistical data analysis are capable of reshaping data from one format to another), whereas unstructured data are information stored as text, images, sounds, vocal records, and other data that cannot be stored in a tabular form.

As written earlier, structured data are tables: we can refer to tables containing medical data, so that any row is an individual patient, and any column is a measure of interest, such as the date of disease onset, age, gender, weight, height, body mass index (BMI), red blood cell count, antibiotic treatment, and so on. In these tables, we aknowledge various types of variables: some are continuous, such as the BMI, and are expressed as a number, some are categorical, such as the gender or the type of antibiotic treatment, which can be expressed by a word, for example, the trade name of the drug used, or the name of its active ingredient (always a preferable option). In a given table, the number of rows times the number of columns is called the *dimension of the table* or even the *size of the table*.

4.1 Continuous Variables

Continuous variables are given as real numbers: indeed, they are measures (age, weight, height, systolic blood pressure, lymphocyte count, and so on), which in most cases are pragmatically given as integer numbers. Thus, we would read of ages expressed as whole numbers of years (to be precise, those who work in demography generally use only age expressed in completed years, whereas in other fields, one may tend to express age with years rounded to the nearest integer), weight in

© The Author(s), under exclusive license to Springer Nature Switzerland AG 2025   31
M. Nichelatti, *Mathematical Tools for Telemedicine*, TELe-Health,
https://doi.org/10.1007/978-3-031-81709-0_4

kilograms, and height in centimeters. A special case is cell counts: here very large degrees of approximation are used: for example, we know that for females, a normal value of red blood cells is 4.6×10^{12} per liter of blood, while for men, it is 5.2×10^{12} per liter of blood. It is obvious that with these magnitudes, the count is strongly approximated, basically to the tens of billions of erythrocytes per liter of blood.

A continuous variable is a quantitative variable, which can take its value within a given range, depending on the variable itself: if the variable measures the age of an adult patient, we would expect it ranging from 18 to 100 or more, and if the variable measures the height of adult patients, we would expect it ranging from about 150 to about 210 cm. The distribution of the values of a continuous variable is expected to be bell-shaped (if the collected data are great enough), with a more high frequency of values around its mean. However, some data (outliers) may be located very far from the mean: these values must be carefully evaluated, since they can have a profound effect on the whole distribution.

Basically, we recognize two types of continuous variables, which are: (1) the ratio variables, which have a predetermined zero value (length, and so on), and in which any ratio between two subsequent values is equal; (2) the interval variables, which also have a predetermined zero value (time, and so on), and in which any interval between two subsequent values is equal. Both types can be analyzed by calculating their mean, median, and standard deviation, and if some data are missing, they can be possibly replaced with the mean or the median.

Among continuous variables, we also find the *composite variables*, which are formed from the combination of two or more variables. They can be additive or multiplicative: we have a case of additive composite variable, for example, when a total score of a questionnaire is calculated by summing the various scores obtained from the single dimensions encompassed by the questionnaire itself. A more complicate additive composite variable is the resting energy expenditure (REE) which gives the minimum enery needs (in kcal/day) of men and women according to the Harris–Benedict equations, first published in 1918,[1] and then revised in 1984.[2]

Technical note. *The Harris–Benedict equations take the form*

$$REE_{men} = 13.397 \times weight\ (kg) + 4.799 \times height\ (cm) - 5.677 \times age\ (ys) + 88.362$$

for men and

$$REE_{women} = 9.247 \times weight\ (kg) + 3.098 \times height\ (cm) - 4.330 \times age\ (ys) + 447.593,$$

---

[1] First published as JA Harris, FG Benedict. A Biometric Study of Human Basal Metabolism. Proceedings of the National Academy of Sciences of the United States of America. 4: 370–373, 1918.

[2] See AM Roza, HM Shizgal. The Harris Benedict equation reevaluated: resting energy requirements and the body cell mass. The American Journal of Clinical Nutrition. 40: 168–182, 1984. https://doi.org/10.1093/ajcn/40.1.168.

for women. Thus, the REE of a 38-year-old man who is 180 cm tall and weighs 78 kg is calculated as

$$REE = 13.397 \times 78\,kg + 4.799 \times 180\,cm - 5.677 \times 38\,ys + 88.362$$
$$= (1045.0 + 863.82 - 215.73 + 88.362)\,kcal/day$$
$$= 1781.5\,kcal/day$$

and the REE of a 42-year-old woman who is 171 cm tall and weighs 58 kg is calculated as

$$REE = 9.247 \times 58\,kg + 3.098 \times 171\,cm - 4.330 \times 42\,ys + 447.593$$
$$= (536.33 + 529.76 - 181.86 + 447.593)\,kcal/day$$
$$= 1331.8\,kcal/day.$$

Note that the coefficients used in the Harris–Benedict equations aren't a dimensional: in both equations, the first coefficient has the dimension kcal/(day × kg), the second one has dimension kcal/(day × cm), the third one has dimension kcal/(day × ys), and the last one has dimension kcal/day.

A very well-known example of multiplicative variable is the body mass index (BMI) given by the ratio between the weight in kilograms and the squared height in meters[3] (so, BMI nominally has the dimension of a pressure), regardless of the subject's gender and age, e.g.,

$$BMI = \frac{\text{weight in kg}}{(\text{height in m})^2}$$

so that if a subject of any sex and any age is 1.78 m tall and weighs 75 kg, the BMI is

$$BMI = \frac{75}{(1.78)^2}$$
$$= 23.67\,m/kg^2.$$

---

[3] See for example, H Blackburn, D Jacobs. Commentary: Origins and evolution of body mass index (BMI): continuing saga. International Journal of Epidemiology. 43: 665–669, 2014. https://doi.org/10.1093/ije/dyu061.

Another multiplicative variable is the Dubois's S,[4] giving the body surface area in cm^2, which is calculated with the formula

$$S = 71.84 \times (\text{weight in kg})^{0.425} \times (\text{height in cm})^{0.725},$$

so that, if an individual (regardless of gender) weighs 82 kg and is 176 cm tall, then the estimated body surface area is

$$S = 71.84 \times 82^{0.425} \times 176^{0.725}$$

$$\approx 71.84 \times 6.51 \times 42.461$$

$$= 19,850 \text{ cm}^2$$

$$= 1.985 \text{ m}^2$$

so the body surface area is just slightly less than 2 m^2.

The distribution of a continuous variable in most situations takes a bell-shape, and in this case, the variable is termed Gaussian or normal. In some other cases, the distribution is not bell-shaped and can take more forms; when a variable shows this behavior, we are dealing with a non-Gaussian or a non-normal continuous variable. Notably, the statistical tests applied to Gaussian variables are defined *parametric tests*, since these are based on some parameters, such as the mean, while the statistical test to be used for non-Gaussian variables is defined *nonparametric tests*, since they are based mainly on the ranks of the variable values.

4.2   Categorical Variables

When dealing with categorical variables, it is mandatory to distinguish between *ordinal* and *nominal* ones. Ordinal categorical variables have a "natural" hierarchical structure, in that its possible values can be aligned in a logical ascending (and thus also descending) order: an example of ordinal categorical variable is the tumor staging (I, II, III and IV), but also the level of schooling achieved is ordinal; in fact, it is obvious to think that a doctorate is superior to a master's degree, and this to a bachelor's degree, and this, in turn, is superior to a high school diploma.

The reason why an ordinal variable cannot be treated as a continuous variable is that "jumps" from one value to another are not equivalent. Assuming that we are evaluating the level of schooling, we quickly find that the jump (understood in the metric sense) from a high school license to a master's degree cannot be thought of as twice the "schooling" jump that exists from the high school license to the bachelor's degree, nor can the jump from the high school license to the bachelor's degree be

---

[4] See D Dubois, EF Dubois. A formula to estimate the approximate surface area if height and weight be known. Archives Internal Medicine. 17: 863–871, 1916.

thought of as equal to the jump between the bachelor's degree and the master's degree. In other words, the passage to a given value to another is not linear, but goes ahead by "jumps." However, working with ordinal categorical variables, it is possible to use a label encoding, say, assigning the value 1 to high school license, 2 to bachelor's degree, 3 to master's degree, and 4 to doctorate, but when elaborating the data, one must always remember that the variable is ordinal and not continuous: some statistical software require different commands when dealing with continuous or with ordinal variables.

The approach to nominal variables is quite different: here we don't find any specific natural (or artificially imposed) hierarchical order, e.g., there are no reasons to think that a given value is better or worse than another one. Some examples are the ZIP code, the tax identification number, the VAT number, but also the hair color and the shape of the auricle, are nominal, as well as the gender, as well as the the town or region of residence. Assume we are dealing with a bunch of subjects living in five distinct cities, say, A, B, C, D, and E, identified by their ZIP codes. We could fill a single column named "ZIP" and let there write the values, say, "101," "102," "103," "104," and "105," respectively, but we preferably would have to define five *dummy variables* called with the same values of the ZIP codes. In practice, noting that the ZIP codes are *mutually exclusive* (that is, nobody may have two different ZIP codes), as a first approximation, the table could be presented in a simpler form like

Patient	ZIP code
1	103
2	104
3	101
4	105
5	102
6	105

but il will be much more convenient if we decide to arrange the table, to get the data in the more readable form

Patient	ZIP101	ZIP102	ZIP103	ZIP104	ZIP105
1	0	0	1	0	0
2	0	0	0	1	0
3	1	0	0	0	0
4	0	0	0	0	1
5	0	1	0	0	0
6	0	0	0	0	1

wich requires an increase of table size, but the table can be better understood. Moreover, this tabular form is the optimal one when working with most of the ML algorithms. However, the meaning of this tabular form is intuitive, since each patient is associated, for each dummy variable representing the zip code, with the value "1" when the zip code is his or her own, while it is associated with the value "0" if the zip code is not his or her own: very simple, indeed.

In some cases, the use of dummy variables is practically mandatory: think of situations in which the values of the variables ain't mutually exclusive, as in the case of therapies with some possible concomitant drugs, which we here simply call A, B, C, and D. In this case, tabulation without dummy variables would look almost horrible (incidentally, with this method it is also easier to make mistakes when introducing data into the table) and completely unusable even for a trivial descriptive statistical analysis

Patient	Drugs
1	A, D
2	B, D
3	C
4	None
5	A, B, D
6	A, C

whereas rearranging the data with the dummy variables, will produce a much more readable table

Patient	Drug A	Drug B	Drug C	Drug D
1	1	0	0	1
2	0	1	0	1
3	0	0	1	0
4	0	0	0	0
5	1	1	0	1
6	1	0	1	0

The use of the dummy variables (in some textbooks, this operation is called the *one-hot encoding*) may increase the dimension of the table, but in some cases, when dealing with binary variables, its use may actually reduce the table size. For example, taking the two variables gender and patient vaccinated, we can pass from a possible redundant form

Patient	Male	Female	Vaccinated	Not vaccinated
1	1	0	0	1
2	0	1	0	1
3	1	0	1	0
4	0	1	Not known	Not known
5	0	1	0	1
6	1	0	1	0

to the collapsed form

Patient	Female	Vaccinated
1	0	0
2	1	0
3	0	1
4	1	
5	1	0
6	0	1

where cells referring to unknown values are left blank (in this case, we are dealing with *missing data*). However, in this table we identify four possibilities of combinations, which are: (1) female vaccinated; (2) female not vaccinated; (3) male vaccinated; (4) male not vaccinated. For what aforementioned, the table can be virtually collapsed into an even more concise form.

However, first, if we like to proceed, in most cases we would have to substitute the missing data, by assigning to any possible missing value a value corresponding to mean or median (if data are continuous) or to mode (if data are categorical): in any case, the substitution of missing data is not a simple issue, and must be preliminarily evaluated very carefully, including taking into account how many values are actually missing from the total in a given variable.

4.3 Introduction to Statistical Analysis of Data

Data are analyzed by means of various statistical descriptive techniques, which allow to get a synthesis of the information contained in the data. When working with descriptive statistics of continuuous data, we obtain the measures of central tendency and measures of variability (or dispersion). The former are the mean, median, and fashion, while the latter are essentially the variance, standard deviation, range, and interquartile range (IQR), which is the distance between the 25th and 75th percentiles of a continuous variable.

When we are dealing with categorical data, that is, discrete variables, using descriptive statistics we will obtain frequency tables that will give the percentage distribution of each individual value of a categorical variable.

This method is used to summarize and describe the characteristics of a continuous variable. Measures such as mean, median, mode, range, variance, and standard deviation can be calculated to give a sense of the central tendency, variability, and distribution of the data.

Inferential statistical analyses, on the other hand, are dedicated to extracting information not immediately deducible from simple observation of data. The most widely used inferential techniques are the analysis of variance (ANOVA), which allows us to see whether the mean value of a continuous variable is the same within two or more groups identified from the database: for example, ANOVA can be used to see whether mean blood glucose values are similar in three independent groups of normal-weight, overweight, and obese patients. It should be added that if there are only two groups to be compared, the ANOVA can be replaced by Student's t-test. In some cases, if one wants to compare a continuous variable in two (or more than two) groups, adjusting for the behavior of some other variables, then the analysis of covariance (ANCOVA) must be preferred. Notably, ANOVA, t-test, and ANCOVA are parametric tests, e.g., they can be used only if continuous data are Gaussian: if not, the nonparametric equivalents to be used are respectively the Kruskal–Wallis test, the Mann–Whitney U test, and the Quade nonparametric ANCOVA.

Regression analysis is a technique that is used when one wants to look for the effect of one or more variables, called independent variables, on another variable, called the dependent variable. There are various types of regression, the best known and simplest being ordinary least squares linear regression (OLS regression), in which in the simplest form, we want to see if the continuous values of a dependent variable y are affected by the continuous values of a variable x, using a formula such as $y = a + bx$, where a and b are two unknown coefficients, of which the regression will allow us to calculate the values; OLS regression allows us to work with many independent variables (the number of which, however, depends on the number of subjects available in the database), so that the formula will be $y = a + b_1 x_1 + \cdots + b_n x_n$. Another widely used type of regression is the logistic regression, in which one wants to see how a dependent variable that can only take on two values (typically 0 and 1) is influenced by one or more continuous or discrete independent variables: for example, we can evaluate if blood glucose, age, and body mass index are able to predict whether the patient is hypertensive or not; in other types of logistic regression, the dependent variable can be categorical ordinal (ordinal logistic regression) or categorical nominal (multinomial logistic regression).

Correlation Analysis can be used to calculate the possible association between two continuos variables: the Pearson correlation coefficient r is used when searching the correlation between two Gaussian variables, whereas the Spearman's ρ and the Kendall's τ are used when the variables ain't Gaussian.

The survival analysis is used to analyze the time it takes for an event to occur: for example, the time for light bulbs to burn out in a building, or the time for deaths from a disease to occur in a population. The various survival analysis techniques are largely used in medicine.

Other techniques widely used are the Time Series Analysis (in which one is interested in the change of a continuous variable over time: it can be useful to evaluate the variations in the sales volume due to any advertising investments or more simply due to the season) and the Principal Component Analysis (PCA, used to search for possible patterns and "latent" variables, to try to reduce the dimensions of the dataset).

When working with categorical data, the possible association between variables is evaluated by using the Fisher's exact test (which can be always used) or the Pearson's χ^2 test (which can be used when some assumptions are obeyed).

In some cases, the comparison to be carried out is not between two or more groups, but rather within a single group: this is the situation typically faced when conducting "before vs. after" studies. For example, it may be necessary to test whether the use of a certain drug was able to reduce blood glucose in a group of patients: for this purpose, Student's t-test for paired data, or Wilcoxon's test will be used (respectively, whether the data are Gaussian or not); if the measures within gruops are more than two, one will have to use the Repeated Measures ANOVA, or the Friedman test (again, respectively, whether the data are Gaussian or not). For categorical data, the McNemar test is one of the most widely used options).

The strength of the association between variables is measured by the p-value, which is calculated using the appropriate statistical test for the analysis one wishes to conduct. In general, the association is assumed to be statistically significant if $p < 0.05$ and not statistically significant if $p \geq 0.05$ (see a next section).

4.4   Null Hypothesis and Alternative Hypothesis

When planning an experiment, we are facing mainly two possible scenarios: (1) we don't know what will going to happen, so that we just do "something" to the sample we are studying, and we wait to see the effects of this "something"; (2) we hypothesize a possible effect that the "something" we are doing to the sample, and we want to test whether this effect actually occurred.

An example of the first scenario can be an experiment in which we subject lymphocytes to different frequencies, say four, of radio waves, and see if at any (or none, or all) frequencies, the lymphocytes' in vitro immune activity (maybe measured by the production of a given molecule) increases, or decreases, or remains constant: in this case, we did not make any assumptions: we simply performed the experiment on the lymphocyte sample in vitro and measured the results.

An example of the second scenario requires more complex reasoning. Pretend we are studying a disease for which there is a gold standard treatment (a gold standard drug), and that a new treatment claims to be better than the gold standard: let us call A the gold standard and B the new drug. We want to compare treatments A and B, and to do so we must plan an experiment: we know that drug A has a 60% probability of clinical success, so we would expect, say, at least a 70% of clinical successes with the drug B. For first, we must define a *null hypothesis* that we call H_0, and this null hypothesis must be conservative (or even pessimistic, if we want), so that to say: H_0 = {drug B is not better than drug A}. We would have to define also an *alternative hypothesis* H_A; in our case, the alternative hypothesis is H_A = {drug B is better than drug A}. Of course, on the basis of our assumptions, we can also write that "drug B does not reach a 70% of clinical successes" (null hypothesis) and that "drug B reaches 70% of clinical successes" (alternative hypothesis). Note that null hypothesis and alternative hypothesis are mutually exclusive. Not just: null hypothesis and alternative hypotesis are exaustive, e.g., nothing can happen outside of these hypotheses, and we expect that one (and only one) of the hypotheses will surely be realized, since *tertium non datur*.

To make a comparison with a criminal trial, in the clinical trial we are planning, drug B is "accused" of working better than drug A, and the null hypothesis amounts to the phrase "every defendant (in this case: drug B) is innocent until proven guilty."

One may ask why drug B must reach 70% of successes to be considered better than drug A: 65% or also 61% of successes would not be sufficient, if the rate of successes with drug A is just 60%? It depends on several factors, but mainly it depends on the clinician's experiences and knowledges about the disease. For example, the doctors may say that a fraction of successes until 69.9% is not clinically meaningful (because perhaps they feel that from the point of view of clinical success rate, a difference is irrelevant unless it is at least 10%), so that they want to reach at least a 70% of successes to convince themselves that drug B is significantly better (from a clinical viewpoint) than drug A.

At this point, we can arrange an experiment: we take a given number of patients and randomly assign each one to receive drug A or drug B: this is going to be a randomized controlled clinical trial (RCT), where we use a control drug A to statistically verify if actually the experimental drug B is better. After some days, we will be able to count clinical successes in both groups and to compare them.

4.5   Errors, Power, Sample Size, and *P*-Value

In an experiment like the one we're planning, we may commit two kinds of mistakes. Maintaining the assumption to study a drug, the first error is the α *error*, which is a false positive error: in other words, it is the error we make when we attribute to a drug a clinical efficacy that the drug actually does not have. The second error is the β *error*, e.g., a false negative error we make when we do not attribute to a drug the clinical efficacy that the drug actually does have.

Returning to the metaphor of the criminal trial, already mentioned in the previous section, we can say that α error corresponds to convicting an innocent person, while β error corresponds to acquitting a guilty person. It is intuitive that an α error is much more serious than a β error: indeed, if we continue the metaphor related to the criminal trial, we find that convicting an innocent person also means letting the guilty person go free. In the case of a clinical trial, one must be sure that the probability of an alpha error, i.e., the probability of a false positive, is small; in general, one makes sure that the alpha error is always not more than 5% (say, it must be $\alpha \leq 0.05$), while the β error can be tolerated up to a value of 20% (e.g., it must be $\beta \leq 0.2$).

The concept of *statistical power* must also be defined: this is given by the $1 - \beta$ value, and corresponds (and here we return to the court) to the probability of convicting a guilty person, thus the probability of being in the right. If the β error can have a maximum value of 0.2, then the statistical power must always be worth at least 80%, that is, for the power to be $1 - \beta \geq 0.8$.

The comparison between drug A and drug B, since the aim of the study is to measure the rate of healing (clinical successes) will have to be done using a Fisher's exact test. Using a fairly simple computational algorithm, in which we ask how many patients are needed to verify that a cure rate of 70% (that of drug B) is actually higher than the cure rate of 60% (that of drug A), with an α error of at most 5% and a power of at least 80% (e.g., with at most $\beta = 0.2$), we obtain that 750 patients will need to be enrolled, of whom 375 will be treated with drug A, and 375 with drug B; assignment of a patient to treatment with either A or B will be done by randomization. A numerical check will show that for the design used, the true alpha error will be about 0.041 (thus less than 0.05) while the true power will be 0.801 (thus more than 0.8).

It is remarkable to note that only if we compare two groups of (at least) 375 patients each can the expected 10% difference (i.e., the difference in the proportions of clinical successes between the two groups) be statistically significant. With two groups of lower numbers (say, 100 and 100), the difference in clinical successes would not have been statistically significant, and thus could be attributed simply to chance. But then, we have a need to measure a difference to see whether it is indeed statistically significant: this necssity is carried out by the *p-value*.

When using a test to test a hypothesis (in this case, we used Fisher's exact test) we define the p-value as the probability—assuming that null hypothesis is true—of having results equal to or even more extreme than those obtained using the test. In practice, the p-value tells us whether the difference between the expected and observed outcome is due to chance alone, or whether it is significantly attibuable to an actual difference between the data collected in the (two or more) groups analyzed, and thus, the difference is unlikely to be attributable to chance alone, i.e., unlikely to be attributable to random differences due to sampling during data collection.

The definition of p-value seems a bit complicated, but this definition serves to prevent p-value from being misunderstood. In fact, it should be clarified that the p-value is not the probability that the null hypothesis is true, so that 1 minus the p-value is not the probability that the alternative hypothesis is true: indeed, this is a very easy misinterpretation to make. Say, if $p = 0.02$, then $0.02 = 2\%$ is not the probability that the null hypothesis is true, so that we are not allowed to reject it in favor of the alternative hypothesis, which then should be 98% true. Moreover, the significance level (i.e., the α value) and the p-value are different things: the former is decided a priori by the experimenter, the latter is calculated by statistical testing.

To better explore all these aspects, it is recommended to consult a book specifically devoted to inferential statistics.

References

1. Hays W. Statistics, 5th edn. Orlando: Harcourt Brace; 1994.
2. Stuart A, Ord K, Arnold S. Kendall's advanced theory of statistics, Volume 2A: classical inference and the linear model, 6th edn. London: Arnold; 1999.
3. Zar JH. Biostatistical analysis, 4th edn. Upper Saddle River: Prentice Hall; 1999.

A Note on Bayesian Probability

Put in simple terms, the definition of frequentist probability of an event is, on the long run, the ratio of the number of times a defined event has occurred to the total number of all events that have occurred. Thus, by rolling a die, we know that after a sufficiently large number of rolls (say, 10,000), it is expected that the number of times the result of the roll will be 5 (or any other result between 1 and 6) will have to be about equal to $\frac{1}{6} \times 10{,}000 \approx 1{,}667$, so face number 5 will have come out about 1,667 times, as is also expected for the other faces, because the die has 6 faces, and each result has the same probability of occurrence.

The set of all possible outputs of an experiment is called the *sample space* (or the *outcome space*), so for a die toss, the sample space is the set $\mathbb{S} = \{1, 2, 3, 4, 5, 6\}$, while for a coin toss, the sample space is $\mathbb{S} = \{\text{heads,tails}\}$.

The probability of an event varies between 0 (if the event is impossible, that is, if the event cannot happen) and 1 (if the event is certain, that is, if the event will definitely happen). So, we say that the probability $P(A)$ of an event A will be always between 0 and 1 including extremes (and in mathematical notation, we will write $0 \leq P(A) \leq 1$).

We would have no reason to believe that if we repeated the experiment of rolling the die tomorrow, things might change, and thus, we would then expect to get the same results: in the long run, the frequency with which the faces of the die would occur would be the same as on the previous day, i.e., about $\frac{N}{6}$, N being a sufficiently large number of rolls.

However, there are situations in which the probability may change over time, for example, if the information we possess about the system we are studying does change.

M. Nichelatti, *Mathematical Tools for Telemedicine*, TELe-Health,
https://doi.org/10.1007/978-3-031-81709-0_5

5.1   What is the Probability, in Simple Words

To begin with, let us say that to any given event A, we can associate a real number $P(A)$, which we call the probability of A. The concept of *probability* is very intuitive, but it is not very easy to explain. In general, each event A can be associated with the probability $P(A)$ of that event occurring; for this purpose, the first interpretation of probability could be the ratio

$$P(A) \approx \frac{n_A}{n} \qquad (5.1)$$

where n_A is the number of times the event A occurred, while n, which is always expected to be reasonably large, is the total number of experiments we carried out. So, we can plan a simple experiment: we roll a die n times and measure the probability to obtain the event $A = 3$: if n is sufficiently large, then we expect $P(A = 3) \approx 1/6$ (so, we understand that probability is a number). Moreover, if we call $n_{\bar{A}}$ the number of times the event did not occur, plus the number of times it occurred, we can also write $n = n_{\bar{A}} + n_A$, and

$$P(A) \approx \frac{n_A}{n_{\bar{A}} + n_A},$$

so, we may also define $\phi(A)$, e.g., the *odds* of the event A, which is the number of times A occurred divided by the number of times A did not occur: in other words,

$$\phi(A) = \frac{n_A}{n_{\bar{A}}},$$

and, for our experiment, on the long run, we expect to have $\phi(A = 3) \approx \frac{1}{5}$.

However, the definition (5.1) is not the best one, since—for example—there are situations in which an experiment cannot be repeated as many times as we want.

To solve this problem, let us first think to any possible outcome of our experiment, and let us consider the list of outcomes as a set $\mathbb{S}$ (this is the sample space, which we met just earlier), so that $\mathbb{S}$ is, in general, the set containing all the possible outcomes of an experiment: as we have seen before, if we toss a coin, then $\mathbb{S} = \{\text{heads,tails}\}$, or if we roll a die, $\mathbb{S} = \{1, 2, 3, 4, 5, 6\}$, or, again, if we are searching for a given point along a real line, then $\mathbb{S} = \{\mathbb{R}\}$, where $\mathbb{R}$ is the set of all real numbers, e.g., the numbers going from $-\infty$ to $+\infty$. Each element of $\mathbb{S}$ will be called the *sample point*: if a specific sample point is the realization of an experiment, then that sample point is the *realized outcome*; hence, if our experiment is the roll of a die, and if the result of the roll is 3, then 3 is the realized outcome of the roll.

The elements of $\mathbb{S}$ are mutually exclusive, and so, there cannot be two different outcomes with a single roll of a die, and since $\mathbb{S}$ is the list of all events we should expect, then $\mathbb{S}$ is also exaustive, which means that after a die is rolled, no results other than those listed in the sample space can be obtained, or (which is the same), it means that the sample space contains all possible results that can be obtained by rolling a die. Hence, we can write $P(\mathbb{S}) = 1$ to say that the result of an experiment is certainly contained in the sample space defined for that experiment.

The relations seen earlier, namely $0 \leq P(A) \leq 1$ and $P(\mathbb{S}) = 1$, are the first two axioms on which the definition of probability rests.

The third axiom says that if two events A and B are mutually exclusive (i.e., if the occurrence of A prevents the occurrence of B, and vice versa), then their intersection $A \cap B$ is an empty set, i.e., a set that contains no elements, while the probability $P(A \cup B)$ of their union $A \cup B$ is given by the sum of the individual probabilities, i.e., $P(A \cup B) = P(A) + P(B)$.

Before continuing, it is necessary to explain what the intersection and union of two sets means. We can give a simple example by considering a set $A = \{1, 2, 3, 4, 5\}$ and a set $B = \{3, 4, 5, 6, 7\}$.

We define the intersection $A \cap B$ as the set of elements shared by the two sets, so in our case we will have the intersection $A \cap B = \{3, 4, 5\}$. If, on the other hand, we had two sets $C = \{1, 2, 3, 4\}$ and $D = \{7, 8, 9, 10\}$, it is evident that no element of one is shared by the other: no elements of C belong to D, and no elements of D belong to C. Therefore, C and D have no elements in common, so their intersection $C \cap D$ contains no elements, so we write that the intersection set of C and D is the empty set, which we define with the notation $C \cap D = \{\emptyset\}$.

We define the union $A \cup B$ as the set of all elements contained in set A and set B, so we will write $A \cup B = \{1, 2, 3, 4, 5, 6, 7\}$, and also $C \cup D = \{1, 2, 3, 4, 7, 8, 9, 10\}$.

To finish this brief unraveling of the concept of probability, we must also define the space of events Ω. We define it with a practical example: if for the roll of a die in which $\mathbb{S} = \{1, 2, 3, 4, 5, 6\}$ we define the set of outcomes with A and B, such that $A = \{1, 2, 3\}$ and $B = \{4, 5, 6\}$ (we say that A and B are subsets of $\mathbb{S}$) then the space of events Ω is the set $\Omega = \{A, B, \mathbb{S}, \emptyset\}$, so the sample space and the empty set are also part of the space of events [1].

5.2 Conditional Probability

Rolling a die, we may try to evaluate the probability of an even outcome (say, 2, 4, or 6): in this case, since

$$P(2) + P(4) + P(6) = \frac{1}{6} + \frac{1}{6} + \frac{1}{6} = \frac{1}{2}$$

we infer that the probability to get as outcome an even number is $\frac{1}{2}$, e.g., 50%. But, what happens if we condition the event E "even number" to the conditioning event C "number greater than 2"? We are dealing with the conditional probability of the event E conditioned by the (sometimes preceding) event C as follows:

$$P(E|C) = \frac{P(E \cap C)}{P(C)}$$

where $P(E|C)$ reads "probability of the event E, given the event C," while $P(E \cap C)$ is the probability of the intersection of E with C; means which outcomes E and C have in common: if the sample space of E is $\{2, 4, 6\}$ and that of C is $\{3, 4, 5, 6\}$, then $E \cap C = \{4, 6\}$.

Indeed, C is an information received about the size of the sample space. Of course, it must be $P(E), P(C) > 0$.

In the denominator, we easily find that the probability $P(C)$ of a result greater than 2 is

$$P(C) = P(3) + P(4) + P(5) + P(6)$$
$$= \frac{1}{6} + \frac{1}{6} + \frac{1}{6} + \frac{1}{6}$$
$$= \frac{4}{6} = \frac{2}{3},$$

since the possible outcomes greater than 2 are 3, 4, 5, and 6, thus we have four outcomes among the six possible ones. In the numerator, we must calculate the probability of the intersection $E \cap C$: we have seen that $E = \{2, 4, 6\}$ and $C = \{3, 4, 5, 6\}$, thus $E \cap C = \{4, 6\}$ and therefore the probability of the intersection $E \cap C$ is

$$P(E \cap C) = P(4) + P(6) = \frac{1}{6} + \frac{1}{6} = \frac{1}{3},$$

so that, in this case we have

$$P(E|C) = \frac{P(E \cap C)}{P(C)} = \frac{\frac{1}{3}}{\frac{2}{3}} = \frac{1}{2}.$$

In few words, writing $P(E|C)$ we are looking at the probability of E in a reduced sample space $\mathbb{S}' = C$, provided $P(E|C)$ is a probability measure obeying the three axioms we saw earlier. Moreover, we must have

$$P(E|E) = \frac{P(E \cap E)}{P(E)} = \frac{P(E)}{P(E)} = 1,$$

and, since we are working in the "shrunk" sample space C, for another event F conditioned by the same event C, we have

$$\frac{P(E|C)}{P(F|C)} = \frac{P(E)}{P(F)}.$$

5.3 Bayesian Probability

Earlier we mentioned situations in which the probability may change over time, and we said that this may happen when the information we have about a system does change.

Diagnostic reasoning is a typical situation in which available information may vary (in this case, it is more likely to increase, rather than decrease). Certainly at the time when a physician sees a patient for the first time, there will be little information available: the patient will provide symptoms, perhaps not in a systematic way, perhaps not remembering well when they first occurred: he or she may be vague even in defining the intensity of the pain, and in any case will be imprecise in the information provided to the physician.

For this reason, the physician will have to ask precise questions and write a history that will contain all the information about the patient and his or her family, so as to put otherwise fragmentary or anecdotal information in order. For pain intensity, the physician will have the patient indicate a point on a visual analog scale (VAS) that varies between 0 and 10 (0 will be equivalent to "no pain" and 10 will be equivalent to "the most pain you can think of"). The VAS scale score will give a rough but generally credible quantification of the painful sensation experienced by the patient [2].

After this initial data collection, which will also contain anthropometric and clinical measurements (age, weight, height, blood pressure, heart rate, and so on), some other examinations previously performed, if available, and data from the medical record (if available), the physician will begin to develop a list of possible pathological conditions afflicting the patient, and (even without intending to) sort them according to their probability, that is, according to the probability established by the physician based on the information collected. The diagnosis that the doctor will put first on the basis of his or her experience will still (and even for the doctor himself or herself) have a margin of uncertainty; therefore, the possibility of the doctor accurately identifying the diagnosis at the first glance is quite rare, and the doctor will have to take this into account [2, 3].

Bayes' theorem, in our medical interpretation, says that the probability $P(D|T^+)$ of a certain disease D, given the event T^+ (say, a diagnostic test resulting positive), is equal to the probability $P(T^+|D)$ of event T^+, given the disease D, multiplied by the probability $P(D)$ of disease D, and divided by the probability $P(T^+)$ of event T^+. But $P(T^+)$ is the total probability of the event "being positive for the test," so we will have to take into account that

$$P(T^+) = P(T^+|H)P(H) + P(T^+|S)P(S),$$

where H (healthy) denotes healthy subjects and S (sick) denotes sick subjects.

In formula, we have

$$P(D|T^+) = \frac{P(T^+|D)P(D)}{P(T^+)}$$

$$= \frac{P(T^+|D)P(D)}{P(T^+|H)P(H) + P(T^+|S)P(S)}.$$

So let's take an example: the doctor defines the diagnosis of disease D, knowing that performing the diagnostic test T in the actually sick subjects of disease D will have a positive rate of 85% (true positives) and on the other hand in the healthy subjects will have a positive rate of 5% (false positives), and thus, it will be $P(T^+|D) = 0.85$ and $P(T^+|H) = 0.15$.

If the physician gives the diagnosis an a priori probability $P(D)$ of 75% and the E test is positive, then we will have

$$P(D|T^+) = \frac{0.85 \times 0.75}{0.85 \times 0.75 + 0.25 \times 0.05}$$

$$= 0.9808$$

which is the posterior probability of having the disease D, once one has tested positive for E. In practice, $P(D|T^+)$ tells us which is the probability that one who tests positive is really sick: this probability is named *positive predictive value* (PPV). Its counterpart is the negative predictive value $P(D^-|T^-)$, e.g., the probability that individuals who test negative on the diagnostic test are actually healthy [2].

Remember that conditional probability narrows the possible outcome of an event: an example we might have from the roll of a die. If we are looking for the probability that the outcome of the throw is a multiple of 3, we will write P(outcome of the throw | the outcome is a multiple of 3) $= 1/3$ because out of the six available outcomes, we consider only those that are multiples of 3, that is, 3 and 6. Without the conditioning event, the probability would have been P(outcome of the throw) $= P(\mathbb{S}) = 1$.

5.4   Diagnostic Tests

A diagnostic test is characterized by the following situation

	Actually sick	Actually healthy	
Testing positive	*true positives*	*false positives*	Total positive
Testing negative	*false negatives*	*true negatives*	Total negative
	Total sick	Total healthy	Grand total

In this table, we recognize the sensitivity of the test given by the ratio

$$\text{sensitivity} = \frac{\text{true positives}}{\text{total sick}},$$

and the specificity of the test given by the ratio

$$\text{specificity} = \frac{\text{true negatives}}{\text{total healthy}},$$

together with the accuracy of the test given by the ratio

$$\text{accuracy} = \frac{\text{true positives} + \text{true negatives}}{\text{grand total}}.$$

For example, with a test showing these numbers:

	Actually sick	Actually healthy	
Testing positive	125	18	143
Testing negative	14	97	111
	139	115	254

we have a sensitivity

$$\text{sensitivity} = \frac{125}{139} \approx 0.899 = 89.9\%,$$

and a specificity

$$\text{specificity} = \frac{97}{115} \approx 0.843 = 84.3\%,$$

with an accuracy

$$\text{accuracy} = \frac{125 + 97}{254} = \frac{222}{254} \approx 0.874 = 87.4\%.$$

Now, looking back at equation defining the conditional probability

$$P(E|C) = \frac{P(E \cap C)}{P(C)}$$

we note that we also may write

$$P(C|E) = \frac{P(E \cap C)}{P(E)}$$

from which

$$P(E \cap C) = P(C|E)P(E)$$

so that we may substitute the numerator on the r.h.s., to get

$$P(E|C) = \frac{P(C|E)P(E)}{P(C)},$$

which is the formula for the *Bayes' rule*, where we recognize the prior probability $P(E)$, the conditional probability $P(C|E)$, the marginal probability $P(C)$, and the posterior probability $P(E|C)$.

Bayes' rule is of paramount importance in medicine, in particular for what regarding the disease diagnostic process a physician examines a patient: from the symptoms reported to him, the physician forms an idea about possible diagnostic hypotheses, perhaps mentally listing them according to the probability he assigns to each disease. This is the prior probability. After this stage, the doctor will order some instrumental tests to ascertain the diagnosis, and the results of the instrumental tests will be compared with the prior to give the final diagnosis as posterior, which will eventually be able to confirm or not confirm the prior.

The Bayes' rule is very important also in the screening medicine: assume that an epidemic breaks out among a population, and that a diagnostic test is available with known sensitivity, specificity, positive predictive value (PPV), and negative predictive value (NPV).

To be simple:

- Sensitivity is the answer to the question: "I am sick: what is the probability that the diagnostic test will notice, i.e., what is the probability that I will test positive?"
- Specificity is the answer to the question: "I am healthy: what is the probability that the diagnostic test will notice, i.e., what is the probability that I will test negative?"
- Positive predictive value is the answer to the question: "I tested positive: what is the probability that I am actually sick?"
- Negative predictive value is the answer to the question: "I tested negative: what is the probability that I am really healthy?"

In a sense, then, using a simplifying notation, we could say that sensitivity and specificity "look to the future," considering a diagnostic test that is to be done, while positive predictive value and negative predictive value "look to the past," considering a diagnostic test that has already been done.

Using the notation of conditional probability, we can summarize all the possible information by writing

- prevalence of disease: $P(\text{sick})$
- complementary prevalence: $P(\text{healthy}) = 1 - P(\text{sick})$
- sensitivity: $P(\text{test}^+|\text{sick})$
- specificity: $P(\text{test}^-|\text{healthy})$
- false positive rate: $P(\text{test}^+|\text{healthy})$
- false negative rate: $P(\text{test}^-|\text{sick})$
- positive rate: $P(\text{test}^+) = P(\text{test}^+|\text{sick})P(\text{sick}) + P(\text{test}^+|\text{healthy})P(\text{healthy})$

With these info (one must point out that in all these cases, we are dealing with probabilities), we may apply the Bayes' rule to calculate the posterior as follows to obtain the PPV, e.g., $P(\text{sick}|\text{test}^+)$ as follows

$$P(\text{sick}|\text{test}^+) = \frac{P(\text{test}^+|\text{sick})P(\text{sick})}{P(\text{test}^+)}$$

$$= \frac{P(\text{test}^+|\text{sick})P(\text{sick})}{P(\text{test}^+|\text{sick})P(\text{sick}) + P(\text{test}^+|\text{healthy})P(\text{healthy})},$$

where $P(\text{sick})$ is the prior, $P(\text{test}^+|\text{sick})$ is the conditional probability, e.g., the sensitivity of the diagnostic test, and $P(\text{test}^+)$ is the marginal probability. The posterior is the positive predictive value of the diagnostic test, e.g., the probability to be actually sick, given a test positivity. Note that the false negative rate $P(\text{test}^-|\text{sick})$, even if very important to establish the performance of a diagnostic test, does not effect the calculus of the Bayes' probability.

An important consequence of the posterior probability can be retrieved if we think about population screening for a given disease. Assume that the disease is really very serious and makes it important to diagnose it quickly and early.

In epidemiological research, The PPV is very important, so we discuss it in terms of disease screening to understand its role.

Assume that a population of 1 million is affected by an epidemic, and we draw the epidemiological picture using four scenarios: (1) prevalence of 10%; (2) prevalence of 1%; (3) prevalence of 0.1%; (4) prevalence of 0.01%.

For each scenario, we will calculate the positive predictive value $P(D|T^+)$ of a test to which we assign a sensitivity of 99% and a specificity of 98%. It is therefore a very reliable diagnostic test (a theoretical, nonexisting test), because it will accurately diagnose disease in 99% of sick people, and accurately diagnose non-disease in 98% of healthy people.

Let us now look at the behavior of PPV according to the scenarios.

First scenario: prevalence of 10% (100,000 sick people per million population)

The numbers are as follows

so that

	Actually sick	Actually healthy	
Testing positive	990,000	18,000	117,000
Testing negative	1,000	882,000	883,000
	100,000	900,000	1,000,000

$$\text{PPV} = \frac{99,000}{117,000} \approx 0.8462 = 84.62\%;$$

$$\text{NPV} = \frac{882,000}{883,000} \approx 0.99.89 = 99.89\%.$$

Second scenario: prevalence of 1% (10,000 sick people per million population)
The numbers are as follows

	Actually sick	Actually healthy	
Testing positive	9,900	19,800	29,700
Testing negative	100	970,200	970,300
	10,000	990,000	1,000,000

so that

$$\text{PPV} = \frac{9,900}{29,700} \approx 0.3333 = 33.33\%;$$

$$\text{NPV} = \frac{970,200}{970,300} \approx 0.99.99 = 99.99\%.$$

Third scenario: prevalence of 0.1% (1,000 sick people per million population)
The numbers are as follows

	Actually sick	Actually healthy	
Testing positive	990	19,980	20,970
Testing negative	100	979,020	979,030
	1,000	999,000	1,000,000

so that

$$\text{PPV} = \frac{990}{20,970} \approx 0.0472 = 4.72\%;$$

$$\text{NPV} = \frac{979,020}{979,030} > 0.9999 > 99.99\%.$$

Fourth scenario: prevalence of 0.01% (100 sick people per million population)
The numbers are as follows

	Actually sick	Actually healthy	
Testing positive	99	19,998	20,907
Testing negative	1	979,902	979,903
	100	999,900	1,000,000

so that

$$\text{PPV} = \frac{99}{20,907} \approx 0.0047 = 0.47\%;$$

$$\text{NPV} = \frac{979,902}{979,903} > 0.9999 > 99.99\%.$$

From what has been seen earlier, it is observed that PPV decreases progressively as prevalence decreases. With a prevalence of 0.01%, the probability of being really sick if you test positive for screening is less than 0.5%, so fewer than 5 out of 1000 positives will be really sick, or, to put it another way, out of 200 test-positive subjects, at most 1 will be really sick. This must make people think about the desirability of disease screening when diseases are very dangerous but also very rare. In fact, PPV is a function of disease prevalence, so in general, with rare diseases, PPV will be low.

A second problem arises when we want to compare two different tests, that is, when we want to measure the concordance between two tests. The two tests do not have to be of the same type: for example, one test might be based on hemocultures, while the other might be a radioimmunoassay: the important thing is that the two tests serve to diagnose exactly the same disease.

Since we apply both tests to all samples, the table will be as follows

	Positive for test X	Negative for test X
Positive for test Y	*both positive*	*negative for X positive for Y*
Negative for test Y	*positive for X negative for Y*	*both negative*

A first, very crude approach might consider accuracy and evaluate it as the concordance between tests, so as to have

$$\text{concordant results} = \frac{\text{both positive} + \text{both negative}}{\text{all results}}$$

and try to understand why with a thought experiment.

Let's pretend that two people toss two coins simultaneously and record the results after 100 tosses. We are therefore talking about a completely random experiment. The toss of the first coin may represent test X, and the toss of the second coin may represent test Y. We could have obtained, for example, that 27 times the result was HH, 22 times the result was HT, 25 times the result was TH, and 26 times the result was TT.

If we define H the positive outcome, and T the negative outcome, the result of these 100 tosses in the table seen earlier will be

	Positive for test X	Negative for test X
Positive for test Y	27	25
Negative for test Y	22	26

and then calculating this incorrect concordance we will have

$$\text{concordant proportion} = \frac{27 + 26}{100} = \frac{53}{100} = 53\%,$$

so a totally random experiment gives us a 53% agreement between the results. But this cannot be possible, because the concordance between two tests calculated in this way gives us wrong results, because in this way, we have calculated a totally random concordance.

A different method must be used to calculate the true concordance between two tests. When there are two tests, or when there are two assessors, if the tests or if the assessments, are qualitative (yes/no, etc.), the index to be used is Cohen's coefficient K.

Cohen's K measures the agreement that actually exists between two diagnostic tests, cancelling out effects from chance. Cohen's K is thus the concordance that is not due to chance. Thus, let us rewrite our table using also the marginal totals and the grand total, since we need these additional data: hence,

	Positive for test X	Negative for test X	Total
Positive for test Y	27	25	52
Negative for test Y	22	26	48
Total	49	51	100

From this table, we can calculate the expected frequency in the first cell of the principal diagonal as the product of the marginal totals of the row and of the column to which the cell belongs, divided by the grand total, so that

$$\text{expected value in the first cell} = \frac{49 \times 52}{100} = 25.48$$

and the expected value in the second cell of the principal diagonal is

$$\text{expected value in the second cell} = \frac{51 \times 48}{100} = 24.48.$$

Incidentally, in the same way, we calculate the expected value in the third cell (the first of the secondary diagonal of the table) and in the fourth cell (the second of the secondary diagonal of the table) as follows

$$\text{expected value in the third cell} = \frac{49 \times 48}{100} = 23.52$$

$$\text{expected value in the fourth cell} = \frac{52 \times 51}{100} = 26.52,$$

even if these last two values are not of interest for us, at present.

Now, we can obtain the proportion due to chance given as the sum of the expected values of the first and the second cell, divided by the grand total, e.g.,

$$\frac{25.48 + 24.48}{100} = 0.4996.$$

At this point, we may calculate Cohen's K is as follows.

$$K = \frac{\text{observed concordant proportion} - \text{proportion due to chance}}{1 - \text{proportion due to chance}},$$

where the observed concordant proportion is what we earlier called "concordant proportion": applying the values previously obtained, we get

$$K = \frac{0.53 - 0.4996}{1 - 0.4996} \approx 0.0608$$

Thus, the true concordance between the results randomly generated is extremely low.

A practical translation of the Cohen's K possible values can be as follows:

- $K < 0$: the agreement between the two tests is even lower than that expected if it were governed by chance (maybe there is something wrong with the data)
- $K = 0$: the measured concordance is entirely due to chance
- $0 < K \leq 0.20$: very small concordance
- $0.20 < K \leq 0.40$: small concordance
- $0.4 < K \leq 0.6$: moderate concordance
- $0.6 < K \leq 0.8$: good concordance
- $0.8 < K \leq 1$: near perfect, or even perfect concordance

We can look at a new example, concerning the assessment made by two examiners to a written mathematics exam: the table is as follows

	Examiner A: sufficient	Examiner A: insufficient	Total
Examiner B: sufficient	71	8	79
Examiner B: insufficient	11	30	41
Total	82	38	120

where we immediately obtain the concordant proportion as

$$\text{concordant proportion} = \frac{71 + 30}{120} = 0.842$$

whereas, the expected value in the first cell of the principal diagonal as

$$\text{expected value in the first cell} = \frac{82 \times 79}{120} = 53.983,$$

and the expected value in the second cell of the principal diagonal is

$$\text{expected value in the second cell} = \frac{38 \times 41}{120} = 12.983,$$

thus, the proportion due to chance is

$$\frac{53.983 + 12.983}{120} \approx 0.558.$$

At this point, we get the Cohen's K as

$$K = \frac{0.842 - 0.558}{1 - 0.558} \approx 0.643,$$

which means that there is a good concordance in the judgment of the two examiners.

References

1. Gregory P. Bayesian logical data analysis for the physical sciences. New York: Cambridge University Press; 2005.
2. O'Hagan A, Forster J. Kendall's advanced theory of statistics. In: Bayesian inference. Vol. 2B, 2nd ed. London: Arnold; 2005.
3. Press SJ. Subjective and objective Bayesian statistics. 2nd ed. New York: Wiley; 2003.

Neural Networks

6

In general, we may present the neural networks as a series of operations leading to an output O (a result) starting from a given input I (a set of data). The process goes ahead with the goal of getting a map $f : I \to O$. The learning process of the machine can be supervised or unsupervised: in the first case, the machine is informed about an expected (or desired) result, whereas in the second case, the machine has no information about an expected or desired output [1].

For example, working in the supervised mode, we may give to the learning machine the images of a healthy liver and the images of a diseased liver, while in the unsupervised mode, we can give to the machine some images of the faces of men and women, waiting for the creation of a rule able to actually distinguish the first ones from the second ones.

A neural network would aim to a better reproduction of the functions of the human brain, even we must point out that the "ghost in the machine" (here we guess to deal with a modern computer) and the brain work in a quite different way: the human brain works with a flexible logic, using about 8.5×10^{10} neurons and about 5.0×10^{14} synapses, with a time for data elaboration, which can be estimated in 5×10^{-4} s. On the other hand, a computer generally works with a rigid binary logic with a number of transistors equal to about 8×10^8, and a time for elaboration which can be estimated as 5×10^{-5} s. The speed of the signal in the human brain is about $5 \times 10^2 \, \text{ms}^{-1}$, while in a computer that speed is about three orders of magnitude higher. Despite these marked differences in the performance, the power absorbed by a modern computer is about $60 \, \text{W}$, while the power absorbed by the human brain is about $20 \, \text{W}$ [2].

M. Nichelatti, *Mathematical Tools for Telemedicine*, TELe-Health,
https://doi.org/10.1007/978-3-031-81709-0_6

6.1   What is a Neural Network

A neural network is basically a system based on algorithms developed to identify patterns and make decisions, as the human brain would. The term neural network comes from our knowledge of the way our brains work, as we know it now, by means of the models, we use to interpret the relationships between neurons, their connections, and their interactions.

Neural networks have given a very strong impetus to the development of machine learning and artificial intelligence. A neural network receives inputs, processes them, and turns them into outputs. The nodes, or artificial neurons (sometimes called perceptrons), are disposed in layers and connected by edges, and therefore, we will distinguish the input layer, one or more hidden intermediate layers, and an output layer. Information processing takes place mainly in the hidden intermediate layers, and such "anatomical" organization and related processing mimic those of the brain. Figure 6.1 reports a very simple schematic design of a neural network, with just one hidden layer.

The nodes, or artificial neurons (also called perceptrons), are arranged in layers, whereby an input layer, one or more hidden layers, and an output layer are distinguished: the number of hidden layers will be able to allow the complexity of processing to be predicted, as will the number of nodes within each hidden layer. It is in the intermediate hidden layers that information processing takes place, which will then be transmitted to the output layer. This "anatomical" organization of a neural

Fig. 6.1 Neural network

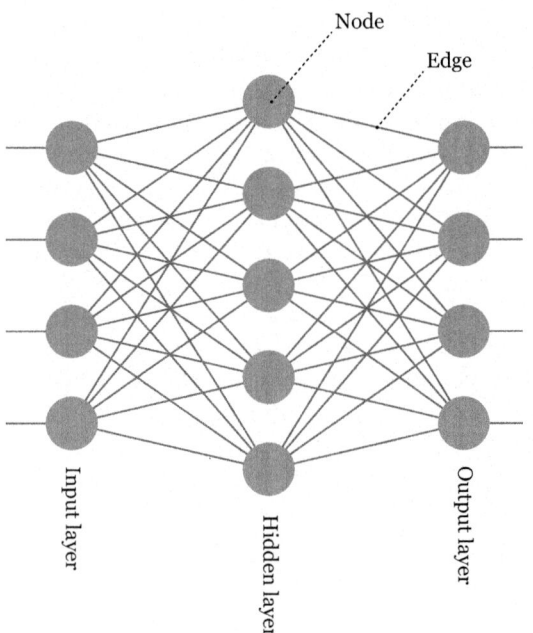

Input layer

Hidden layer

Output layer

network and related information processing mimics the brain's mode of processing and its structure.

Nodes are the units capable of receiving one or more pieces of information from outside (from other nodes), processing it, and transmitting it to other neurons through the edges that connect them. To try to be concrete right away, we could say that a node is an event, while an edge is an implication of that event.

The input of a neural network can be any kind of information, such as a sequence of musical notes, a piece of radio signal, the pixel of a picture, a sequence of words (whether of co-occurring meaning or not), and the output of the neural network will be a decision, which will take the form of a prediction of what is expected at the level of the future evolution of the received signal: thus, the neural network will classify, decide congruently with the received training, returning a response, a reaction, to the received signals. This response may be the title of the song containing the sequence of notes, the author of the lyrics and music, and the year of production, as much as it may be the photographic reconstruction of a face or a message in modern typeface taken from an ancient and deteriorated manuscript.

A neural network needs to be trained: we could ask the network to recognize hand-typed numbers represented as images. Images of handwritten lowercase letters are provided, for example, as images of 16×16 pixels. At each training session, the system will "read" the image of the letter presented as input and "write" its response (the reading) as output. Although the inputs and outputs will always just be vectors, our system will be able to learn from its mistakes and will make fewer and fewer of them.

As we saw, a neural network consists of several layers (which are its building blocks): an input layer, an output layer, and between them, an unspecified number of hidden intermediate layers (and we could think the more, the better). The nodes communicate with each other by carrying a set of information that is transmitted to the nodes of the next layer, and as the information travels to the output layer, the same information is enriched and refined. Making a metaphor, the progression of communication within the neural network may resemble what takes place in an assembly line, where everyone adds his or her own to the piece under construction, but perhaps the neural network works, indeed reasons, in the same way that Sherlock Holmes' deductive thinking reasoned in Arthur Conan Doyle's novels. From the obsevation of a detail (invisible or irrelevant to all but him), the most famous fictional detective of all time would arrive at the deduction that was (invariably) true. To anyone who followed him, deductive reasoning seemed mysterious, but what made it mysterious were just those tiny mental steps from one elementary deduction to the next, and to the next, and to the next again, until the final deduction was reached. The fact that the elementary deductions were hidden steps in the mind of the detective brings us to the possible comparison with what happens in the intermediate layers of our neural network.

Neural networks learn through training, which in a nutshell involves loading the network with a large amount of labeled data. Eventually, as we shall see, the result will not be perfectly the same as the real one, and the difference between expected and obtained data can be measured through the cost function (also called loss function, or again, error function). A neural network also uses backpropagation algorithms to adjust and correct the transmission of information.

To accomplish this task, a neural network uses optimization methods.

6.2   Algorithms

Algorithms are sequences of to-do's to reach a given aim; algorithms are like predetermined orders of things to be done, given as a list to be strictly followed. The algorithms range from cooking recipes, to lists of lab tests to diagnose a given disease, to the assembly sequence of mechanical parts to build a heat engine, and more. The number of instructions of an algorithm must always be finite. Probably, the simplest and easier algorithms are the cooking recipes, but also the instructions for assembling furnitures using a hex wrench are an algorithm, even if not always so easy to understand.

There is no human activity that cannot be programmed with an algorithm: from the shortest route from home to work to how to calculate the derivative of a function, everything can be presented as a sequence of operations. However, when working with objects to build a machine, the algorithms are mandatory.

When dealing with computers, algorhitms gives instructions about data elaboration, by specifying what to do: adding, subtracting, multiplying, and dividing numbers, taking some decisions, doing some tasks, and so on. To be simpler, an algorithm works in three steps: (1) input; (2) computation; (3) output. In this way, algorithms transform data into knowledge, or, better, algorhitms produce knowledge using data as raw material.

A simple example of algorithm is the binary search, which works using the median of a group of numbers or the midpoint of a group of generalized data. We here recall that the median of a group of (increasing or decreasing) ordered numbers is the value of the element that is in the midpoint of that group. In other words, if the list is

$$3, 4, 6, 9, 10, 11, 23$$

we see that there are seven numbers, and that the fourth of them is 9; thus, 9 is the median of the values listed earlier. If, on the other hand, the list contains an even number of elements, such as

$$5, 6, 8, 12, 14, 17, 29, 31$$

where the elements are 8, then the median of these numbers is halfway between 12 (the fourth element in the group) and 14 (the fifth element), so the median is 13. The median is the value that cuts a set of data, ordered in ascending or descending order, into two parts with the same number of elements.

Let's take a set of 10 elements, which contains the first 10 natural numbers: the set will be

$$0, 1, 2, 3, 4, 5, 6, 7, 8, 9.$$

Let's assume that we don't know what elements our set contains, and let's ask ourselves now if the number 1 is contained in the set: since we are aiming to use the binary search algorithm, how will this search proceed? First, the algorithm calculates the midpoint of the number ordered list, obtaining 4.5, e.g., the median of the integers ranging from 0 to 9. As second step, the algorithm compares the midpoint 4.5 with the number we are searching for, e.g., 1; the algorithm will therefore recognize that number 1 is in the left part of the number list, with respect to median, that is to say, 1 is less than 4.5.

Thus, the algorithm will now consider only the values below the median and will again seach the value 1 among the list of the remaining numbers, until it will determine that number 1 actually belongs to the list it had as input.

In the case we were searching for the number 1 in the list

$$0, 2, 4, 6, 8, 10$$

the algorithm would have found that number 1 does not belong to the set.

Algorithms must be efficient and crystal-clear, that is, they must be easy to read and to understand; at the same time, an algorithm must spare memory and must also have a good execution velocity. To gain these characteristics as much as possible, it is mandatory to read its instructions and to modify or correct them. For first, one must count the number of mathematical or logical operations needed to obtain the output after a given input, since this is the rate-determining step of all the job. Maybe, the algorithm may search for a given value x_T by using the binary method we have seen earlier, or maybe, it could search for the same value by checking all the numbers x_i of the input data to find in which case $x_i = x_T$, also seeing that $x_i \neq x_T$.

To get an approximated value of the velocity of execution of an algorithm, it must be put to work in various conditions, e.g., using various inputs, but one must bear in mind that speed of the algorithm depends also on other factors, such as computer speed or its available RAM memory, so the speed depends also on the device where the algorithm runs, and therefore, an algorithm may be more or less fast than a second algorithm depending on the computer and processor on which it is used. It is therefore advisable to test the various algorithms usable for the same purpose on the same machine to determine which is the fastest. It is equally important to think about the type of algorithm to use or suggest if this is implementable on various types of machines, letting the programmers decide which is best for them, case by case.

6.3   Backpropagation

In the field of neural networks, the backpropagation algorithm is widely used for training neural networks. Basically, backpropagation uses the error rate of a forward propagation and moves it backward through the various layers of the neural network for fine adjustment of weights. It calculates the gradient of the cost function with respect to the weights associated with the transmission of information from one node to another in the network. The backpropagation works on the input data transmitted to the next node, thus, obtaining a prediction, after which the algorithm works in the opposite direction by having the network transmit the error in the direction of the previous layers, making the network itself realize the error and correct it by changing the weights assigned to each input, mitigating or reinforcing them. The gradients with respect to the weights, which are calculated by backpropagation, are used by the gradient descent optimization algorithm [1].

Backpropagation is the backbone of the training phase of a neural network. As we have said, it is used to adjust the various weights of the neural network (which are associated with the transmission of inputs from one node to another node in a next layer), with a method that is based on the error rate obtained with the previous iteration. Fine-tuning the weights makes the error rates smaller, while increasing the reliability of the model and the extensibility of its use to more generalized situations.

To apply backpropagation, you do not need to know the neural networks or have previous experience, and programming is easy because it is based only on inputs, without the need to know the characteristics of a specific function, so in summary, its application does not pose too many obstacles.

The backpropagation of a neural network should continue without interruption, but there are methods that allow this algorithm to operate at its full potential.

One of the useful methods for optimizing the process is to provide a lot of data, so that the backpropagation algorithm produces fewer errors in each iteration: moreover, the training data must be cleaned as much as possible (no typographical errors, no conceptual mistakes, no repeated data), so that the input values can be normalized, and the overall process is smoother.

In general, the more data are entered into input, and the more these data have been thoroughly checked and cleaned up, the greater the chance of the neural network having wider experiences and reducing the likelihood of future errors.

Obviously, the learning rate in training is a function of the size of the data, the problem to be solved and a multitude of other factors, large and small, but it should be noted that accelerating the learning rate can be detrimental to optimizing network performance, so in some cases it is better to count on better results, even if achieved with slower learning rates. The whole thing depends on the situation to be faced, the problem to be solved, and the capacity of the programmer. It will be up to this figure, at the end, to test the effectiveness of the backpropagation model using the test set, that is, the data not used during the training phase.

6.4   Optimization: Gradient Descent

In many cases, the simpler ones, however, it is possible to calculate the maximum and/or minimum values of a function (care must be taken, because they are not necessarily both defined: for example, the function x^2 has a point of minimum, but not a point of maximum, while the function $x - 3$ has neither maximum nor minimum), that is, to see for what values of abscissa and ordinate the function is at a point where it changes direction, going from decreasing to increasing values (in the case of minimum) and from increasing to decreasing values (in the case of maximum); thus, a derivative is negative when the function is decreasing and is positive when the function is increasing.

Technical Note Let us see a very simple (and also extremely simplified) example of a derivative, for the function $y = x^2$, which tells us what the surface area of a square is, as a function of the length x of its side.

Calculating the derivative (also called the gradient) of a function $f(x)$ means seeing how fast the function increases after a very small increase dx in the variable x; the derivative of a function is defined as $\frac{\mathrm{d}f(x)}{\mathrm{d}x}$, that is the ratio of the increment d$f(x)$ of the function $f(x)$ to the (very small) increment dx of the variable x. In our case, by increasing the side x by a very small amount dx, we will see that the area of the square will become equal to $(x + \mathrm{d}x)^2 = x^2 + 2x\mathrm{d}x + (\mathrm{d}x)^2$.

Now, since dx is very small by definition, then its value raised to the square $(\mathrm{d}x)^2$ will become extremely small, so small as to be negligible, so small as to be really close to zero. Therefore, the increment $\mathrm{d}f(x) = \mathrm{d}x^2$ of the function x^2 becomes $\mathrm{d}x^2 = 2x\mathrm{d}x$, from which, dividing both sides by dx, we obtain the derivative of x^2 as $\frac{\mathrm{d}x^2}{\mathrm{d}x} = 2x$.

At points where the function is neither increasing nor decreasing, its derivative is zero. In our case, the derivative of the function x^2 is zero when $2x = 0$, and this is true when $x = 0$, that is, when the function x^2 has a point of minimum.

This topic will be addressed in detail in the third part of the book, where we will see how to compute the derivatives in general.

Technical Note A person is holding a rope that is 100 m long and wants to find the rectangle that, given this perimeter, has the maximum area: it then means finding two positive numbers x and y, with $2x + 2y = 100$ (it is a rectangle with base x and height y, so the perimeter is $2x + 2y$), such that the product xy reaches the maximum value.

Let us begin by writing $x + y = 50$, so that $y = 50 - x$, hence $A = xy = x(50 - x) = 50x - x^2$. At this point, we simply calculate the derivative of A as $\frac{dA}{dx} = -2x + 50$, and letting the derivative be zero (e.g., since at maximum and minimum points the derivative of a function is zero), then $2x = 50$, thus $x = 25$. But we already know that $x + y = 25 + y = 50$, so it must be also $y = 50 - 25 = 25$.

We then deduce that given a rectangle with a known perimeter $2p$, the maximum area is reached when the rectangle becomes the square having sides equal to $\frac{p}{2}$.

Maximum and minimum problems are not only speculative, but have very obvious practical applications in all disciplines that involve the need for scheduling and thus in many cases are important for guiding production processes in manufacturing companies and predicting raw material supply needs, both quantitatively and qualitatively [2].

Technical Note A factory needs to produce steel cylinders that are closed only at the base, all of which must contain exactly L liters of water, but the cylinders must be produced while saving as much steel as possible, so the question is: what the container size will be that allowing the minimum quantity of steel to be used. The total surface S of the cylinder (e.g., the quantity of steel needed) is πx^2 (the base surface with radius x), plus $2\pi x h$ (the lateral surface, h being the height of the cylinder, and $2\pi x$ being the base circumference), and its volume is $L = \pi x^2 h$, so $h = \frac{L}{\pi x^2}$. Let us minimize the total surface by calculating $S = 2\pi x (x + h) = 2\pi x^2 + \frac{2L}{x}$, such that $\frac{dS}{dx} = 4\pi x - \frac{2L}{x^2}$, obtaining $\frac{2\pi x^3 - L}{x^2} = 0$. Therefore, $x^3 = \frac{L}{2\pi}$ and $x = \sqrt[3]{\frac{L}{2\pi}}$, while $h = \sqrt[3]{\frac{4L}{\pi}}$. Thus, we can write $\frac{h}{x} = \frac{\sqrt[3]{4L/\pi}}{\sqrt[3]{L/2\pi}} = \sqrt[3]{\frac{4L}{\pi} \frac{2\pi}{L}} = \sqrt[3]{8} = 2$, from which $h = 2x$, so the cylinder with the minimal need of steel is the one in which the height is equal to the diameter of the base.

It has been said that the calculation is easy in the simplest cases, that is, when we are talking about functions of one or two independent variables. Things get complicated if, on the other hand, the independent variables increase, when the calculation is not immediately verifiable, so it is preferable to solve the problem with machine learning.

For this purpose, the so-called optimization algorithms should be used, which manage to find the optimal values of the independent variables, which fed into the function return the values that best approximate the real ones.

There are many optimization algorithms, and they differ in their computational specificities, which make them suitable for various types of machine learning.

Some of the most widely used optimization algorithms, and ones that seem simple enough to understand, are those that use the *gradiend descent* method, which go to estimate the minimum point of the cost function (see below). Basically, one takes any point in the cost function and calculates its derivative at that very point: the calculation will provide the gradient of the curve, again at that point, directing the search for a point of minimum. at which the derivative—as is well known—will be zero.

The best known are batch gradient descent and stochastic gradient descent.

The batch gradient descent calculates the gradient of the cost function using the entire available dataset for computation: however, the method's reliability and accuracy are countered by a relative slowness in computation.

Stochastic gradient descent, on the other hand, calculates the gradient of the cost function for only one sample at a time: in this case, the calculation is much faster, but the learning process is disrupted by a number of background noises, which slow it down.

A compromise between the two techniques is given by the mini-batch gradient descent, which processes only a single sample extracted from the data.

In order to study the function, in the sense of moving along its lines, we have to choose the speed with which we move, which we could define as the length of the steps we take moving over hilly terrain. This choice of speed of movement is called learning speed and is symbolized by the letter a.

The choice of alpha values is very important and very delicate: if it is too large (steps too long), we would run the risk of not being able to appreciate all the undulations of the terrain, which in practical terms means risking not finding all the possible minimum points we are looking for. But choosing an alpha that is too small is also risky: we would move too slowly over the terrain, and this, in our perspective, means increasing the number of calculations needed to find all the minima we are interested in.

Obviously, if we are talking about a more complicated regression model, the calculation will have to be done on the partial derivatives.

6.5   Loss Function

A neural network cannot be a perfect machinery: the output will always present an error, no matter how small. That is: the actual output won't be the target output. Of course, if the error is small, then the performance of the neural network can be acceptable; however, we generally would have to deal with the cost functions governing the error, or—better—giving a number that depends on the total error of the network. There are a variety of cost functions that can be used for neural networks: here we merely mention the simplest ones, while neglecting more complicated ones such as the Hellinger distance, the cross-entropy, and the Kullback divergence [1].

The simplest loss functions we consider are the mean square error (MSE), the root mean square error (RMS), the quadratic error (SE), and sum of squared errors

(SSE). All these cost functions contain the difference between the expected value and the calculated value squared. Elevating a difference to the square (as happens in statistics when we use the formula for calculating variance) serves to prevent adding up the differences between expected and calculated values (some will be positive, some negative) to arrive at a null value for the cost function.

By squaring the positive or negative differences, these differences will always be positive (a negative number squared always becomes a positive number), thus preventing the cost function from becoming zero.

Technical Note   The loss functions (or cost functions, or—again—error functions) most considered are the following ones:

- Mean squared error (MSE) given as

$$\text{MSE} = \frac{1}{n} \sum_{k=1}^{n} (E_k - C_k)^2,$$

  which is the most used cost function, accounting for the squared difference between the output and the expected output
- Root mean squared error (RMSE), which is the square root of the previous cost function, since

$$\text{RMS} = \sqrt{\frac{1}{n} \sum_{k=1}^{n} (E_k - C_k)^2}$$

- Squared error (SE) defined as the MSE, but dividing by 2 instead of n

$$\text{SE} = \frac{1}{2} \sum_{k=1}^{n} (E_k - C_k)^2$$

- Sum of squared errors (SSE) defined by

$$\text{SSE} = \sum_{k=1}^{n} (E_k - C_k)^2,$$

  which is the double of the SE.

The loss functions considered here therefore require the sum of the differences between expected and computed values raised to the square. We must therefore first ask what an expected value is: it is the value E_k expected to be obtained at the end of processing (as the output), while the computed value C_k is obviously the value actually obtained (again, as the output). The value we get by measuring the difference between expected and computed takes the name of the total error of the neural network, and it tells us whether and how wrong the network's work was in processing the information introduced in the input layer. Since we know the expected values, then we are working in a supervised training mode.

At each evaluation of the cost function, that is, at each training session, the $E_k - C_k$ difference will be calculated, which then will be the specific difference for that specific session. Then the total error measured with a cost function after n training sessions will be given by a formula like

$$(E_1 - C_1)^2 + (E_2 - C_2)^2 + \cdots + (E_n - C_n)^2 = \sum_{k=1}^{n} (E_k - C_k)^2,$$

in this case corresponding to the sum of the squared errors (SSE). Thus, the sum here obtained is the sum of the local errors observed after each training session.

This, however, is only a very small part of the picture: in fact, a neural network consists of a great many nodes, each of which has an input and an output, and each node will also have a local error.

So we need to solve a problem, since we need to understand how the total error is unfluenced by the values of w within the layers, and then we need to change the values of w so that the error is minimized.

To do this, we will have to calculate the derivatives of the error with respect to the individual values of w, i.e., we will have to see how the error varies with respect to a minimal (i.e., small as desired) change in each individual w_k, assuming that the error depends on w_k (i.e., that the error is a function of w_k).

6.6   An Introduction to Chain Rule

We need to give a brief description of what happens when a function is compounded, because understanding this will be critical to understanding how values can be changed, correcting them.

We say that a function z is compound if it depends on a variable y, which in turn depends on another variable x.

In this case, we can write

derivative of z with respect to $x =$

$= $ derivative of z with respect to $y \times$ derivative of y with respect to x

This is called *the chain rule* and can be extended to an arbitrary number of function.

6.7   The Node in a Neural Network

We can consider a "Boolean" (yes/no, 1/0) node as the first basis to discuss about a generic node in a neural netwok: we assume a node receiving Boolean binary signals and transmitting a Boolean binary signal; the sum of all incoming signals x_k (where $x_k = 1$ or 0) should be grater than a given threshold value $T > 0$, and in this case, the output of the node is $z = 1$, whereas, if the sum of incoming signals is below this threshold, then the neuron output is $z = 0$. In other words, the output can be only 0 or 1.

The evolution of the binary neuron is the *node*, in which all inputs x_k are multiplied by real-valued weights w_k, with a threshold, which is set to zero.

The nodes may learn via a process of error correction allowing the fine-tuning of the weights by adjusting them and learning, which is the impact of a given input on the output, such that a weight at "time" t is $w_t = w_{t-1} + \Delta$, being Δ the difference between predicted and measured values.

However, the node alone is unable to deal with nonlinearity, so that any of the output signal is multiplied by an activating function A, which introduces the nonlinearity in the decisional process managed by the node. A node of an output layer, with its incoming information, is presented in Fig. 6.2.

The most crucial aspects to consider in defining a neural network are the number of input and output nodes and the number of nodes that make up the hidden layers, obviously taking into account the weights.

Fig. 6.2 Node of an output layer

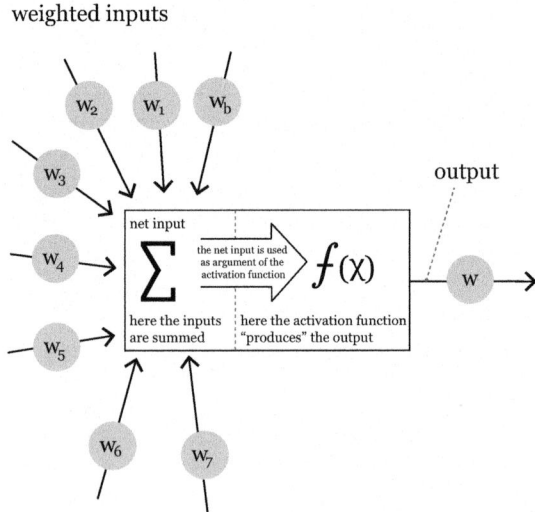

6.8   Neural Network Architecture

A neural network is a machine learning algorithm that takes inspiration from the human brain works; aims to solve problems in a similar way. A neural network is part of the deep learning: it solves problems by learning from examples instead of executing instructions from programming; it is a set of a large number of interconnected nodes working in parallel [1, 2].

The parts of a neural networks are layers of nodes (artificial neurons), where we identify an input layer formed by input neurons (tipically, one neuron per component), plus one (or more: the more, the better) hidden layer formed by an unknown number of nodes, and a layer of output neurons, producing the final output. We recognize one specific output neuron for any possible output produced by the output layer. In the hidden layer, each k-th neuron receives one or more inputs x_k from the neurons of the preceding input layer and transmits an output z_k to the node of the next hiddden layer. Any input or output is characterized by a synaptic weight w_k: synaptic weight represents the degree of influence exerted by one node on all nodes immediately following it: the signal from the node upstream of the next layer is thus mediated, and modified, by synaptic weight. The node in the next layer receives information from each active node in the previous layer, and the information received is also mediated by the respective synaptic weights. Thus, synaptic weight is effectively a way of defining the influence exerted by one node on the following ones.

The total weight entering the node is obtained from the sum of the various weights arriving from the nodes that are active at that time. If the total weight is greater than the weight needed to turn on the node that is receiving, then the same node is turned on, whereas if the threshold for turning on is greater than the incoming weight, the node will not turn on.

The neural network is trained in two successive times: the training human evaluates the behavior of the node after providing an input, while the second time of training is instead devoted to modulating the synaptic weights based on the result obtained during the first phase. With a null output and an expected nonzero output, the strategy will consist of a constant increase in the incoming synaptic weights at the node, which should increase its probability to respond positively during the next training session, while with a null expected response and observed nonzero response, the adjustment process can take place following the reverse path.

Assume that we are observing the inputs arriving from the leftmost layer (the layer of the input neurons) and going to the rightmost layer, the output layer: this kind of propagation is called *forward propagation*. The net input arriving at a given j-th node, belonging to a hidden or to an output layer, may be represented by the sum

net input arriving $=$ sum of inputs coming from the preceding layers $+$ bias;

the bias coming to the node we can assume is arriving from a node in its own right: let's call it a bias node; an unbiased arriving signal has bias equal to zero.

In turn, any single input from the preceding layer is

single input arriving = input from a preceding node × synaptic weight.

thus

net input arriving = sum of all (inputs coming from a preceding node × synaptic weight)

+ bias × bias weight .

This can be resumed in a very syntetic model, by writing the net input arriving at j-th node as

$$S_j = x_1 w_1 + x_2 w_2 + \cdots + x_n w_n + B w_B$$

where B is the bias arriving from a bias node (for example, we may assume that $B = 1$), while $x_1 w_1$ is the input arriving from the first node of the preceding layer multiplied by its specific synaptic weight, $x_2 w_2$ is the input arriving from the second node of the preceding layer, again, multiplied by its synaptic weight, and so on.

Input layer nodes receive information that they themselves turn into numbers: a sequence of musical notes becomes a series of frequencies (for example, an A, becomes 440 Hz), an image becomes a series of pixels in gray scales, a series of words can become numbers, and so on.

More correctly, we will say that the input layer nodes work with vectors. Without going into too much detail (we will discuss vectors in the third part of the book), we can say that a vector could be defined as a "multidimensional number."

Let us take the case of some patients with characteristics described in a database: let us assume four patients of whom we know three variables, as follows

Patient	1	2	3	4
Height	176	165	174	170
Weight	70	50	58	55
Age	58	60	34	46

so that each patient carries an information, being associated to three characteristics, e.g., to the values of three variables. In this case, we may define any patient as a vector (generally, vectors are indicated by a lowercase letter in boldface), so that

$$\mathbf{p}_1 = \begin{pmatrix} 176 \\ 70 \\ 58 \end{pmatrix} ; \ \mathbf{p}_2 = \begin{pmatrix} 165 \\ 50 \\ 60 \end{pmatrix} ; \ \mathbf{p}_3 = \begin{pmatrix} 174 \\ 58 \\ 34 \end{pmatrix} ; \ \mathbf{p}_4 = \begin{pmatrix} 170 \\ 55 \\ 46 \end{pmatrix} ,$$

where any single number in the vector is called a dimension. So in our case, for the neural network, four patients become four three-dimensional vectors ($\mathbf{p}_1$, $\mathbf{p}_2$, $\mathbf{p}_3$ and $\mathbf{p}_4$), because each vector contains three numbers, that is, because each patient is characterized by three variables, so our four patients are carrying twelve numbers in total.

Well, if this information is passed to the input layer of a neural network, then we will have to expect this input layer to contain at least 12 nodes, since each node will handle only one of the values contained in the vector. In this case, four vectors containing three values each implies that 4×3 nodes will be needed in the input layer. This is actually an extremely simple example that serves to make people understand what a vector is. Situations are generally much more complicated: for example, if we want to send a 64×64 pixel image to the input layer of the neural network, the amount of nodes in the input layer becomes 4096, since the image carries 4096 dimensions.

The hidden layers are the part where most of the work of a neural network is done: a hidden layer can have very many nodes, and a neural network can have a very large number of hidden layers. In general, one tends to have the same number of nodes in each hidden layer. Each node in the first hidden layer receives information from each node in the input layer through the edge and then transmits its processing to each of the nodes in the next layer, and so on. Each received signal and each transmitted signal are "modified" by the weight, which we have already heard about and will discuss in more detail.

After passing through the various hidden layers, the processing carried out by the neural network arrives at the output layer, which is the output that provides the neural network's response. As with the input layer, the output layer also uses vectors, and each individual node in the output layer will contain a dimension of the response vector. If, for example, the desired response is the recognition of one of 26 handwritten letters of the alphabet transformed into an input vector, then the output layer will consist of 26 nodes, in which the recognized letter among the 26 possible ones may have a binary code of 1, while the 25 unrecognized letters will be identified with zero.

6.9 Activation Functions

Now, a node can send its output to a next node, but the output of the j-th node is not the S_j value, since the S_j value is transformed by an *activation function* A,, which takes various possible forms. The activation functions are necessary to introduce the nonlinearity in the layer behavior. We must also know that the argument of the activation function (whichever activation function) in a node is the net input summed inside the same node, and thus, if the net sum of the weighted inputs is $S_j = \theta$, then the activating function will be $A(\theta)$, which will be also the output of the same j-th node.

The schematic graphs of some common activation functions are presented in Fig. 6.3.

Fig. 6.3 Examples of
activation functions

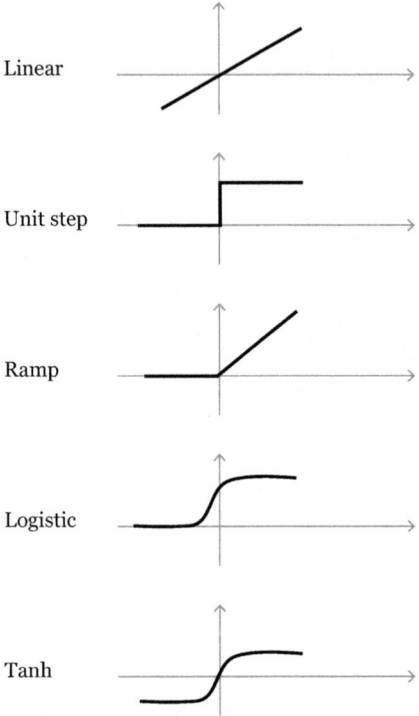

A first possible activation function is a linear transformation multiplying the net
sum θ of the inputs by a scalar λ, so that the activation function is linear, with the
form

$$A(\theta) = \lambda\theta,$$

with the special cases $A(\theta) = \theta$, if $\lambda = 1$, and $A(\theta) = 0$, if $\lambda = 0$.

A second case is the unit step (or Heaviside) activation function, which is given
by

$$A(\theta) = \begin{cases} 1 \text{ if } \theta \geq 0 \\ 0 \text{ if } \theta < 0 \end{cases}$$

thus, in this case, the net output of the node is binary: it is a constant equal to 1 if
the net input is greater than or equal to 0 (or greater than or equal to a given quantity
a), or the output is null if the sum of the inputs is less than 0, or less than a given
quantity a): note that with the unit step the node output is always a constant, since
any value of $\theta \geq 0$ is flattened to 1, and any value of $\theta < 0$ is flattened to zero.

A third case of activation function lies somewhere between the previous two, in
that the function is a ramp, defined by the equation

$$A(\theta) = \begin{cases} \theta \text{ if } \theta \geq 0 \\ 0 \text{ if } \theta < 0 \end{cases}$$

where the output is equal to net input θ if that net input is greater than or equal to 0 (or greater than or equal to a given quantity a), or the output is null if the net input is less than 0, or less than a given quantity a).

In the case of a logistic activation function, the nonlinearity is introduced into a neural network with the formula

$$A(\theta) = \frac{1}{1 + e^{-\theta}},$$

where e is the basis of natural logarithms ($e \approx 2.7182818284$): the logistic curve has a very recognizable S-shape and is bounded between its minimum value at 0 and maximum value at $+1$.

The second activation function that introduces nonlinearity is the hyperbolic tangent $\tanh(\theta)$, whose formula is

$$A(\theta) = \tanh(\theta) = \frac{e^{\theta} - e^{-\theta}}{e^{\theta} + e^{-\theta}};$$

in this case, the net input of the node is introduced in a formula that is quite a bit more complicated than the previous one but has the same S-shape, where the lower limit is -1 and the upper limit is $+1$.

With the logistic and the hyperbolic tangent activation functions, the nonlinearity forces the output of the node to have real values between 0 and $+1$ and between -1 and $+1$ respectively, so the nonlinearity of these two activation functions "squeezes" the output by forcing it to stay within a limited range, no matter how large the net input arrived at the node might have been.

There are many reasons for introducing nonlinearity into a neural network: the first reason is what we have just seen, that is, limiting the output, which not only prevents the network from reaching outputs that are too high (which with linear activation functions might continue to grow) but also produces limited variations in the output even in the case of very large values of the net input arriving at the node; the second reason is that nonlinearity helps in solving nonlinear problems, for example, in the case of classification problems.

Another activation function, specifically used for classification problems, is the softmax, which gives the probabiliy to each class, e.g., by calculating

$$P(k) = \frac{\exp(z_k)}{\sum_{i=1}^{N} \exp(z_i)}$$

which tells how likely it is that a certain classification k is the true one among N possible classifications.

The softmax activation function deals with classification problems where each class has a given input: the softmax reads the corresponding logits and gives the probability distribution of the various classes, that is, softmax assigns the probability of each classification output; in other words, softmax accepts input as a vector with N dimensions and returns a different vector with N dimensions where the components add up to 1; thus, the components can well be defined as probabilities. For example, if one wants to recognize a given handwritten number, then in aforementioned equation $N = 10$, since we have 10 numbers ranging from 0 to 9: for example, we could have an output, which can be represented by the vector like

$$\mathbf{p} = \begin{pmatrix} 0.001 \\ 0.092 \\ 0.001 \\ 0.001 \\ 0.900 \\ 0.001 \\ 0.001 \\ 0.001 \\ 0.001 \\ 0.001 \end{pmatrix}$$

(note that these values, as well as their vector representation, are completely invented, and are only used to give an idea of what the output of a softmax function might look like, and note also that all ten components of the vector $\mathbf{p}$ add to 1); in this case, the highest probability value is assigned to "4" (the first row gives the probability of "0", while last one is representing the probability of "9"), whereas the second highest value is given to "1" (which in some ways may actually resemble a badly written "4"). The great power of the softmax activation function resides in the ability to distill probability values from scores, so that it can be used in cases where classifications are the main goal, like

- handwritten numbers
- handwritten characters, both lowercase and uppercase
- in general, quite all image classification systems, since the softmax activation function is very effective in classifying heterogeneous images, for example, distinguishing between female and male faces, between photos of lions and zebras, between bicycles, cars, and airplanes.
- natural language processing
- speech recognition, since softmax is the basis of some systems that use a feature analysis of the voice signal
- sentiment analysis, which has various applications in marketing for commercial companies.

6.10   Chain Rule in Neural Networks

Working with a neural network, we assume to have found a total error $\mathcal{E}$, which tells us the difference between expected and calculated output. This errror will be the sum of all the local errors cumulating at each node; errors observed during the training sessions: therefore, the next step is to verify how single weights affects the total error, and this must be done by taking the derivative of the error with respect to this specific weight.

Thus, if we are in the output layer, and if we want to know how a weight w_n, arriving to the output layer from the immediately preceding layer, we must calculate the change of $\mathcal{E}$ with respect to a (small) change of w_n, but holding constant all other k values of w that are not w_n arriving to the output node of interest. The result of this operation will tell us exactly how much the total error varies when a change in the w_n weight occurs.

However, we know that the total error was computed using a cost function, and bearing in mind the chain rule, we may also see that the influence of the weight w_n on the total error $\mathcal{E}$ is "mediated" by the influence of that weight on the computed output C: therefore, we write

$$\text{change of } \mathcal{E} \text{ with respect to a small change of } w_n =$$

$$= \text{change of } \mathcal{E} \text{ with respect to a small change of } C$$

$$\times \text{change of } C \text{ with respect to a small change of } w_n.$$

However, we know that the output C is the result of applying an activation function $F_n(T_n)$ on the total local input T_n of the output node, so we will be able to evaluate the effect on C of a small change in the function F_n, so we will write that

$$\text{change of } \mathcal{E} \text{ with respect to a small change of } w_n =$$

$$= \text{change of } \mathcal{E} \text{ with respect to a small change of } C$$

$$\times \text{change of } C \text{ with respect to a small change of } F_n$$

$$\times \text{change of } F_n \text{ with respect to a small change of } w_n$$

This action can be repeated an indefinite (but integer) number of times. In particular, this chain-rule-based reasoning can also be applied to the hidden layers of our neural network.

Considering a hidden node in a hidden layer: the error $\mathcal{E}$ will change on the basis of a small change of a weight wk arriving to the node nk of the k-th layer as

$$\text{change of } \mathcal{E} \text{ with respect to a small change of } w_k =$$

$$= \text{change of } \mathcal{E} \text{ with respect to a small change of } F_k$$

$$\times \text{change of } F_k \text{ with respect to a small change of } w_k.$$

thus, being F_{k+1} the activation function of the following layer, we have

change of $\mathcal{E}$ with respect to a small change of F_k =

= change of $\mathcal{E}$ with respect to a small change of F_{k+1}

×change of F_{k+1} with respect to a small change of F_k,

and defining G_k the output of the node in the following layer, then

change of F_{k+1} with respect to a small change of F_k =

= change of F_{k+1} with respect to a small change of G_k

×change of G_k with respect to a small change of F_k,

then

change of $\mathcal{E}$ with respect to a small change of w_k =

= change of $\mathcal{E}$ with respect to a small change of F_{k+1}

×change of F_{k+1} with respect to a small change of G_k

×change of G_k with respect to a small change of F_k

×change of F_k with respect to a small change of w_k.

This set of operations based on the chain rule for derivatives can be iterated for an indefinite number of times, so that to obtain the derivaive of the error with respect to any weight in the layers.

6.11   Overfitting

A neural network can utilize a dataset as a training data (to adjust the various synaptic weights) during the operations (about the 60% of the total dataset). Overfitting in machine learning is a type of error that is observed if the model works accurately and gives reliable predictions when working with training data, but fails instead when using new data. So with overfitting, the model is not reliable when you make it work with data other than training data, and its predictions can become very inaccurate. In practice, overfitting relies excessively on training data and cannot be generalizable.

Overfitting also consists of giving excessive (or exclusive) importance to a certain component of the dataset: if we analyze data on the occurrence of acute myocardial infarction based on data collected—for example—only in very elderly female patients, we cannot expect the model to perform well by predicting the probability of the occurrence of an infarction in a young male patient. In this situation, overfitting acts by decreasing the accuracy of the calculation and reducing the reliability of the model, since this is limited to only a portion of the population that the model would like to study.

Overfitting can occur if the training data are too limited quantitatively, but also if it contains some redundant or excessive, or trivial, information that diverts the model's attention, directing it to unhelpful situations. For example, we might want the model to learn to distinguish men's faces from women's faces: if the set of images we provide contained more or less similar backgrounds (house facades, or trees, or whatever), our algorithm could also associate faces with certain backgrounds, making their analysis an integral part of the recognition process.

Overfitting can be avoided or reduced by using certain strategies, such as limiting the training phase, or eliminating superfluous and reasonably useless data: if we are looking for a predictive model on the possible occurrence of myocardial infarction, some variables such as dietary habits might be indicative of a certain risk, but others—such as the type of car owned—might be completely useless, so it may be necessary to inform the algorithm that some of the variables collected with should be processed. In practice, to avoid overfitting, one should train the model to be more data-aware and less sensitive to background noise in the dataset.

6.12 Convolutional Neural Networks

The convolutional neural networks (CNN) are a particular type of neural network, involved in image recognition (graphic charachters, handwritten digits or letters, faces, animals, and so on), and are based on a different network architecture, in which the dominant feature is the presence of three kinds of layers that are not used in the "normal" neural networks.

We must start by explaining what convolution is: it is an operation (conducted through the calculation of an integral) that allows us to produce a new function starting from two others. The operation consists of making (so to speak) "interpenetrate" the two initial functions, turning one and sliding it backward on the other. This may be enough for the moment: we will talk more about convolution in the third part of the book.

A convolution neural network contains three specific layers: (1) the convolutional layers; (2) the pooling layers; (3) the fully connected layers.

The convolutional layers do the majority of the job: in the convolutional layers, the convolution is put at work, starting from an image to get its first characteristics, say, edges (which would be like translating an oil portrait on canvas, turning it into a pencil sketch, as many filters associated with the software used to manage images do), then using blurring and sharpening techniques, to highlight the most relevant characteristic of the image. The first convolutional layers do the coarsest work, starting with highlighting the profiles and edges (for example, of a face), while as you go deeper into the convolutional layers, the work becomes more and more refined, due to the application of increasingly sophisticated filters. At this level, the images introduced have been processed so that the final layers are able to obtain even the most complex information.

After the convolution, the ramp activation function, which we have already encountered previously, is generally applied. This is a function that generates nonlinearity in the neural network and is often defined as Rectified Linear Unit (ReLU), also given by the equation $f(x) = \max(0, x)$, which means that this activation function is equal to zero if $x \leq 0$, while it is equal to x when $x > 0$.

Pooling layers follow the convolutional layers and capture their outputs by acting in such a way as to reduce their dimensions, that is, to restrict their width and height, so as to reduce the computational burden and reduce the risk of overfitting. Pooling layers work on small portions of the image and do so generally by selecting and keeping the pixels with the highest value, while the other pixels are eliminated. The data thus processed are transmitted to the subsequent convolutional layers.

The fully connected layer is found at the end of the processing chain in which the image features are extracted and uses the information deriving from the work of the previous layers to classify them. Pooling layers follow the convolutional layers and capture their outputs by acting in such a way as to reduce their dimensions, that is, to restrict their width and height, so as to reduce the computational burden and reduce the risk of overfitting. Pooling layers work on small portions of the image and generally do so by selecting and preserving the pixels with the highest value, while the other pixels are eliminated. The data thus processed are transmitted to the subsequent convolutional layers.

The fully connected layer is found at the end of the processing chain in which the image features are extracted and uses the information deriving from the work of the previous layers to classify them. The result is extremely interesting and important because the analysis of diagnostic images activated with CNNs is used to find the possible pathologies.

A classical and widely known source of data for putting a CNN at work is the MNIST (Modified National Institute of Standards and Technology) dataset,[1] which contains 70,000 images, of which 60,000 are for training and 10,000 for testing, of handwritten numbers (containing all the digits between 0 and 9), organized into 28×28 antialiased pixel images. Together with this database, the Fashion-MNIST[2] is also available (indeed, There is a lot of data available to test CNNs and fine-tune them): it also contains 70,000 images of fashion products, belonging to 10 categories; even in this case, the training set has 60,000 images, while the test set has 10,000 images.

Data must be downloaded and prepared for analysis, maybe normalizing the gray scale of pixels. The standard CNN can be designed with an input layer, whch will receive the images, followed by at least two alternate convolutional and pooling layers plus, again, a second again convolutional and pooling layers. In the first couple of layers, the image is decomposed in smaller pieces by 32 3×3 filters and then the result is used as argument of a ramp function to be trasmitted at the pooling layer, where the filtering continues, this time using 2×2 filters to reduce the size

---

[1] see https://yann.lecun.com/exdb/mnist/.

[2] see https://www.tensorflow.org/datasets/catalog/fashion_mnist.

of the image. In the second passage between the two consecutive convolutional and pooling layers, first double the number of filters (64 vs. 32) are used, which is then sent with a ramp activation function, followed by a new reduction in the size of the dimensions. At this sequence of activities, the maps expressed as two-dimensional matrices are transformed into one-dimensional vectors in a new specially designed layer.

The information extracted from the images in all these steps is then analyzed and interpreted by the fully connected layer, which passes the information to the output layer, formed by 10 nodes, i.e., as many as the 10 digits from 0 to 9. Using a softmax activation, the output layer will provide the answer in probabilistic terms for the 10 digits to be recognized.

The CNN must then compiled to start the training session: thus, it is the part of the CNN assessment corresponding to the instruction phase, thus using the training set to fed the CNN, followed by the validation using the testing set.

6.13   Recurrent Neural Networks

The recurrent neural networks (RNNs) are a special kind of neural networks that are able to analyze data in sequence, and thus are suitable, for example, in time series forecasting, but their utility is also proven in translations from one language to another, or also in other situations in which sequences of data are to be processed.

The RNNs have the capability to retain a memory of their activity: more precisely, there are activity loops maintaining the results of the preceding pass, and using these results as a part of the input of the next pass, thus allowing to capture the dynamics of data and their possible time-dependency: in other words, RNNs are able to detect the time-dependent properties of data. To this we must add the fact that in the RNN are used the same weights and the same bias for all time steps, so an RNN can use the same dynamics learned in all sequences, Thus, the learning efficiency becomes greater than that of a normal neural network.

However, the training phase of an RNN is quite complicated, not to say difficult, because of the errors that can be generated and propagated backward as the various time sequences pass, and because the long-term correspondences and associations that exist between signals in input tend to fade away as the same signals processed pass through the successive layers. To remedy this situation, a special version of the RNN, called Long Short-Term Memory Recurrent Neural Networks (LSTM RNNs), where the flow of information is regulated by the presence of gates (namely, an input gate, a forget gate, and an output gate) that allow the network to discriminate between relevant and non-relevant information and use the former for the learning process. The input gate decides whether to let new information pass through the system, just as a house gate can let people who ask to enter. The forget gate decides whether old information is no longer important and can be deleted, just as the head of a library service decides to throw away old math books because they are conceptually or educationally outdated. Finally, the output gate decides whether to keep the data and use it in the current time step and therefore corresponds to the librarian who decides which old math books to keep because they are still current, which would fade during the passage through the various layers, with a gradient (calculated in the training phase) that vanishes or explodes when they overlap the information propagating back at each time step. This does not happen with LSTMs as they can use the first data entered even in later processing steps.

The applicability of RNNs to translation methods between two different languages is due to the fact that in RNNs the length of input and output can vary, which is typical for translations from one language to another, where the length of the sequences of letters and words in language A is practically never equal to that of language B.

6.14   Solitonic Neural Networks

In the computers we use every day, when it processes a piece of data, the processor has to read it into memory: in the so-called neuromorphic approach (exploiting the same topological properties of the nervous system), on the other hand, data processing and memory are located in the same place, as they are in our brains.

The possibility of devising neural networks based on solitons was brought about by the possibility of a signal propagating self-confiningly, as if it were constrained within a waveguide such as those that characterized early microwave spectroscopes, in which such electromagnetic waves were "locked up."

In this case, the radiation produces its own dielectric waveguide and is not subjected to scattering, nor diffraction. This is the basis of solitonic neural networks. Solitons, are in essence solutions of certain nonlinear partial derivative differential equations that appear in the description of many kinds of physical phenomena. A classic example of a soliton is a tsunami (tidal wave that propagates even thousands of kilometers across seas and oceans), but solitons are also involved in many biological phenomena, such as nerve impulse propagation and DNA replication. In solitons, dispersive and nonlinear effects mutually elide each other.

Solitons have been applied for information transmission along optical fibers, but more recently, they have been used for signal processing.

An early development was the conception of photonic neural networks, which proved capable of unsuspected (at first glance) mathematical abilities, to the point of being able to solve differential equations. Solitonic signals can change the refraction of the medium in which they move, and paths can be created in which they move without scattering and diffraction [3].

Executing artificial intelligence algorithms with soliton-based hardware and using the neuromorphic approach enables ultrahigh processing speeds in machine learning with very short latency times, which are then able to meet the ever-increasing demands in terms of analytical power that medicine, physical sciences, and engineering sciences require.

References

1. Aggarwal CC. Neural networks and deep learning. Cham: Springer Nature; 2018.
2. Grossberg S, editor. Neural networks and natural intelligence. Cambridge: MIT Press; 1988.
3. Bile A. Solitonic neural networks. Cham: Springer Nature; 2024.

Machine Learning and Deep Learning 7

Machine Learning (ML), which is also often referred to as "software 2.0" is the ability—by a machine—to learn from the data it is given and the output obtained from processing these data.

If there is a possible model, whether simple or complex, that transforms input data into output data, then the ML is able to obtain it using a progressive learning process. Once the model, i.e., the mathematical law governing the transformation of input data into output data, has been obtained, then the ML will be able to apply the same model to new input data to verify that the learning has taken place correctly and to check whether indeed the extracted model passes the challenge of being applied to new data as well.

Machine Learning is nothing but a type of artificial intelligence, just as the eagle is a type of bird. Therefore, the question arises as to what is the specific quality of machine learning within artificial intelligence, because if all machine learning is also artificial intelligence, not all artificial intelligence is machine learning [1–3].

The most noticeable difference lies in the type of algorithms that a machine uses to learn from experience. In machine learning, the algorithms are less rigid: they come from a human instructor with a lot of information that allows the machine to be trained using a relevant number of sources, images, or other information, which are needed for the machine to learn from experience, so in a sense it is the algorithm that allows the machine to learn, or rather, the learning, as an end result, is partly due to the algorithms, partly to the experience.

There are two main families of algorithms used in machine learning: one is based on statistical techniques, the other on neural networks.

With statistical methods, the human trainers provide the machine with information about some objects by mean, for example, of their images (such as, say, airplanes, cars, and bicycles), without addding any other information (like the specification "this is a bicycle", and so on), so that the machine should be able to memorize the shapes of the various images, and to frame them in the appropriate cluster, and so—this clustering, which does not involve any additional

© The Author(s), under exclusive license to Springer Nature Switzerland AG 2025
M. Nichelatti, *Mathematical Tools for Telemedicine*, TELe-Health,
https://doi.org/10.1007/978-3-031-81709-0_7

information—should, in the long run, enable the machine to classify as airplanes, cars, and bicycles the new images that will be shown to it by the human in the second part of training [2, 3].

If, on the other hand, the vbased algorithm on neural networks is used, the human instructor provides the machine with additional information, e.g., by showing the machine a picture of a bicycle, a car, an airplane, with the additional information "here is a bicycle," "here is a car," "here is an airplane," so the machine learns using the proposed examples, i.e., in our case, a picture associated with a label or a flag.

The image instruction associated with the label continues for a very long time, so that the machine can then recognize a new image by itself, specifying, at the request of the human instructor, whether what is represented is an airplane, a car, or a bicycle.

Of course, the classes can be far more than three. The important thing is to understand that machine learning is not significantly different from the way we use to learn. For example, many of us, on the basis of received instruction (books read, television broadcasts, movies, and more) and on the basis of accumulated experience, are able to recognize dog breeds: and, if not all of them, at least the most common ones [2, 3].

Machine learning should be able to find even the hidden pattern in a data set. For example, assume that we are studying the extremely symple system with a single input and a single output like

Input, p	Output, q
5	19
6	29
7	41
8	55
9	71
10	89
⋮	⋮

from the data in the table, we see that the accepted input values are the integers greater than or equal to 5. In turn, we see that for a given input p_n, the corresponding output is given by the equation $q_n = p_n \times p_{n-1} - 1$ (always provided the input is an integer greater than or equal to 5), so that, for example, $71 = 9 \times (9 - 1) - 1$.

The difference between ML and statistical data analysis is very simple: in statistics, the input and the model are known, while the output is unknown, whereas in ML, the input and output are known, while the model is unknown.

For example, we potentially may create an ML system able to calculate the pattern existing from the characteristics of a group of cars (fuel consumption per km, country where the car is produced, maximum speed, type of engine, number of cylinders, and so on) to their respective sale prices. Once the pattern is determined, it can be used to predict the price of other new cars by the knowledge of their characteristics. In any case, data are essential, and they must have a reasonably large size. The data used to learn the pattern are the *training data*, whereas the data where we will apply the learned pattern are the *unseen data*. Obviously, training data and unseen data must share the same pattern: this is the case of the car price problem; however, it is evident that we cannot use the car price learned pattern to predict the value of the stock market.

Therefore, in our definition, the *machine learning* is the product of a sequence of algorithms and methods, allowing a machine to learn from data and to adapt its behavior in a fully autonomuos way, remembering the past experiences, and changing its future behavior just on the basis of what happening in the past. In this situation, a machine can therefore learn without the need of an explicit programmation, only using a suitable set of mathematical and statistical information.

7.1 Predictions

Prediction is the process allowing to estimate a future result, like the next value of the stock market of the company XYZ, the winner of next NBA championship, the sales volume of a given tuna fish can, the clinical result after 1-week administration of a drug in obese patients, and so on. Of course, data collected 2 years ago can be used to predict the results obtained 1 year ago (and to compare these theoretical results with the actual results) [2].

However, all ML systems may do some mistakes due to some problems in algorithm definition; other possible mistakes may derive from non-updated information and from changing patterns. For example, the prediction of consumption orientation in a population requires that unemployment rate, median income, ethical beliefs (for example, vegetarianism), and most other information (and, maybe, also new information), be constantly updated, to obtain reliable updated predictions: in this case, we are dealing with *continual ML*.

7.2 Supervised Learning

Supervised learning is used when it is believed that it is necessary to give information to the system in such a way that this information suggests to the system the desired outcome. Basically, it involves asking the system to obtain a function that is able to map the information and arrive at the desired result. In general, classification problems are solved using supervised learning [2].

One method of analysis that generally requires supervised learning is regression, which allows the behavior of a given variable (dependent variable) to be obtained from the knowledge of one or more independent variables.

In short, we enter the known values we want to simulate (we call them "labels"), along with other information that we think is important, into a given database that contains the "training data," and give the machine some instructions in the form of examples and/or hints, for processing the data. For example, suppose we have some retrospective data on a group of patients, and those data were collected when the patients were all 40 years of age, and we add to the data an information about the age of death of each patient; then all of the patients' data go back to when they were 40 years old, except for the date of death. The database might look something like this (given here in an extremely simplified way: in particular, the number of subjects must be much greater than five)

Gender	SP	CH	TG	BG	BMI	*Age at death*
M	145	260	150	126	25.3	*74*
F	135	240	160	110	28.2	*78*
F	165	210	245	135	37.8	*65*
M	140	240	190	130	26.9	*69*
M	150	190	150	119	20.5	*82*
...	...	...	...	...	...	...

The variables entered (collected when the subjects were all 40 years of age), are sex, systolic blood pressure (SP), total cholesterol (CH), triglycerides (TG), and body mass index (BMI). The label column (slanted numbers) contains the age at which the various subjects died.

The goal is to obtain a predictive model that can estimate the mortality of a 40-year-old subject based on the information collected at the time. Obviously, for reasons of space, here we have a table that contains very few variables, but the principle is the same. The machine, based on the information provided by the supervisor, will be able to build a risk model, which it can then improve, for example, by changing the risk "weights" for each variable, to adjust the model's reliability. In our example, the machine will search for a function g like

$$\text{age at death} = g(\text{gender, SP, CH, TG, BMI})$$

which will approximate the true function $f(\text{gender, SP, CH, TG, BMI})$, returning the expected age of death from the knowledge of the collected variables (note that the system does not actually know f). The approximation g will be evaluated by using a new set of data, called the "test set," again given by the supervisor: the test set and the training set are different. The machine will be able to produce its own prediction for each subject involved, and each prediction is compared with the result provided by the supervisor for the test set. If the number of the exactly predicted output reaches a predetermined value, then the model is accepted.

7.3 Unsupervised Learning

Unsupervised learning is used in cases where you want the system to search on its own, without having information about the desired outcome, for a possible result by analyzing the data. This is a situation in which the result is not "driven" by prior knowledge. This includes clustering problems, which could then refer to searching for and identifying groups that are not explicitly defined among the subjects whose data we have collected. Thus, in this situation, it is a matter of identifying the elements of a population based on their functional "closeness," which is measured by using a certain metric [2].

In this case, the table of training data could be (again, the actual number of subjects must be much greater than five)

Gender	SP	CH	TG	BG	BMI	*Cluster*
M	145	260	150	126	25.3	?
F	135	240	160	110	28.2	?
F	165	210	245	135	37.8	?
M	140	240	190	130	26.9	?
M	150	190	150	119	20.5	?
...	...	...	...	...	...	...

Here we would like to know if, for example, we can separate the subjects in two or more clusters, depending on the data. In this case, we have no labels to insert and the machine will have to do the entire job, without help. The unsupervised learning is useful even if we would need to reduce the number of variables by eliminating the redundant ones.

7.4 Semi-Supervised Learning

Semi-supervised learning is a hybrid of supervised and unsupervised learning. Training is done through data that are largely unlabeled and a small part labeled, so that regression and classification methods can be used. These are methods that are used if obtaining fully labeled data is very costly in terms of time and resources, so it is convenient to use these mixed-type data.

7.5 Reinforcement Learning

The reinforcement learning is based on a trial-and-error process: is a type of training that involves reward and punishment, as might be the training of a dog that receives a cookie if it correctly performs what it is asked to do, while not receiving it if it does not correctly perform the task assigned to it (here we refuse to think that a dog can actually be physically punished).

The system works as follows: it receives as input all the information needed to achieve the goal: the feedback received regarding the response the system has sent, whether right or wrong, will be rewarded or punished: more precisely, the feedback will be used to modify the response. The strategy used by the system to learn is called "policy," which can be deterministic or stochastic. The set of all the various situations in which the system may find itself constitute its state space, while the set of all the possible activities that the system may perform constitute its action space: the reward is commensurate with each activity performed by the system (which depends on the state the system itself is in) by means of the reward function, while the value function controls the cumulative reward achieved by the system.

Reinforcement learning is used for some computer simulations (role-playing games) and for training some robots that must learn to perform specific tasks.

Reinforcement learning involves an interaction between the machine and the environment that helps the machine make a decision regarding a certain problem. The system studies the information from the environment and decides what initiative to take in response to the stimuli. This could be the management of food and water resources to be distributed during a famine to animals raised on a farm: the system decides what to do and how to distribute the food, perhaps based on the caloric requirements of individual species and their resistance to thirst. The environment will align with these arrangements and give feedback on the effects of the decisions made, which can be communicated as a virtual cash reward. On this basis, the system will be able to vary some of the decisions made and communicate them to the environment, which again will make a judgment with a reward. Eventually, the system will have reached a virtual money sum, the maximization of which is the purpose of reinforcement learning.

Starting from the same basis of reasoning, reinforcement learning can be used to generate treatment recommendations: here the environment is the patient, from whom the system learns to prepare the best treatment strategies based on the feedback it receives from the patient.

7.6   Some Fields of Application of Machine Learning

Wanting to be concise, let us say that machine learning (or more precisely its algorithms) is about learning from data and improving one's learning performance. It was the English mathematician Alan Turing who first hypothesized that a machine might be able to learn using training algorithms: machines of this type have been called "Turing machines."

As we have seen, machine learning can be put to work using various instruction and learning techniques, starting with deep learning, which aims to simulate human learning methods through the use of neural networks arranged in successive layers (input layer, several hidden layers, output layer).

When, on the other hand, data arrive sequentially, we speak of online learning, a situation in which elearning occurs as data become available, so that the output is continuously updated and the learning process up to the time immediately before the arrival of new data determines subsequent learning, until new input data arrive.

Machine learning does not only find use in the area of scientific research, nor in healthcare applications alone, as one might have imagined. Machine learning and its applications are part of our daily lives even if we do not realize it. First of all, in smartphones, machine learning is used for voice recognition of the owner/user, as is the case with many home automation applications, and as is especially the case in text dictation processes, where it is initially required to give time to the machine to learn to recognize the user's way of speaking, although by now this phase of instructing the system is no longer so necessary (think of the dictation methods of Office products by Microsoft), or of automatic translators, to which texts can be dictated directly.

User profiling of several websites is another application of machine learning: in general, the user is asked whether to accept all cookies or only those that are indispensable: the acceptance of all cookies is the choice that allows the site exact profiling and thus the sending of online (or e-mail) advertisements related to the possible interests of those who are browsing the site, whose online browsing is tracked by collecting information from, for example, search engines. Similarly, machine learning intervenes to protect our privacy by filtering out possible spam or other potentially harmful messages and placing them in a special folder in our inbox [3].

The same happens when, after making a purchase of a book, or an item in an online auction site, we immediately receive a message with the information "you might also be interested in..." in which we see a book appear that presents and discusses a similar topic as the book we just purchased, or an item with similar use, or more, up to those messages that alert us that the same item we want to buy in the site where we are (and that we have not yet paid for) is available at a lower price in another e-commerce site.

Then there are the same search engines that, based on unsupervised machine learning algorithms, use the keywords we input, a name, a topic we are interested in, or something else, to index a series of keyword-generated answers that enable us to find the answers to our questions. Machine learning algorithms are widely used by banks and in finance to classify users of credit cards or loyalty cards (e.g., from supermarkets), whose purchasing habits, such as our favorite brand of beer, and how often we access the store near our home or work, are recorded. Unusual buying behavior, or a very expensive purchase of a kind that is completely infrequent for us, can be monitored to check that the buyer is always the same and that, for example, the credit card has not been stolen from the actual holder.

Machine learning is finding a very important use in the transportation sector: for a company involved in transportation and shipping (but also in home delivery or again, in public transperto networks), it is essential to minimize costs and wear and tear on means of transportation by tracking the routes (air, sea and road) that are most economical (it is a concrete answer to the generalization of the old "traveling salesman problem," which everyone involved in operations research and logistics knows), best implementable, and also least trafficked.

However, in the area of transportation, probably the most important application and the most harbinger of progress is, in the automotive sector, automated car guidance, which is currently being tested: it involves a series of algorithms based on reinforcement learning, and which, thanks to cameras and sensors built into the body of the car, may 1 day be able to juggle itself even in the midst of heavy traffic and even on roads that are not continuously maintained, or made slick by rain or made dangerous by a snowfall, deciding whether and when to accelerate, whether and when to brake, and deciding how to avoid a pedestrian crossing the road, and not necessarily on a crosswalk. The evolution of machine learning algorithms will, in time, make it possible to get there, in the style of 1970s science fiction TV shows.

References

1. Bishop C, Bishop H. Deep learning foundations and concepts. Cham: Springer Nature; 2024.
2. Huyen C. Designing machine learning systems: an iterative process for production-ready applications. Sebastopol: O.Reilly Media; 2022.
3. Theodoris S. Machine learning, a Bayesian and optimization perspective. 2nd ed. London: Academic Press; 2020.

Artificial Intelligence

8

With Artificial Intelligence (AI), we define the capability of a machine (a computer) to perform by itself an analysis and to give by itself an answer to a question. In other words, the machine must be able to learn and to give judgments, showing intelligence, e.g., the machine must show the capability to learn, the capability to understand, and then, the ability to judge and produce an opinion by means of the reasoning.

According to World Health Organization (WHO), the definition of artificial intelligence is as follows[1]

> *"Artificial intelligence" generally refers to the performance by computer programs of tasks that are commonly associated with intelligent beings. The basis of AI is algorithms, which are translated into computer code that carries instructions for rapid analysis and transformation of data into conclusions, information, or other outputs. Enormous quantities of data and the capacity to analyze such data rapidly fuel AI*

Thus, the aim of AI is to produce machines capable of simulating human reasoning, capable of automatic learning, capable of understanding the human language, and capable of sensory perception.

We know that artificial intelligence is the ability of an instruction-accepting machine (computer, robot, or otherwise a device capable of reasoning, and learning from its prior experience), to perform tasks that generally only intelligent beings can perform [1, 2].

Some applications have become very efficient and are capable of equaling, if not exceeding, human capabilities (at least in terms of the time elapsed between making a request and receiving a response) and thus have become of normal use in many areas of human activities, including, in particular medicine, although we all have to deal with artificial intelligence when we interact on the phone with automated

---

[1] Ethics and governance of artificial intelligence for health: WHO guidance (page 4); ISBN 978-92-4-002920-0 (electronic version); ISBN 978-92-4-002921-7 (print version)—© World Health Organization 2021.

© The Author(s), under exclusive license to Springer Nature Switzerland AG 2025
M. Nichelatti, *Mathematical Tools for Telemedicine*, TELe-Health,
https://doi.org/10.1007/978-3-031-81709-0_8

answering systems, when we argue with a chatbot, or when we make a query to a common search engine.

8.1   More About AI vs. ML

It happens that in various situations, AI and machine learning are used without noticing the inherent difference between the two concepts, and so even in newspaper and magazine articles, the two terms have become almost synonyms, but they are not, and the only thing they have in common is the scope of use.

Artificial intelligence is a set of software that is used in computers: the purpose of artificial intelligence is to make the computers that have it capable of performing predetermined tasks. In other words, the car needs fuel to move and to get people from one place to another, but the car can also function without the fuel, for example, if it is used only as a passenger compartment to shelter from the rain. Thus, AI enables the computer to perform certain complex tasks just as fuel enables a car to move. AI is not a solid, material object; AI is a computer program.

Machine learning is different from AI because it is a component of it: to use (very casually) a term from many years ago, we could write that machine learning is a "set of subroutines" formed by algorithms that are applied to data to bring to light the patterns that govern the production of outputs based on the inputs that have been introduced.

Quoting the same WHO report again, on the same page, we find a sharp description of machine learning as follows:

> Machine learning, which is a subset of AI techniques, is based on use of statistical and mathematical modeling techniques to define and analyze data. Such learned patterns are then applied to perform or guide certain tasks and make predictions.

Therefore, machine learning algorithms are needed to perform AI, but it is not correct to confuse the two terms because they stand between them as felines (a family) stand to the tiger (a species), and then we can simplify it by saying that machine learning is a type of artificial intelligence. Even better, if artificial intelligence is the technology that wants to create a reasoning and problem-solving structure similar to that of the human brain, machine learning is a method utiilized by AI to achieve its purpose. Just as machine learning is a subset of artificial intelligence, it is worth mentioning that, in turn, deep learning is a subset of machine learning in which artificial neural networks (designed to mimic the behavior of the brain) are employed to perform analysis and reasoning processes that occur without human intervention [3].

8.2   The Logic Theorist

The term AI was firstly used during a Workshop held at Dartmouth College (New Hampshire, USA) in 1956: at that time, computers (as we understand them today) did not yet exist, but already participants had begun to discuss computer systems programming. After a short time, Allen Newell and Herbert Simon developed a program, called *Logic Theorist* (LT), capable of producing demonstrations of mathematical theorems, and doing so using logic.[2] One of LT's best known successes was the proof of many of the theorems shown in Chapter Two of the book "Principia Mathematica" by Bertrand Russell (1872–1970) and Alfred North Whitehead (1861–1947). Notably, some theorems were proved particularly brilliantly: theorem 2.81 was proved by LT using 22 steps (Russell and Whitehead had used 37 steps), while theorem 2.85 was proved by LT using 9 steps (Russell and Whitehead had used 22 steps).

The Logic Theorist worked using *heuristic search*: in a nutshell, if one wants to cook a homemade pizza, one could choose whether to work with an algorithm (the recipe) or to arrive at the final result through a trial-and-error process (heuristic search) so that to improve the result from time to time. With the heuristic search, LT started with an initial hypothesis and arrived, using various branching processes based on logic, at the theorem sought, then eliminating unnecessary branches. In other words, LT knew how to cut unnecessary branches in order to find the most convenient path. Further, major developments of AI were due to the machine learning and to the birth of neural networks.

As we saw, artificial intelligence can be defined as the ability to perform tasks attributable to an intelligent being when those tasks are instead performed by a computer directly or through a robotic system. The term Artificial Intelligence thus has to do with systems capable of handling processes that require human-like intelligence, and thus the ability to reason, the ability to interpret textual or verbal information, the ability to learn from experience, to generalize, and to make predictions about the future evolution of a system [3].

Computers are programmable by means of certain instructions in a certain language, and with those instructions are able to perform complex tasks (proving theorems, like LT did, playing chess), although not always having the flexibility and imagination of human thought. However, artificial intelligence has already found many applications in the medical field (diagnosis) as well as in activities that we perform quatidaily without almost realizing it, such as in the use of web search engines or as in the automated customer service response systems of almost all commercial companies.

---

[2] See L Gugerty, Newell and Simon's Logic Theorist: Historical Background and Impact on Cognitive Modeling. Proceedings of the Human Factors and Ergonomics Society Annual Meeting. 50: 880–884, 2006.

8.3   AI and Patient's Needs

The demand for health is one of the most necessary constants, especially as the average age of the Western population rises. In particular, the demand for health is increasingly associated with the demand for care at different times and places and is also associated with the need for the memory of each individual's past illnesses and treatments.

The need for timely diagnosis, especially for oncological diseases, as well as the capability of prediction of a new disease based on some laboratory data, has also become crucial. For this aspect, artificial intelligence has learned, and is still learning, to build predictive mathematical models that are able to use pathophysiological and genetic information, as well as to process data regarding the spread of new and/or recurring infectious diseases.

For oncological diseases, it has often been the case in the past that the correct diagnosis (by tomography or other similar techniques or by laboratory diagnostics) was made only when the size of the tumor had reached values that—although still relatively small—made it difficult to set up an immediately effective treatment. Thanks to deep learning and its recognition algorithms, imaging has made a considerable leap forward.

We have been living with artificial intelligence for a long time, particularly since we need telephone assistance related to a purchase, or when we chat with a "robot" to get information about our banking conton. But artificial intelligence is now everywhere: Amazon has long put out Alexa, which is able to answer questions asked verbally in real time, just as new AI-based search engines give us our query results by sorting and personalizing them according to our priorities.

8.4   Artificial Intelligence and Language Processing

A considerable part of artificial intelligence has been devoted to computers' understanding of human spoken language. The work of these AI applications is very difficult, because the complexity of speech is very great and is made up of verbal nuances, accents, and ways of expressing words (with joy, or with anger, or with irony, or with sarcasm) that the system should be able to grasp quickly, already at the level of perception, in the voice dictation systems, with which many applications are equipped that are capable of listening to what is being said and turning it into a text file, with a decided saving of time compared to what it would take to write the file using the keyboard [2, 3].

Voice communication with a computer is handled by Natural Language Processing (NLP). However, true human–machine communication is not resolved by text dictation alone, of course, but must rest on a more solid foundation: it must learn the linguistic differences, for example, those between agglutinative languages (including Hungarian, Finnish, Korean, and Japanese), which construct words using multiple morphemes strung together, and inflectional ones (such as most Indo-European languages), as well as other types of language. Therefore, we can easily imagine the complexity of a translation from Chinese to Estonian, or from Hungarian to Korean.

What's more, a human talking to a machine may get parts of the message wrong, for example, it may have a mismatch between genders and word endings, or it may express itself using dialect jargon, or more, so the complication is even greater. In communication of this type, words are treated as vectors with high number of dimensions, and the similarity between words will be representable as a similarity between vectors. In addition, the emitted word itself can be likened to a soliton (i.e., speaking in extremely simplified terms, a self-propagating wave preserving its amplitude characteristics).

It is not only about extrapolating the meaning of a speech that can be fumbling and poorly articulated, it is also about making, for example, evaluations of how much words are used to judge a product, the chapter of a book, based on the words chosen, so as to understand whether a new brand of potato chips is positively accepted or not, whether it is too salty, and so on. This part of human–machine communication is evaluated with the tool of sentiment analysis.

In some cases, interaction systems can quickly answer specific questions by gathering the most important information and assembling it into a comprehensible, easy-to-read discourse by understanding each word that makes up a sentence. In still other cases, NLP systems called "virtual assistants" can converse verbally with the user and can respond, for example, in a humorous way to questions asked in the same tone: "let me listen to a Frank Sinatra song," or "tell me a joke," or "give me a quick recipe for dinner," or "give me the weather forecast for tomorrow in Warsaw" are among the questions that can be asked verbally to these virtual assistants, now widely publicized on the Web and television. Chatbots can behave similarly, assisting customers and providing information on how to use a given product or collecting any complaints.

8.5   An Experiment with ChatGPT

One artificial intelligence application now within everyone's reach is ChatGPT, with which we can converse in real time, and from which we can have answers that are mostly reliable to many of our (simple) questions. ChatGPT is a language model developed by OpenAI, Inc. (San Francisco, USA), based on a Generative Pre-trained Transformer (GPT) architecture. In general, ChatGPT can interact with humans by answering questions and starting a conversation, but its activity is not limited to that, since it uses Natural Language Processing (NLP) to individuate the context of the question: for example, it can distinguish between the two meanings of the word "wind," based on the other words that form the question, so that the answers will always be consistent and appropriate to the questions asked. the ChatGPT app is trained in two different phases: the pre-training phase consists of having the system learn the next word to a given word within a sentence; in the second phase, the fine-tuning phase, the system is trained with human feedback to certify and improve its performance by working on specific topics. The training uses a large number of documents from the web (articles, books, etc.: for example, it is useful to compare the answer to a question asked in ChatGPT with the Wikipedia entry devoted to the same question). Training allows ChatGPT to master lexical terms, slang modes, and the ability to reason from its learning sources.

Thus, ChatGPT could and should potentially be able to pass the Turing test, which assesses the capability of artificial intelligence: the Turing test would be passed when in the conversation between machine and human, a trained observer would no longer be able to distinguish who is the human and who is the machine.

It should be made immediately clear that ChatGPT is not capable of learning during a normal conversation, but at present, ChatGPT is widely used in the areas of customer service, tutoring, and for generating drafts of projects. ChatGPG can also be used to generate text for scientific articles (but the ethicality of this activity could be questioned) or technical articles, such as user manuals for specific devices and instruments. However, great caution is needed in the dissemination of texts created by ChatGPT because the app cannot guarantee the accuracy of responses. In particular, the check must be very accurate when using ChatGPT to generate mathematical or physical queries, where the check is essential, indeed. The chances of generating some possible error could perhaps be directly proportional to the complexity of the topic being addressed.

Just out of curiosity, let's see how ChatGPT responds to the request to solve a simple algebraic equation of the second degree: here we asked to solve the equation $x^2 - 7x + 3 = 0$.

Question to ChatGPT:

Solve $x^2 - 7x + 3 = 0$

Answer from ChatGPT:[3]

To solve the quadratic equation $x^2 - 7x + 3 = 0$, we can use the quadratic formula:

$$x = \frac{-b \pm \sqrt{b^2 - 4ac}}{2a}$$

Here, $a = 1, b = -7$, and $c = 3$.
Plugging in the values:

$$x = \frac{-(-7) \pm \sqrt{(-7)^2 - (4)(1)(3)}}{2(1)}$$

---

[3] Disclaimer: the following text in slanted characters has been generated by ChatGPT (OpenAI, Inc., San Francisco, USA).

Simplify the expression:

$$x = \frac{7 \pm \sqrt{49 - 12}}{2}$$

$$x = \frac{7 \pm \sqrt{37}}{2}$$

So, the solutions are:

$$x = \frac{7 + \sqrt{37}}{2} \quad and \quad x = \frac{7 - \sqrt{37}}{2}.$$

Thus, everything seems clearly explained, and no steps are omitted in obtaining the solution.

However, let us try to get general information from ChatGPT on a problem with clinical application by asking about telemedicine.

Question to ChatGPT:

Tell me about telemedicine

Answer from ChatGPT:[4]

Telemedicine is the use of digital technologies to deliver medical care, consultation, and health services remotely. It allows healthcare providers to evaluate, diagnose, and treat patients without requiring an in-person visit, making it a powerful tool for increasing access to care, especially in underserved or remote areas.

Key Aspects of Telemedicine:

*1. **Types of Services**:*

*- **Teleconsultation**: Virtual visits with doctors via video conferencing, phone calls, or messaging platforms.*

*- **Telemonitoring**: Remote monitoring of patients' health data, such as blood pressure, glucose levels, or heart rate, often through wearable devices or mobile apps.*

*- **Telepharmacy**: Remote prescription of medications and consultations with pharmacists.*

*- **Teleradiology**: The transmission of radiological images (like X-rays, CT scans) for interpretation by a radiologist who is not physically present.*

*2. **Technologies Involved**:*

*- **Video Conferencing**: Platforms like Zoom, Microsoft Teams, or specialized healthcare apps.*

*- **Mobile Apps**: Apps designed for managing patient data, appointment scheduling, and virtual visits.*

---

[4] Disclaimer: the following text in slanted characters has been generated by ChatGPT (OpenAI, Inc., San Francisco, USA).

- **Wearable Devices**: *Smartwatches, fitness trackers, and other devices that track and transmit health data.*

- **Electronic Health Records (EHRs)**: *Systems that store and share patient data among healthcare providers.*

3. **Benefits**:

- **Increased Access to Care**: *Particularly useful for people in rural or remote areas where healthcare facilities are scarce.*

- **Convenience**: *Patients can consult with doctors from the comfort of their homes, which is especially valuable for those with mobility issues or busy schedules.*

- **Cost-Effective**: *Reduces travel costs and time and can decrease the need for emergency room visits.*

- **Better Management of Chronic Diseases**: *Continuous monitoring can lead to better outcomes for patients with chronic conditions.*

4. **Challenges**:

- **Technology Barriers**: *Not all patients or healthcare providers are comfortable with or have access to the necessary technology.*

- **Regulatory Issues**: *Licensing and credentialing can be complicated, as telemedicine often crosses state or national boundaries.*

- **Privacy Concerns**: *Ensuring patient data security and confidentiality is critical, given the digital nature of the services.*

- **Reimbursement**: *Insurance coverage and reimbursement for telemedicine services vary and can be a hurdle for both providers and patients.*

5. **Impact of COVID-19**:

- *The COVID-19 pandemic significantly accelerated the adoption of telemedicine, as it became a crucial tool for maintaining continuity of care while minimizing the risk of virus transmission. Many countries and healthcare systems rapidly expanded telemedicine services during this time, leading to broader acceptance and integration into regular healthcare practices.*

6. **Future of Telemedicine**:

- **Integration with AI**: *Artificial intelligence could enhance telemedicine by offering diagnostic support, personalized treatment plans, and predictive analytics.*

- **Hybrid Care Models**: *A combination of in-person and virtual visits, creating more flexible and patient-centered healthcare.*

- **Global Reach**: *Telemedicine has the potential to bridge gaps in healthcare access worldwide, especially in low-income regions.*

Telemedicine is likely to continue evolving, with ongoing improvements in technology, regulatory frameworks, and patient engagement strategies.

A disclaimer has been associated with both (verbatim) citations of ChatGPT responses, warning, precisely, that the text was generated by this system, lest someone reading it might run into errors, or imperfections that can be contained in ChatGPT-generated text, perhaps believing that the same text is instead the product of human intelligence.

The question remains, therefore, whether it might be possible to distinguish text created by a human from text created with ChatGPT or with other tools based on artificial intelligence. The answer, at the moment, could be summed up by the words "maybe, but it's not very easy."

There are tools that can help determine whether a text was generated by a human or through artificial intelligence, but these tools are themselves based on artificial intelligence.

OpenAI, i.e., the same producer of ChatGPT, has launched *AI Text Classifier*: it is estimated that this system can work well on texts created with ChatGPT, since it should know the "way of reasoning," but the answer will never be exact, because the probability that the text was generated by artificial intelligence will be expressed with a five-value score: (1) probable; (2) possible; (3) uncertain; (4) unlikely; (5) very unlikely.

The *Giant Language Model Test Room* (GLTR) system works by using the complexity of language: each individual word is analyzed and classified with a four-color code (green, yellow, red, and purple) that documents their complexity (in terms of the possibility of their being used in common language). The more "rare" a word is, the more complex the text will be, and the less likely it will be an elaborate one produced with the AI.

The *ChatGPTZero* system uses a series of algorithms that evaluate a variety of parameters, producing a two-dimensional vector from which you can tell how likely it is to be AI-generated text.

Another evaluation system is *GPT-2 Output Detector*, which reasoning in much the same way will provide a similar answer.

So the systems are there, but they do not seem to be able to give absolute answers, since they make judgments in terms of probabilities: in particular, those who use them will rarely be able to be absolutely certain that a text is fake.

8.6 Big Data

Technology, research, and all other human activities produce an enormous amount of available data every day. According to an estimate by SG Analyitics, in 2020, new bytes of information entered into the network was equivalent to 2.5×10^{18} every day (and the size of the amount of data available doubles approximately every two years). Let us rewrite it: this is a whopping 2.5 billion new bytes every day, which are derived[5] from, for example, messages exchanged via Whatsapp (about 700 million messages every second), phone and video calls (about 23 million every second), email (about three billion every second, of which, about two billion are spam messages), and many other types of communication, such as videos: by way of example only, every second YouTube disseminates about 700 thousand hours of video.[6]

---

[5] Source: https://financeonline.com.

[6] Source: https://www.wyzowl.com.

Hand in hand with the growth of available data, the appetite of hackers is also increasing, with more than 450 thousand new malware and potentially unwanted applications (PUA) and potentially unwanted programs (PUPs) entering the Internet every day.[7] Note that PUAs and PUPs are a group of completely useless software that collect confidential information and generate advertising screens or invitations to pay certain amounts for unspecified reasons or may download some other unsolicited or malicious applications. In other cases, they hack into the user's search engine and alter its parameters (e.g., the main page), or they may even change the search engine itself; all without requesting consent. They are software on the borderline of malware and often hide behind freeware that one downloads from certain sites. PUAs and PUPs make up to about 20that 450 thousand new malicious software introduced to the Web every day.

The availability of health data is also very large, and processing it is not always easy: one can use neural network algorithms in supervised learning to obtain the abilities to predict the generation of a given output from the related input, or one can use those in unsupervised learning (such as clustering) that allow one to extract order from chaos, that is, to find the hidden laws underneath the data that underlie the generation (or rather, discovery), laws that are the "underground" processes, the hidden dynamics, that perhaps we would not expect to find.

Healthcare big data contain a lot of information, from biomedical data of patients, to tomographic images, to genome sequencing, to information from clinical trials. From this mass of information, artificial intelligence (particularly with neural network algorithms) will play a predominant role in determining the next most important developments in medical science in the service of curing disease.

Big data, precisely because of its size, allows for more complete answers than can be obtained with standard data holds, because in big data the information content is greater. The potential for answers is greater, and this can mean a greater likelihood of getting problem-solving.

There is no defined amount of information contained in a database that can be a threshold value for understanding that we are dealing with big data, so we may define big data as a set of structured or unstructured, homogeneous or nonhomogeneous data, such that it needs to be analyzed by specific ad hoc (statistical or other) processing methods to obtain the desired information.

So, for the time being, let's be satisfied to say that big data are extremely large sets of information and that they come from a variety of sources, and that such data exceed the management capabilities of usually used databases and the processing capabilities of generally used software for "normal size" data.

Big data must conform to what has been defined as the "3V model"[8] (i.e., volume, velocity, and variety) of data. The term "volume" means, as one might guess, the amount of data that becomes available every second (of which we have already defined the quantities). The term "variety" refers to the different types of

---

[7] Source: https://www.av-test.org/en/statistics/malware/.

[8] As defined by the financial analyst Doug B. Laney.

data (numerical data, video, text, and so on) structured (the usual tables arranged in rows and columns), semi-structured (composed of documents in which fixed information and variable information alternate), and unstructured (data presented as text files or in some other non-tabular way), that are made available. The term "velocity," on the other hand, refers to the speed at which data are generated and the speed with which it reaches the machines that are to analyze it.

For the sake of completeness, we add that in recent times, two more "Vs" have been added. The first of these is "veracity", which refers to how truthful the data are and thus what their reliability is in terms of their use for analysis; using unreliable data will inevitably reduce the quality of the results, so it may be useful to quantify (as a percentage value or as a scale value) the truthfulness of an information before introducing it into the processing model. The second new "V" is "value," i.e., the ability of data to translate into economic value,[9] as well as the value of the necessary investments.

Big data enable good results, but it also takes away resources: an analyst, as well as a statistician, may spend up to half of his or her working time cleaning up, correcting, and validating data, and validation, in some cases, can be more complex and difficult than data eleboration and interpretation of results.

But added to this is the fact that the results must be rendered in such a way that those who have to use them can understand them, so along with the analysis log, it will be necessary in most cases to produce a report that translates and interprets the log and renders the results in an easily readable form for those who will have to find solutions to problems.

A successful data analysis and a report that can be used by those who have to solve problems and make strategic decisions will be the best way to make investments made in big data pay-off.

A practical and logistical problem, which also requires investment, is the physical space to be devoted to big data. Storage in a server would always require a gradually updated backup of the data to be kept (and the backup would in turn have to be kept in a different physical space than the original data), again bringing to the forefront the problem of hacking. One can also turn to the cloud, which has the advantage of being able to increase the available space as needed without the need to purchase new hardware, but again, attention must be paid to data security.

8.7 Data Mining

Data mining is an efficient system of extracting information from big data. It is a set of techniques able to transform large volumes of data into useful information. Data mining is used to describe data and to produce eventual predictions about their evolution, using possible correlations between variables and employing a series of

---

[9] "Data is the currency of the twenty-first century", according to Douglas Laney's website (https://www.douglasblaney.com/).

models of future behavior. Also typical of data mining is the possibility of obtaining classifications of data and analyzing them with regression models that associate the behavior of one or more variables with the occurrence of a given event or with the behavior of a target variable [2].

Data mining is carried out according to a certain sequence of actions, which start with the collection of data and go through the ordering of the data to make it possible or to improve its visualization. The stages of organizing and applying data mining absolutely must include defining the objectives that the process sets: in fact, it is impossible to think of conducting data mining without knowing clearly, and from the outset, what result is to be obtained, just as it is impossible to believe that a house can be built without a blueprint.

As in the case of the design of a house, goal definition can be the most difficult part of the whole process: just think of the fact that the available data will have to be able to provide the answers, once scrutinized. It is indeed intuitive, but not always easy, to know whether big data will be able to contain all the information that will actually be needed to achieve the desired goal.

The definition of the objective must be followed by the collection of the data (and the choice of the source from which the data are taken), their organization and sorting to make them effectively the raw material to be used in data mining, and finally, the application of the analysis algorithms decided upon while defining the objectives: the algorithms, if carefully chosen, will provide the answers to the questions that the experimenters had set themselves. Of course, one must check that the answers are consistent with the questions.

Defining the goal to be achieved does not arise by chance: instead, it arises from the need to solve a problem (say, I have a problem, and therefore, I need to achieve this goal in order to solve it), and the problem must therefore be uncovered by careful analysis of the situation and must also be defined along with the list of information needed to know in order to solve the problem and achieve the goal. This is a very critical phase that requires a great deal of attention and must be studied using all the collaborative possibilities available in the healthcare corporate structure.

Once the problem has been clarified and the objectives needed to solve it have been defined, the datasets, from among those available, that might contain the information needed to achieve the objectives sought must be found. The databases found must first be cleaned up to remove information that is useless for the purpose (the type of car owned is completely useless if one is looking for information on the spread of influenza) or redundant (e.g., year of birth and age are redundant), or, again, that would violate the subject's privacy (home address, phone number, and so on).

When the data have been cleaned, work must be done on quality control: it is necessary to make sure that the values assumed by the variables are reliable (123 years of age and 270 cm of height are unreliable) and that the data are free of erroneous information (the date of diagnosis cannot be earlier than the date of birth). Missing data can be substituted using various procedures (like inserting the median value for the variable).

Where the errors cannot be easily corrected, and are not attributable to data typing errors (123 years of age could mean that the person who entered the data actually wanted to write 23, but his finger, inadvertently touched the "1" key before touching the "2" key), the irreparably wrong values should be eliminated, i.e., deleted leaving the cell blank. Deletion is also essential when faced with duplicate data, whereby the exact same subject has had data entered multiple times: deletion will serve to maintain only one entry per subject.

The second data cleaning operation should be done by preserving important variables and eliminating unnecessary ones, i.e., the number of dimensions subtended by the dataset should be reduced. The goal is to keep the really important data and increase the speed of performing the analysis.

At this point, it becomes possible to search for the most important relationships among the remaining variables: they will be manageable rules with regression analysis, or more simply of correlation calculations, but to a large extent the study triggered by data mining will appropriate the techniques of artificial intelligence, using supervised or unsupervised learning, to classify the available information, or to obtain a prediction about the evolution of the system represented by that data.

Data mining can use various algorithms and techniques to analyze data: it can use neural networks to eleborate deep learning algorithms, working according to what we have seen, with the various nodes to which the "weighted" information that is produced by the nodes in the previous layer is afferent, and which is reprocessed by the node that produces "weighted" outputs in turn and destined for the nodes in the next layer, simply by using the total input as the argument of the activation function.

The results obtained must then be interpreted, particularly to verify that they are novel findings. The knowledge that can be derived from data mining can then be used to decide on new strategies for approaching the patient and continue to improve the goals that we had set out to achieve. In practice, if we have achieved the goal of figuring out how to improve services to the patient, we will now set ourselves the goal of improving it again, after gaining experience using the improvement determined by data mining.

Another useful algorithm is the K-Nearest Neighbor (KNN), which measures data on the basis of their topological proximity, evaluated with a specifically decided metric (this could be Euclidean distance, or a Taxicab-type distance, but we are not so interested in this at the moment), but the distance sought must be such that similar data lie close together on the hyperplane containing them [3].

Data mining can also base its work using decision trees: again using classificatory or regressive methods to predict the outcomes of a given set of decisions, representing them as a tree diagram.

8.8   Some Thoughts on Sentient Machines

Anxiety and lack of confidence in the future have always been the backdrop for the development of new technologies. In many science fiction stories, the interaction between humans and robots is mentioned. In this regard, emphasizing that the robot was in the service of man, the scientist and writer Isaac Asimov (1920–1992) had developed his famous three laws of robotics, which say verbatim: *(1) a robot may not injure a human being or, through inaction, allow a human being to come to harm; (2) a robot must obey the orders given it by human beings except where such orders would conflict with the First Law; (3) a robot must protect its own existence as long as such protection does not conflict with the First or Second Law.*[10]

We also remember that the neural-network-based SkyNet system became sentient in the celebrated film "The Terminator" (and later in the related franchise), directed by James Cameron, based on a plot by Cameron himself and Gale Anne Hurd, and starring Arnold Schwarzenegger. Moreover, the supercomputer HAL 9000 was able to lie and to kill humans in Stanley Kubrik's unsurpassed masterpiece "2001: A Space Odyssey", based on the short story "The Sentinel" written by Arthur C. Clarke (1917–2008).

But are such events actually possible? In particular, could an AI system actually become sentient and achieve self-consciousness? For a number of years, a branch of ethics has been developing that aims to study artificial intelligence and the relationship between it and humans. In that field, there is talk of a possible, looming singularity, one in which an AI characterized by an intelligence far superior to that of humans will be able to escape our control unless governed and limited.

Although the hypothesis is not current and is probably far off in time, it is certainly appropriate and reasonable to come up with systems that will help to understand when AI will eventually reach consciousness.

The problem is by no means negligible: if an AI system achieved self-awareness, a series of ethical and moral evaluations would open up. What rights could a self-aware AI have? And above all, would a self-aware AI possess its own ethics? And what ethics could it possibly be: respectful of human life, respectful of the laws of nature, or perhaps it would be respectful only of itself and aimed only at protecting and preserving itself, perhaps at the expense of everything else. And then, in legal terms, would the self-conscious system have rights? And if so, what ones?

Therefore, that of AI self-awareness is a problem that is by no means insignificant, especially since the companies dealing with these systems do not study it or implement it in their products, except in a marginal way. This must have been on the minds of the 19 researchers and scientists (neurologists, computer scientists, psychologists, ethicists, philosophers, and others) who developed a kind of questionnaire (better, a checklist) that should allow them to assess whether an AI system has achieved self-awareness or at least a reduced form of it. The prepared paper has been posted on the arXiv server,[11] so it is not yet a peer-reviewed scientific publication, but it is already capable of provoking debate or at least scientific curiosity. More recently, other articles have appeared that have done

---

[10] Isaac Asimov: *Runaround*, a short story featured in the periodical "Astounding Science Fiction", Street & Smith Publisher, March 1942.

[11] P. Butlin et al. Consciousness in Artificial Intelligence: Insights from the Science of Consciousness. arXiv:2308.08708v3.

more multifaceted analyses,[12] where the more purely ethical part of the topic is analyzed, starting with the various assumptions that could justify the concept from AI self-awareness using the human brain as a reference.

We understand from these readings that this risk is currently absent, if, the reading shows, none of the models of AI functioning may be able to match the higher functions performed by the human brain. This does not detract from the fact that a day may come in the future when AI activities will be such and so complex as to bring these machines closer to a possible state of self-awareness, but at present, there is no need to worry. If anything, it will be a case of figuring out how to identify, on that future day, the realization of the possible self-awareness of machines.

8.9 An Ethics for Artificial Intelligence

One application of artificial intelligence that perhaps can approach these problems of machine self-awareness lies in military applications, where the ethical problem is clearly manifested. Already now we have drones, i.e., armed airplanes that are remotely guided with a joystick: the absence of pilots in the cabin makes drones safer for aviators, and for a variety of circumstances means that the size compared to a normal military fighter plane is reduced, so the drone will be difficult to detect and hit.

Weapons can easily be incorporated within systems that use AI (they are called killer robots); their purpose is to achieve surgical precision in eliminating the enemy and thus also reduce the number of civilians who are killed, but these systems, precisely because they are potentially almost painless for civilians, may risk local and global conflicts being triggered more easily. In addition (which is no small thing), it may come to the condition where the AI can decide for itself whether and when to use weapons.

This unfortunately is not all, because the use of artificial intelligence imposes questions that impact all of society.

Just as the robotization and automation of assembly lines have cost the employment of large numbers of prosution workers in many manufacturing areas, so artificial intelligence applied to the processes of production of tangible and intangible goods (bureaucracy, services, and so on) will lead to a reduction in employment, with the risk of triggering very dangerous social problems. More seriously, the unintended (hopefully) introduction of bias into AI systems (a bias generated by an algorithm or even by biased data) could make the social consequences even more severe. One wants to avoid thinking that the bias can be interpretive, that is, that it can be determined a posteriori by those who must interpret and apply the results. When an algorithm has been finished, the problem is not closed, because the biases may lie hidden or concealed in the instructions, and may only come to light in the

---

[12] M. Farisco, et al. Is artificial consciousness achievable? Lessons from the human brain. arXiv:2405:04540v2.

long run. It therefore necessitates that the system and its results always be carefully monitored.

Ways to reduce the risks of bias in the operation of AI-based systems are based on mechanisms to be used before and after.

One must start with the data, which are the raw material of analysis. The data must be cleaned, verified, and validated: the existence of duplicates or out-of-context values must be checked, and all variables, which must always have different, self-explanatory names, must be checked so that validation is easier. For example, categorizing sex as a number (1 vs. 2) might make it difficult to interpret, and then better to categorize with a string (M vs. F), or use a dummy variable that explains the categorization, for example, naming the sex variable as "bad," so that it equals 1 in males and equals 0 in females. The same is obviously true for other variables that can be expressed as dummies, such as "sick," in this case coded 1 if a subject has a disease, and 0 if the subject is healthy.

First, provision should be made for algorithms to be designed to be easily readable and equally easily corrected, so that continuous rereading as they are written allows for continuous surveillance of their contents. An algorithm, before it is used, must be put to the test to see how it works.

The process of generating an algorithm should possibly be followed by more than one person, and by more than one person, the check on how it works should be done. And if people with different experiences and cultures in terms of artificial intelligence participate in the construction of the algorithm, it will probably be easier to detect bias during the construction.

References

1. Boden MA. Artificial intelligence: a very short introduction. Oxford: Oxford University Press; 2018.
2. Mitchell M. Artificial intelligence: a guide for thinking humans. London: Peli- can Book; 2020.
3. Russell S, Norvig P. Artificial intelligence, a modern approach, 4th edn. Harlow: Pearson Education; 2022.

Part II

Telemedicine

Systems

In simple terms, a system is a set of things that enable a process to function. From medicine, we know of the existence of the respiratory system of the circulatory system and other systems and apparatuses each of which consists of a collection of organs and tissues that allow taken individually and taken all together the organism to function properly and survive.

A system can be viewed in many different ways: for example, we might be interested in studying the anatomical structure of the circulatory system, but we might instead be interested in understanding how it works, for example, to get information about how the heart rate is regulated, or how the circulatory system can function improperly, for example, due to an anomalous rise in systemic blood pressure.

In general, by studying the circulatory system or any other physiological system, we will obtain information about the position of individual organs on their size and functioning: in general, we could define a set of inputs that reach the system producing a set of outputs that can either self-regulate the system or that can be directed to other districts of our body, thus becoming in turn inputs to some other organ or system. In any case, the study of a system must look at its components and study its behavior through the evaluation of certain variables at the input and other variables of output.

Of course, there are many other examples from the real world that we can consider systems: an automobile is a system, the circulatory system a system, the solar system is a system, a rail transportation network is a system, a telecommunications network for radio or television is a system, the Roman Empire was a system. In all cases, we are talking about a set of objects that enable the operation regarding some activities that are indispensable at the economic and managerial level.

In general, a system is thus a set of real objects connected to each other (not necessarily connectedness occurs through physical contact), which contribute to the performance of a given collective task [1].

M. Nichelatti, *Mathematical Tools for Telemedicine*, TELe-Health, https://doi.org/10.1007/978-3-031-81709-0_9

In general, a system can be described as a set of components, each of which has its own tasks to perform. The collective task is to receive something as input and transform it into something else as output (as an example, one could easily think of what happens in the digestive system).

9.1   What Does a System Do

A system reacts to external stimuli (input variables) by producing output variables; internally, a system is characterized by a number of state variables that govern its behavior and determine the translation of the various received inputs into outputs. In some cases, systems are very basic, like a vending machine: simplifying as much as we can, we can say that the inputs of the vending machine are the coins and the signal that comes in by pressing the button to choose the drink one wants to buy, while the outputs are the drink itself (the "physical" drink), plus the eventual change in coins. State variables describe the characteristics of the system, so they contain all the information about what condition a system is in at a given instant. In our case, the state variables definitely include a binary one (machine on/off) plus the one that calculates the difference between coins received and cost of the various choice options (coffee, cappuccino, tea, other) to calculate what change is to be dispensed to the buyer. To these state variables will have to be added those that control the temperature of the drink being dispensed and the volume being placed in the plastic cup. A schematic description of system examples is given in Fig. 9.1.

It should be added that during the process of preparing and dispensing the drink, the machine is unable to accept orders, so the next customer will have to wait until the machine has finished serving the previous customer and has given change, if any.

In general, it should be possible to predict the behavior of a system, that is, to know what response the system will issue in output knowing the signals received as input.

9.2   Characteristics of a System

State variables describe the characteristics of the system, so they contain all the information that allows us to know what condition a system is in at a given instant. In some cases, information about state variables is particularly important so we are interested in studying the system as if it were a glass box, the contents of which we can explore and know in terms of state variables: in this case, we speak of a white box model. In other cases, knowledge of the state variables, and thus knowledge of what is happening inside the system, may not be necessary, and we may be interested only in knowing the input and output, that is, what output we get from a given input: in this case, we are studying the system as a black box. This is the case with the vending machine: no client will feel like knowing the internal behavior of the machine and will regard it as a black box, because he or she will only be interested

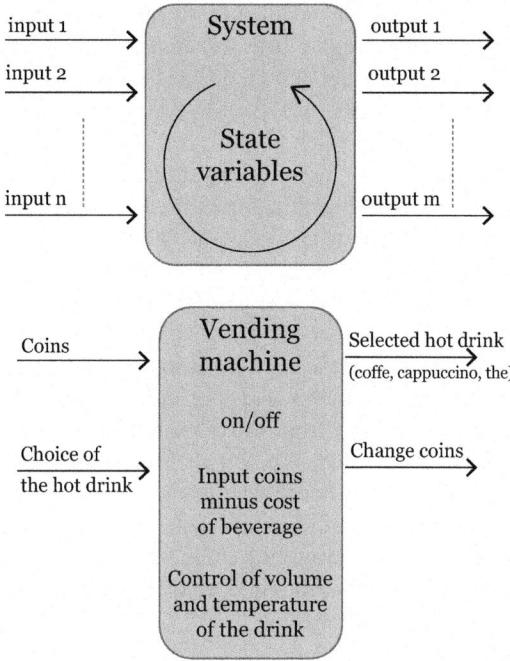

Fig. 9.1 Simplified examples of systems

in verifying that by inputting coins and choosing the desired beverage, he or she will actually get what he or she requested and any change coins.

Systems are classified in various ways: probably, the most important distinction is between *linear* and *nonlinear* systems. A system is said to be linear when, given an input x_1 that produces an output y_1, and an input x_2 that produces an output y_2, if the input is the sum of the two inputs $x_1 + x_2$, then the output will be the sum $y_1 + y_2$. If not, then the system is nonlinear. In a linear system, we then speak of superposition of effects, and in general, we may write that an input $x_1 + x_2 + \cdots + x_n$ will produce an output $y_1 + y_2 + \cdots + y_n$.

The behavior of a system is generically determined by a transition function that evaluates the state of the system at a given time t based on the evaluation of the system itself at time zero and the set of inputs that always arrive at time zero; the transformation function, on the other hand, calculates the value of the output at a generic instant t based on knowledge of the inputs and the state of the system always at time t. If the transition and transformation functions of a system allow the outputs from the system to be obtainable in a determinate way, then the system is called deterministic; if, on the other hand, the results of at least one of the two functions can be affected by some random fluctuations, then the system is called stochastic. A stochastic system is that constituted by virtually all prize games, beginning with the roll of a die whose outcome is affected by a number of probabilistic-type effects that influence the output of the outcome, such as the force with which the die is rolled.

A system is defined as discrete if the system does not recognize intermediate times between the discrete time t_n and the next discrete time t_{n+1}, if the system accepts discrete-valued inputs, and if the transition function and the transformation function are both discrete-valued functions even when their argument is continuous: an example of this situation is the "next integer" function $F(x) = \lceil x \rceil$, in which a function accepts a continuous value x as input, returning a discrete value (the next integer $\lceil x \rceil$) as output, so, for example, we will have $F(1.01) = \lceil 1.01 \rceil = 2$, $F(4.3) = \lceil 4.3 \rceil = 5$, and so on. In case all three characteristics of a discrete system are not verified, then we speak of a continuous system.

A system is called combinatorial if its outputs at a given instant depend solely on the inputs it receives at the same instant (no memory); if, on the other hand, the output values from the system also depend on the previous values, then the system has memory. The result (heads or tails) of a coin toss is clearly a system without memory, because the output head or tail does not depend on the output of the previous toss. A system is dynamic if the state variables of the system can change over time, while it is static if the variables cannot change. If the transition function varies in a system, then the system is called time-varying, while, conversely, it is called time-invariant [1].

9.3   Telemedicine is a System

So far, we can summarize the situation by stating that a system is a collection of objects, elements, individuals, and other things, which are related to each other according to precise and (hopefully) known laws, so that they work together to achieve a predetermined goal. A country's healthcare system is a collection of people (doctors, pharmacists, nurses, economists, engineers, dedicated staff for cleaning and disinfection, and so on), overhead facilities (hospitals, public and private clinics, chemical-clinical testing laboratories, hospices, and so on), emergency-equipped vehicles (helicopters, ambulances, medical cars, etc.), drug distribution and supply systems (regulatory authorities, pharmaceutical companies, and so on), technical equipment (laboratory instrumentation, diagnostic instrumentation, chemical reactants, beds, mattresses, pillows, linen, gowns, wheelchairs, and so on), aimed at treating disease and achieving the highest possible state of well-being for the population of that country. A very simple (and fully theoretical) system aiming to glucose monitoring of a diabetic patient is described in Fig. 9.2.

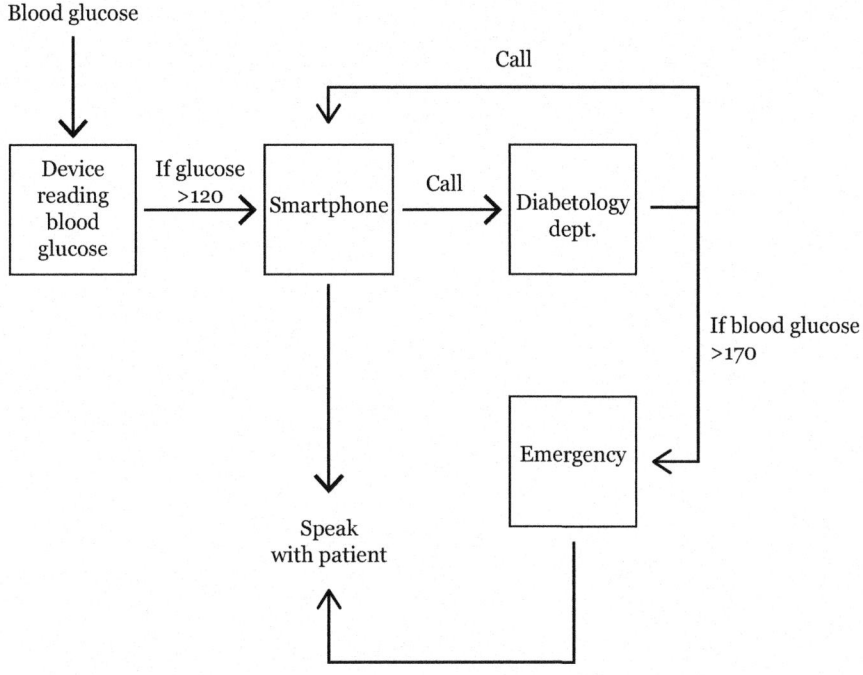

Blood glucose

A simple hypotetical system aiming to constantly monitor the blood glucose of a diabetic patient

Fig. 9.2 A theoretical system for blood glucose

From these very simple introductory concepts, we can already understand that telemedicine is a real health service delivery system that needs strong regulation of its behavior so as to optimize its operation and the results we expect.

Reference

1. Oppenheim AV, Willsky AS, Young IT. Signals and systems. New York: Prentice Hall; 1983.

Telemedicine, e-health, telehealth

10

Telemedicine means delivery of healthcare services and transmissions of medical and biological information through communication technologies, without the need for physical contact between doctor and patient or the simultaneous presence of doctor and patient in the same place at the same time.

The transmission of data between doctor and patient or between a doctor and another doctor is not the only activity encompassed by the definition of telemedicine, because we can distinguish various situations that telemedicine deals with. These are:

- Patient distance education
- Continuing medical education
- Distance medical meetings
- Telediagnosis
- Telematic recipes and telematic medical certificates
- Electronic medical records
- Management and security of the patient's clinical data, with safeguarding and protection of the patient's sensitive information and privacy
- Telehealth networks and systems
- Cloud computing
- Patient movement, remote admission, remote discharge
- Isolation and quarantine of the patient potentially or actually suffering from communicable diseases

Of course, the domain of telemedicine is not limited to what aforementioned, which represents only the main topics in which telemedicine is involved.

In many cases, we see that the term telemedicine is used as an alternative to the term eHealth (or teleHealth), and vice versa: in general, however, people prefer to use the definitions eHealth and teleHealth for the nonclinical aspects

© The Author(s), under exclusive license to Springer Nature Switzerland AG 2025   115
M. Nichelatti, *Mathematical Tools for Telemedicine*, TELe-Health,
https://doi.org/10.1007/978-3-031-81709-0_10

of telemedicine, while the term telemedicine seems more appropriate for remote clinical services [1, 2].

The most important aspect to consider in telemedicine is that of data communication, data communication that needs constant technological updating and also needs constant monitoring of the situation in terms of the security of data transmission.

It is not simple and perhaps not even possible to reason about telemedicine without starting with an essential assumption: providing telematic services to a patient means adapting to provide them according to the patient's ability to receive the services. It makes little sense to transmit services and information in ways that the patient does not access: it makes no sense because it is money and time wasted. It can cost the patient's loss of trust in telemedicine.

Adapting to the needs of those who are less technologically equipped (because they do not have state-of-the-art equipment or because they do not have enough money to equip themselves with it) is what is called the "bottom-up approach."

The bottom-up approach can be described as a hydrodynamic process: imagine a funnel into which we pour water to pour it into another container. The rate at which the water is transferred will depend on the width of the funnel neck, that is, the fluid will flow into the new container at the rate at which it flows through the funnel neck, not at the rate at which we pour the water into the funnel.

Therefore, where possible, use communication tools within everyone's reach: use the telephone for audio communication, use the Short Message Service (SMS), or use messages via WhatsApp, which are widely used communication methods even among the elderly.

The average age of the population in Western countries is rising, so there is a gradual aging of the population, and associated with this is also the increase in life expectancy due to improved care.

In general, the population is aging and birth rates are getting lower and lower so that the almost constant or even increasing value of the number of individuals in a Western population is often due to the increase in life span and life expectancy as well as in some cases also the increase in migration flows. In front of this situation, there is a general improvement in health conditions due to the evolution of research and the creation of new drugs, which, however, have to cope with the conditions of increasing chronic and degenerative diseases that are due to the increase in the average age of the population while also taking into account that these diseases require constant continuous treatments, even throughout the life span. Thus, the reduction of mortality risk leads to an ever-increasing demand for care for the elderly population; this demand is not limited to treatment and medication but also includes everything including patient socialization, thus also the concept of tele-nursing. In fact, the resolution of a clinical problem in an elderly patient, perhaps even suffering from a chronic disease, does not imply the resolution of the care problem as well, because the patient must not only be treated but must also be cared for in such a way that all of his or her needs are met, not only health needs but also relational needs, so that the quality of life of these individuals reaches the highest possible value.

In this area, telemedicine seems to be a particularly appropriate tool, although its applications aimed at facilitating and speeding up all care processes are not limited to the elderly patient but are also easily addressed to the care of the ordinary citizen with particular reference to remote areas where the intervention of traditional medicine is not always applicable as quickly as necessary.

Telemedicine had a great development during the recent COVID-19 outbreak in which it was essential to provide the health services under population isolation (in most of the pandemic-affected states). For telemedicine, the COVID-19 pandemic was probably the most important test case and also the main impetus for its development. During the pandemic, the healthcare system was tested in many countries, and telemedicine won the trust of physicians and patients and certainly set the stage for its further development determined by both the communication techniques and the telemonitoring and telehealth tools that had to be developed and implemented during the most critical periods. Generally, the health feedback from the use of telemedicine seemed positive and also influenced the use of telemedicine even in experimental clinical protocols that showed how successful remote therapy and remote visitation were to the point that telemedicine was developed even for epidemiological conditions that were not necessarily critical such as those observed during the pandemic.

Telemedicine involves many ethical issues because the way in which communication between doctor and patient is set up is different from the way the patient and the doctor themselves have been accustomed to in long years of practice, especially if both the doctor and the patient are elderly. In particular, one problem may be that of the reliability of the relationship between doctor and patient, which with telemedicine could be considered as a technically reduced time, which in general could exclude the various stages of mutual acquaintance that are established between the patient and the family doctor, so it is necessary that the time devoted to telemedicine also contains spaces for dialog and information and thus be seen as a process of natural evolution of health care. Among the ethical aspects, it is also worth mentioning that the communicative closeness and immediacy of connection produced by telemedicine are able to allow the patient to save the time needed to go to the family doctor's office and especially all the waiting time so that in a sense the patient's confidence and trust in the doctor are fostered; furthermore, with telemedicine, also considering the possible time availability of the doctor, it is possible that the patient can access contact with the doctor more easily and more frequently, as long as this does not result in an obsessive demand for care that is not justified by the patient's real health situation.

In the field of telemedicine, we distinguish two basic parts: (1) telediagnostics, that is, the set of all technologies that enable remote diagnosis; and (2) teleconsultation, that is, the technologies that enable video calls between patient and doctor and between doctor and specialists.

Another key part is telehealth, which allows monitoring of certain activities of the elderly patient and immediately defining the occurrence of events such as a fall or fainting and allowing immediate geolocation of the subject: it consists of a small device normally worn around the neck, and which is equipped with some buttons, including an emergency one (usually defined by the acronym SOS), which allows the subject quickly connect to the care center and/or a relative's phone to report a problem in real time.

Mention should also be made of telenursing, generally given by all those technologies that allow nursing activities to be carried out at a distance, including all the activities necessary to educate the patient in the use of technologies so that he or she can be supervised at all times of the day. Similarly, we speak of telemonitoring when certain information about the functioning of the circulatory system is constantly recorded, such as hemoglobin saturation.

Telemedicine is supported in its developments by advances in artificial intelligence and developments in numerous apps that are also available for use with an ordinary smartphone.

Virtually, telemedicine originated with the invention of the telephone and took its cue as early as the 1950s, when an attempt (successful) was made to send X-ray images from Westchester Hospital to Philadelphia Hospital, some 40 km away. Later, television broadcasting techniques were used at the University of Nebraska for lectures to medical and surgical students. Telemedicine was also used very early for the care of the sick at sea on transport ships and naval vessels, enabling the transmission of electrocardiographic signals to remote healthcare centers on land [1].

In later years, technologies useful for telesurgery activities began to develop, initially with tele-mentoring In the early 1990s (see in a later chapter), in which an experienced surgeon is able to communicate remotely with another, less experienced surgeon, providing him or her with the assistance and information needed to perform a given operation, and by responding in real time to questions asked of him or her.

These, first experiments in guiding surgeries (initially urology with laparoscopy) were performed with video and audio monitoring. Subsequent laparoscopic mentoring experiments showed good results, fully comparable to those obtained by inexperienced surgeons trained in attendance conventionally: probably, the most sensational experiment for those times was the use of surgical mentoring to guide from Honolulu an eye surgery performed in Manila, Philippines.

The use of telemedicine went to situations where the patient was aboard ships: in particular, the U.S. Navy created a telemedicine system that connects naval ships sailing in the Pacific Ocean with a base in California [1].

In the mid-1990s, the first telesurgery experiments were done in which a robotic arm was able to guide the endoscope, while a telestrator highlighted the most important things so that the surgeon could focus his attention on those.

The telestrator (or video marker) is a technological invention that has proved extremely useful in telemedicine. It is a device that is equipped with a touch-sensitive screen (like that of smatphones or tablets) on which an operator can trace hand drawings, or lettering, that is superimposed on a photographic image or video. It is a technology that is widely used in weather forecasting broadcasts, or even in sports broadcasts, to analyze plays used during basketball, football, and soccer games, making it an almost indepensable system for describing what happens during team sports competitions.

The telestrator is also used for educational purposes to comment on scientific films or to enhance the visibility of particular aspects of a photographic image under a microscope (cells of a tissue) or X-ray and is therefore very suitable for implementation in a medical teleconference or during surgical tele-mentoring.

Telemedicine is also finding wide use in countries where widespread poverty in urban or rural areas makes it almost impossible to have medical facilities or experienced doctors: experiments of this kind were developed in the late 1990s in Ecuador.

10.1 The Organization of Telemedicine

It is necessary, before invoking the use of telemedicine, to define exactly which patients will actually (and advantageously) benefit from it, and this means knowing the true needs of the patient: therefore, telemedicine must be tailored to the needs of the patient. If the needs for hospitalization outweigh the needs to be able to be cared and treated at home, then hospitalization will certainly be preferred to telemedicine.

If, on the other hand, the reasons for telemedicine will prevail based on the patient's needs, then it will be time to consider which telemedicine services are best suited to the patient's situation, keeping in mind that telemedicine does not repudiate traditional hospital care, but replaces or supplements it when appropriate. Therefore, telemedicine and traditional medicine are not in conflict.

We are facing a kind of epochal change in the delivery of healthcare services, but this, as is already intuitable for all areas of medicine, does not mean that telemedicine is applicable to all patients, especially pediatric patients, because of the great variability that can be expected in these individuals.

Inclusion and exclusion criteria must therefore be defined, depending on the variability of the subject and the availability in the area, which can be traced back to screening, training and education for patients, nonemergencies, follow-ups, monitoring of subjects with wearable or implanted devices, and teleconsultations between healthcare personnel [1, 2].

A basic requirement for all telemedicine activities is the audio and video recording of all sessions that took place remotely, both for the sake of keeping track of what was said and done during the connection and, in the case, for possible availability of the same at the forensic level. Obviously, someone within the hospital or point-of-care facility will be responsible for recordkeeping.

If desired, a follow-up of patient satisfaction would also be recommended to see if the service provided is working as it should, or if there are some aspects to be improved, in particular the way the patient perceives (also characteristically, emotionally) the contact with the doctor should be probed, and not only, therefore, the mere effectiveness of the telematic communication, so a satisfaction questionnaire could be structured to assess the various dimensions of care.

One can also ask whether telemedicine can be adapted, or tailored, to emrgency situations, in which telemedicine is, even temporarily, the preferred resource. These options need to be foreseen in advance, and equally in advance, organizational, resource, and matrial flows will need to be anticipated.

Telemedicine is a key tool at the disposal of public and private healthcare to deliver services that must be rapid, effective, and available to all actual and potential patients; but to do this, telemedicine needs strong integration both at the territorial level (think rural districts, for example) and at the level of the complex of healthcare services that must be made available to the population. The economic aspect (cost of services), the financial aspect (finding the economic resources to meet the same costs), and the commercial aspect (companies producing the goods needed for telemedicine, which can offer products at a reasonable cost, while obtaining a good margin that allows them to invest in new products and continue to respond to individual and collective health needs) have a strong relevance in this area.

Other problems that arise are technological as well as actual health issues, and they go hand in hand with the problems arising from making the service accessible to everyone, including those who live far from hospitals and those of an age that does not make compatible the use of detection systems that are not extremely simple in the processes of activation, connection, and shutdown. This whole set of collective and individual interests results in the need to match technology (efficient and available low-cost networks, wearable tools for recording biomedical parameters, and so on), people (physicians, technicians, engineers, and so on), and organization (political-economic structure of the healthcare organization, commodity-producing enterprises, and relationships between them and healthcare institutions), having a clear goal of serving any patient by providing him or her with what is needed, leaving no one behind: resource allocation, governance of the entire sector, and preparation for adverse events of collective concern, such as earthquakes, floods, and other disasters of various origins. This means designing optimal resource allocation, planning for governance of the entire sector, and preparing early responses to all possible adverse events of collective concern, such as earthquakes, floods, and other disasters of various origins. Therefore, telemedicine is also an emergency medicine that must be able to enable the intervention and rescue of people displaced in places momentarily inaccessible to ordinary medicine.

Thus, a health economic system that is not able to target these goals would risk bringing down the whole castle of telemedicine without even being able to make it express its great potential. Without explicit recognition of these challenges and without targeted strategies to address them, any telemedicine initiative risks not expressing its full potential, so it is essential to take into account the problems that telemedicine poses to the health system in a way that defines them in their economic and organizational dimensions in order to be able to address and overcome them.

The first and most obvious problem is that telemedicine requires that the patient and the healthcare facility to which the patient is referred are not in the same (and, in some cases, not even at the same time), which is the basis of ordinary healthcare delivery. By the problem of unfeasible in-person linkage, we mean all those who are prevented from moving to a hospital or physical place where health care is dispensed. Here we can include not only rural dwellers but also military personnel engaged overseas, maritime laborers, emigrants, and tourists, who would have to pay even substantial sums of money to access health care in the host country.

Then, in Western countries, the average life span is always increasing, and with it, the incidence of chronic noncommunicable diseases, compounded by the reduction of available health personnel (doctors, nurses, social and health workers). This means having to increase the overall health budget to meet the ever-increasing demand for health. In addition, one should not forget the effects of migration flows that create groups of disadvantaged individuals whose demand for health care may also be different from that of the original population. Thus, the main need is availability of communication technologies that are able to ensure reliability in the exchange of data and information, including but not limited to real time.

Because of what has been said, it is essential to identify the variables that need to be considered when embarking on a challenge to give telemedicine the chance of success that will lead it to represent a practical reality in providing an answer to the need for health.

It follows that telemedicine must be the result of a project that is well defined in all its aspects, in which at the strategic level, but also at the local level, its strengths and weaknesses (which relate to the project itself) as well as its opportunities and threats, which instead relate to the socioeconomic, health, and political environment, are analyzed. In particular, while one opportunity (among many) of telemedicine is to help and stimulate the growth of data transmission technologies (perhaps, in particular, for the miniaturization of wearable sensors, problems may arise from the need to keep the telemedicine project abreast of the times, and this is something that affects not only patients but also doctors and nurses. A key social and health problem is the reduction in the healthcare workforce that technology upgrades will have to address.

Immediately identifying weaknesses in care and threatening factors to the long-term survival of telemedicine must therefore be a priority strategic choice by all those who share the need to provide quality service. Strategic choice means recognizing right away the priorities on which to intervene, assuming that an intervention cannot be carried on several floors simultaneously. Of course, such work cannot be considered conclusive: challenges to development continue over time, and so must be equally continuous surveillance of telemedicine behavior and ever-changing expectations.

This work does not appear to be particularly complicated because it may be sufficient to collect statistical data on the utilization of available health care resources and to poll dedicated focus groups formed by those who work there, in the health services.

10.2 The Design of a Telemedicine System

Designing telemedicine is not conceptually different from designing a building: one will have to know from the outset whether the building will have to meet the housing needs of affluent people, or whether it will be a dwelling destined to become a social housing, or again, whether the building will house a supermarket, or whether it will be a whole shopping mall. Depending on the intended use, the building will have to be served by some infrastructure, so if we are talking about a commercial center, high-density connecting roads and multistory parking lots will be needed, while if the intended use is ordinary housing, then normal roads and open or covered parking spaces for the inhabitants can be provided [1, 2].

It will also be important to decide on the basis of the state of affairs: a shopping center will fill a need in the area, that is, it will provide an answer to the demand for available and nearby stores in a neighborhood where stores are lacking, so people have to travel long distances to do their shopping: it would be unthinkable to build a new shopping center next to an existing one.

Similar to the design needs of a building, telemedicine also has needs and demands to be met. If a telemedicine system is to be designed, it is essential to know from the outset the goal that the system is to achieve, that is, the health needs that the system is going to meet.

At this point, the project may start on the basis of the acknowledged needs and on the funding available. Focusing on the impact of the new system on the currently existing situation, so as to identify any opportunities to hinge on the previous system to the new one.

At this stage, too, it will be essential to hear the contributions of all stakeholders, especially those of family physicians, whose care role may be changed (or may appear to be changed): the available technology of telemedicine does indeed entail a different, at least partial, approach to the work of family physicians, but their role in health care would not be diminished; on the contrary, it would be positioned even more centrally [1, 2].

The success stories observed in the area of care and healthcare innovations tell of optimal incorporation of therapeutic and technological innovations into a frame of established reliability obtained through years of previous management experience. Thus, development goes in the direction of integration and not in the conflict between old (however reliable) treatment habits and novelties introduced perhaps forced into the preexisting system. So it is a matter of changing processes, gradually and without forcing, so that the transition between old and new care organization takes place osmotically, without cultural trauma. In this regard, and just citing it as an example, AGENAS (the Italian national agency for regional health services) recently published a monographic issue of its Monitor magazine dedicated to some aspects of the integration of telemedicine services in the Italian healthcare system (the issue can be downloaded totally free of charge.[1]

But not only will the role of the physician (family doctor, but also hospital) change: it will involve redesigning the tasks of all the actors participating in the innovation, as well as creating new figures adapted to the new specific needs of telemedicine and equipped with different and previously unforeseeable professional

---

[1] www.agenas.gov.it/images/monitor-47_stampa.pdf.

skills. New professionalism will be particularly necessary to anticipate the needs dof practical instruction of patients in the use of instruments and their maintenance.

It would be enough to think about the possibility of evaluating the new service, after a pilot test period, in terms of reduction (or cancellation) of waiting times in the outpatient clinic, savings in costs and transportation time from the home to the doctor's office, with the understanding that clinical outcomes would certainly not be any worse than before.

In few words, a number of performance indices will need to be considered, which should be taken into account when evaluating the impact of telemedicine on the social and health fabric.

10.3 Performance Indicators

Performance indicators are normally used in all sectors to assess whether and how a given project is progressing toward planned expectations, whether costs are able to be borne by profits, and for all that is relevant and pertinent.

No telemedicine system would be able to survive if, for only 100 contacts per year with treated patients, it involved—for example—the employment of 20 physicians, 40 nurses, and 10 pharmacists: staffing costs would be prohibitive and make the project unsustainable.

Various systems can be envisaged to analyze the performance of telemedicine: one can analyze the size and complexity and duration of service delivery, cost-effectiveness, clinical effectiveness, and satisfaction at the organizational level and satisfaction of needs by providers and patients.

The size of the service is easily measured by the number of users followed in the last 12 months and the total number of annual accesses that users have generated; whether the service is growing or declining will be fairly easily understood by doing the ratio of the number of users and the number of accesses in the last 12 months to the number of users and accesses in the previous 12 months.

For example, if users and accesses in the last 12 months compared with those in the previous 12 months give a ratio greater than 1, the service will be found to be growing. Assume that we had 627 users in the last 12 months, and 569 in the previous 12 months: the ratio will be equal to

$$\frac{627}{569} = 1.1019$$

and thus, the number of patients is up by 10.19%. An entirely similar calculation can be made using the number of accesses, rather than the number of patients.

Obviously, it will be important to check whether the number of patients followed with telemedicine covers an important fraction of the totals afferent to the territorial system. Thus, it will be necessary to know how many patients are affected by disease A, and among them, how many actually access telemedicine services. In particular, it may be very useful to calculate the average number of accesses (per year, per month, per week: it depends on the nature of the disease) for each patient of those traditionally cared for, compared with the average number of accesses for those cared for with telemedicine, in order to compare the two ratios. It is also essential to provide a time trend of the number of patients assisted and the number of accesses (for example, on a quarterly basis): this will also allow monitoring the dynamics of patients flowing from one system to another. It is also important to keep track of the mortality and quality of life observed with the two methods of care, although these indices are not clearly associated with care, as many other variables (e.g., those related to the patient's family, and those related to social relationships with family members and neighbors).

The efficiency of the telemedicine system is concerned with the economic and financial aspects and is obtained by calculating the average annual cost of the service, incusing overhead costs, personnel costs, equipment purchase and depreciation costs, and so on.

More complex and multifaceted is the evaluation of effectiveness, which instead concerns the clinical and curative spheres. Effectiveness is measured in many ways: since these are clinical evaluations, failures will have to be measured, which can be determined by various factors, such as the length of stay in the hospital, or the number of re-hospitalizations needed for the patient, and also by measuring quality of life through appropriate validated multidimensional questionnaires (not created extemporaneously to have a simple collection of information) [2].

Again, the comparison will have to be established toward the effectiveness of the treatment delivered by conventional care. Should the comparison also concern mortality, it will be important to remember and take into account all possible factors that may influence it. For example, if an elderly patient cared for years by the conventional system is transferred to care through temedicine, and if this patient dies a few months after his transfer, his death should not go to telemedicine, unless weighted correction factors are used that know how to impute his death correctly.

Indicators related to care complexity will take into account the average number of professionals involved in the care process: the hours of service of the professionals involved per month-patient of care will then be calculated: for the response to the individual care demand, the response time for each professional figure will have to be calculated, until the specific response for that individual care demand is provided.

The measure of client (patient or caregiver) perception is obtained directly from the measure of patients who voluntarily drop out of care through telemedicine: every single dropout amounts to a failure of telemedicine, and it will be good to check the reasons as soon as possible. A more graduated measure of satisfaction will be obtained by administering suitable questionnaires.

References

1. Choudhuri T, Katal A, UM J-S, Rana A, Al-Akaidi M, editors. Telemedicine: The computer transformation of healthcare. Berlin: Springer Nature; 2022.
2. Eren H, Webster JG, editors. Telehealth and mobile health. Boca Raton: CRC Press; 2015.

3. Gogia SB, editor. Fundamentals of telemedicine and telehealth. New York: Academic Press; 2019.
4. Khandpur RS. Telemedicine: technology and applications (mHealth, TeleHealth and eHealth). Dehli: PHI Learning; 2017.

Computer Networks

11

A computer network is a system that enables the communication and transmission of data, relying on hardware machines, the software that manages its data transmission processes, and a transmission channel consisting of wiring (a "physical" transmission channel) or a wireless system, given by a transmitting antenna and a receiving antenna.

There are various types of networks, such as the local area network (LAN),which allows the connection between processors located in a limited area, where data transmission is generally through a physical channel. Some schematic examples of LANs are presented in Fig. 11.1.

11.1 Bits and Bytes

Think of a binary experiment, like the flip of a coin, to obtain head (H) or tail (T). The coin is assumed perfect, thus flipping the coin is a fair game, and realization of the event H has the same probability of the realization of the event T; clearly, the probabilities are $P\{H\} = P\{T\} = 0.5 = \frac{1}{2}$, thus, before any flip, we expect that the event H and the event T have both a 50% probability of realization. Now, how much information can we retrieve from the realization of the event H as a "binary event"? Assume now to find a specific codon during a genetic analysis: again, how much information can we retrieve from the realization of the event "ACC" (adenine, cytosine, cytosine) among the possible 64 codons of our DNA?

The elementary unit of information is calculated starting from the probability of realization of the binary event, and its unit of measure is called *bit* (from term *bi*nary dig*it*): one bit is by definition the information we get when a binary event that has a 50% probability (such as precisely the coin toss) occurs; mathematically speaking, 1 is the absolute value of the exponent that must be applied to the denominator of the fraction denoting the probability of the binary event with a 50% probability.

© The Author(s), under exclusive license to Springer Nature Switzerland AG 2025
M. Nichelatti, *Mathematical Tools for Telemedicine*, TELe-Health,
https://doi.org/10.1007/978-3-031-81709-0_11

Fig. 11.1 Some LAN's

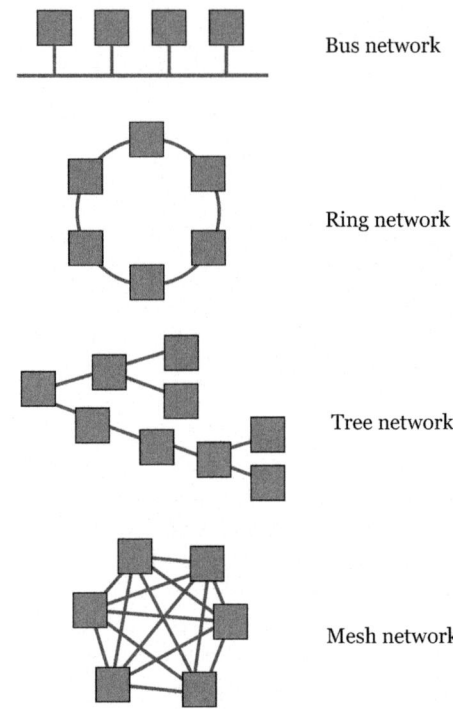

Bus network

Ring network

Tree network

Mesh network

Thus, when flipping the coin, we expect to have

$$P\{H\} = \frac{1}{2} = \frac{1}{2^1} = 2^{-1},$$

that is, the information is $|-1| = 1$ bit, and the probability to find the codon ACC in a given position during a DNA sequencing is

$$P\{\text{"ACC"}\} = \frac{1}{64} = \frac{1}{2^6} = 2^{-6},$$

so that the information carried by a codon is $|-6| = 6$ bits. Of course, here we assume that all possible 64 codons have the same probability. Well, we could have found the same result by remembering that there are 4 possible nucleotide bases in DNA, e.g., adenine (A), cytosine (C), guanine (G), and thymine (T), so each base carries 2 bits of information ($\frac{1}{4} = \frac{1}{2^2} = 2^{-2}$), so the 6 bits of any codon are the sum of the contributions of 2 bits each from the three nucleotide bases that make it up.

As an additional curiosity, we can check how much information is contained in a single amino acid. Since these total 20, we find that for each individual amino acid we have

$$\frac{1}{20} \approx \frac{1}{2^{4.32}} = 2^{-4.32},$$

therefore 4.32 bits. Again, we assume that all possible 20 amino acids have the same probability. Very interestingly, to encode an amino acid carrying on average 4.32 bits of information, we need a codon carrying on average 6 bits of information, so translating the genetic code from DNA to proteins costs the loss of about 1.68 bits of information per every single amino acid that will be assembled in the protein. Indeed, this fact should be very interesting to those who study thermodynamics.

Obviously, information is also contained in the words and letters that make them up. Choosing one letter from among the 26 of the alphabet (let us assume that we are dealing only with lowercase letters, and that all have equal probability of choice) yields information of about 4.7 bits. Similarly (but we here should take into account spaces between words and punctuation), we can estimate that a line of text on the page of a book or document contains information approximately between 700 and 750 bits.

A *byte* (B) is an amount of information equivalent to a sequence of 8 bit (its name should derive from *binary octette,* although it is believed to be a way of recalling the term "bite" by modifying the spelling). The byte is the best known and most widely used unit of measurement in computing, in particular with the multiples kilobyte (kB), meagbyte (MB), gigabyte (GB), and so on, respectively defined as 10^3, 10^6 and 10^9 B. The old tradition of expressing byte multiples as powers of 2 (e.g., 1 kB $= 1024 \, \text{B} = 2^{10} \, \text{B}; 1 \, \text{MB} = 2^{20} \, \text{B}; 1 \, \text{GB} = 2^{30} \, \text{B}$) must therefore be abandoned.

The concept of bits and bytes will soon be superseded by the large-scale introduction of quantum computers, one of the momentous advances in computer technologies.

In fact, in quantum computers, they are not limited to bit values 1 and 0, because they use *qubits* (i.e., quantum bits) that can take on many states according to the superposition principle of quantum mechanics. In a nutshell, quantum computers will be able to reason in multidimensional terms, being able to simultaneously analyze various distinct evolution possibilities of a system. We can only imagine what enormous benefits will accrue to the ability to quickly produce designs, for example, in earthquake-resistant building construction, or in the design of safe and mechanically resilient automobiles, or in the design or discovery of new molecules with pharmacological activity, or in the programming of new commercial software for use in research or day-to-day operations.

In this way, the speed at which information is processed will increase so dramatically that current computer technology will quickly become obsolete, and the quantum algorithms used in machine learning will become much more selective and efficient, particularly when quantum technology is used in big data analysis.

11.2 Frequency and Bandwidth

Regardless of the system we are observing, the signal is transmitted using a certain frequency of oscillation, that is, the frequency at which the wave is sent, represented by the number of wave crests arriving at the receiver every second (think, for example, of counting how many sea waves break on the shoreline every second).

This unit of frequency measurement is called hertz (the symbol is Hz), in memory of the German physicist Heinrich Rudolf Hertz (1857–1894), who had demonstrated that an electrical signal could be transmitted through the air (thus giving the theoretical basis for the invention of radio).

In practice, the frequency of 1 Hz corresponds to one wave (one oscillation) every second, and each of us has certainly heard of the mutiple kHz (1000 Hz, i.e., 1000 oscillations per second), MHz (one million oscillations per second), and GHz (one billion oscillations per second), so when we read that our microwave oven works by emitting an electromagnetic wave at 2.5 GHz, we know what it is. Obviously, the higher frequency corresponds to a lower width (i.e., a smaller distance between two ridges) of the wave: in the case of the microwave oven frequency, the electromagnetic wave has a length of about 12 cm. For any wave, the relationship between wavelength λ (in meters) and frequency f (in hertz) can be calculated using the equation

$$\lambda = \frac{v}{f}$$

where v is the speed (in meters per second) at which the wave propagates.

An electromagnetic wave can transmit information only if it has a way of changing its characteristics as it is sent and only if the receiving station is able to sense these changes.

The signal can be modulated by changing its amplitude (in which case we speak of amplitude modulation), that is, by acting on the wave height, and thus increasing or deminishing the difference between the maximum value and the minimum value of any single wave, but keeping the distance between the peaks of the wave constant, or by changing its frequency (and in which case we speak of frequency modulation), keeping the difference between maximum and minimum constant, but varying the distance between wave peaks. In either case, a wave carrying the signal, called the carrier wave, is modulated by a second wave, called the modulating wave. A third possibility for varying a wave signal is phase modulation.

The information to be transmitted is contained in the modulating signal, while the carrier signal is basically the vehicle that enables transmission and allows specifying at what frequencies the modulation takes place [1, 2].

Amplitude modulation (AM) is used in the transmission of radio signals and for the video component of television signals, although the latter application has been abandoned for some years. It is a transmission technique that has had, and still has, widespread use and wide commercial success, partly because, from a technological point of view, receiving an AM signal is very easy, requiring very simple circuits, but it has the disadvantage of being very sensitive to noise, something that each of us has probably experienced by listening to an AM transmission with a car radio. With AM signals, power is transmitted through the modulating wave.

Frequency modulation (FM) is the system used with great application in the transmission of a radio signal. The frequency of the transmitted signal is made to vary according to the amplitude of the carrier frequency. Frequency modulation

Fig. 11.2 Amplitude modulation and frequency modulation

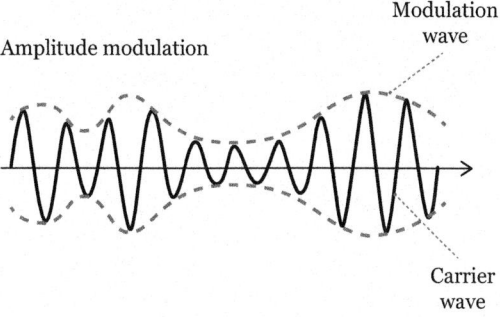

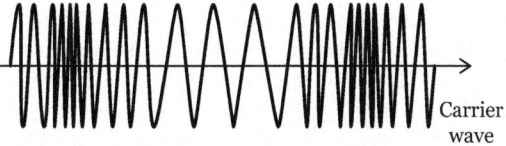

involves varying the frequency of the signal to be used for transmission by making it directly proportional to the amplitude of the signal to be transmitted. The efficiency of FM transmissions is much higher than that of AM transmissions, both because the power carried by the carrier is largely suifficient for transmission and because MF is much less sensitive to noise.

The graphs representing a carrier wave in the case of amplitude modulation and frequency modulation are given in Fig. 11.2.

Compared with amplitude modulation, frequency modulation has the advantage of being less susceptible to noise and allowing better quality transmission. It also has much greater efficiency—compared with amplitude modulation—because the power of the FM-modulated signal is given solely by the power of the carrier and does not require additional power to be transmitted.

A possible point of weakness in FM transmissions may be the need for the receiving equipment to be equipped with an antenna (ham radio), the construction of which, however, is quite simple, since these radios are also sellable in kits for home assembly. A second problem was the increased complexity of the circuits, which, however, does not reverberate on the cost of a radio, since the same circuits have reached extremely low costs for the user.

The bandwidth is a method of explaining what amount of data can be transmitted with a connection between transmitter and receiver: if the connection allows 1 byte per second to be transferred, we will say that the transmission rate is 1 Bps.

Given transmission speed, we can then define bandwidth as the set of frequencies that a transmission system is capable of handling: bandwidth allows us to understand what and how many signals can be transmitted: the wider the bandwidth, the greater the possibility of transmitting and receiving data of various kinds (phone calls, videos, and so on). The bandwidth is a method of explaining what amount of data can be transmitted with a connection between transmitter and receiver: if the connection allows 1 byte per second to be transferred, we will say that the transmission rate is 1 Bps.

Given transmission speed, we can then define bandwidth as the set of frequencies that a transmission system is capable of handling: bandwidth allows us to understand what and how many signals can be transmitted: the wider the bandwidth, the greater the possibility of transmitting and receiving data of various kinds (phone calls, videos, and so on). Bandwidth is generally measured in MHz (or even in octaves: if a frequency goes up an octave, then the frequency is doubled; if it goes down an octave, the frequency is halved).

Bandwidth is a fundamental concept when talking about data transmission rate: it is the frequency band that a signal occupies when it is sent through the transmission channel, and it is defined as the maximum frequency minus the minimum frequency of the signal, so if the maximum frequency were 10 kHz and the minimum frequency were 900 Hz, then the bandwidth would be 9.1 kHz (in fact, $10,000\,Hz - 900\,Hz = 9100$ Hz): however, the maximum rate r of data transmission for a channel having bandwidth W is $r = 2W \log_2 n$, in which n is the number of levels used by the signal (this equation is the Nyquist theorem).

When transmitting with a twisted pair, the bits 1 and 0 are represented by two values V_1 and V_2 of the voltage (e.g. we will have $V_1 \neq V_2$ to distinguish 1 from 0), while with the fiber optic the signal that propagates is a light pulse (here we will have a series of switches between "on" $= 1$ and "off" $= 0$) that travels potentially at the speed that light has in the medium of which the interior of the cable itself is made (and thus at a speed less than 300,000 km per second, which is the speed of light in a vacuum): fiber optic cables are made internally of glass, which provides the best performance in terms of transmission speed, or of plastic material, which is much less expensive. The curvatures of the fiber optic cable do not hinder the transmission of the light beam, since the beam is reflected by the fiber envelope.

11.3 LANs and WLANs

LANs are those normally used to connect computers that are located in the same place (a hospital, a manufacturing enterprise, the administrative office of a munic-ipality, a private home, and so on). Networking is the connection existing between local area networks, between which communication takes place in general via electromagnetic or optical signals: the sources and destinations of the transmitted data are the hosts. Between the transmitting host and the receiving host, the signals (the data packets) pass through a series of switching nodes traveling through a physical channel or through a physical channel or, increasingly, using a wireless connection (using radio waves, in general, between 2.4 GHz and 5.0 GHz), and in this last case, we are dealing with a WLAN (Wireless LAN). In many cases, a LAN can be flanked by a WLAN [1–4].

Among WLAN technology, one of the most commercially exploited is the *Wi-Fi* (perhaps the term comes from a contraction of the words "Wireless Fidelity", but there is no certainty about that). The distance at which a Wi-Fi signal can travel is of the order of magnitude of a hundred meters (but this also depends largely on the presence of possible obstacles), at a speed of about 100 Mbps (Megabits per second). Note that a normal infrared (IR) wireless transmission (for example, connecting a computer with a printer) works between 100,000 GHz and 200,000 GHz, at a speed of about 16 Mbps, and with a range of less than 10 m.

Coming back to LANs, we may distinguishing two main features: (1) the broadcast transmission, i.e., the connection of all hosts with the communication line, and (2) the geometric arrangement of the hosts themselves. For the latter characteristic of LANs, we speak of a BUS network, in which the hosts are connected to the same cable segment, a ring network, if the various hosts are connected to a cable that runs a closed path, a mesh network if each host is connected to all the others, and a tree network if the hosts are on a branched path.

Reasoning in terms of applicability to telemedicine, we can define wired communication as more reliable and more economical when communicating for a short time and over a short range, while in other situations, wireless communication is definitely preferable; moreover, this last ensures the advantage of portability (and the absence of cables that, due to the well-known law of increasing entropy, will "spontaneously" tend to tangle), which a LAN cannot offer. Indeed, we shall see that in the vast majority of cases, wireless technology is the one preferred and used in telemedicine applications.

However, cabling is still an important part of data transfer technology. In the context of telemedicine, we can forget the coaxial cables used for television transmissions (from the receiving antenna to the monitor), while the old twisted pair and fiber optic cable have not yet been abandoned. In both cases, the signal is transmitted in binary code as a series of variations of an electrical voltage for the twisted pair, and a light beam in the case of the fiber optic cable. With fiber optics, the signal can also be carried with solitons, which are pulses or stable waves that represent an exact solution for a wave equation [2, 3].

The essential structure of a WLAN formed by one or more access points (APs) arranged to cover the area inrerested for data reception and transmission: the larger the area to be covered, the greater the number of APs needed must be. To the APs are added one or more mobile clients (MCs), whose task is to keep the connection to the network active by passing through the APs. In general, the MCs will automatically connect to the nearest AP or at least the one where the signal is strongest. Wireless devices have an additional access port, called a hotspot, that can easily connect to a computer.

The popularity, spread, and wide availability of Wi-Fi technology have made it very easy to use for remote patient monitoring, for transmitting and receiving data for those treated at home after hospital discharge, and for those who need constant or seasonally driven mobility, such as during vacations.

As technology progresses, the demand for transmission capacity, i.e., bandwidth in telemedicine becomes greater and greater, and for these needs, in addition to

5G technology, the Wi-Fi 6 standard is making inroads, which enables optimized power utilization and higher signal transmission speed. Devices compatible with previous Wi-Fi standards can also be used with Wi-Fi 6, but the connection requires the purchase of new hardware, so the cost to the healthcare facility of upgrading its systems to Wi-Fi 6 is considerable, so this issue may actually slow down the deployment of Wi-Fi 6 in the healthcare setting.

The winning feature of the Wi-Fi 6 standard is Orthogonal Frequency Division Multiple Access (OFDMA), which is particularly efficient in hospital environments, where the request for connectivity is high, one of the key requirements is to reduce transmission latency times. OFDMA technology allows several different devices (up to 30) to share the same transceiver channel, so the need to stand by for one's transmission shift is abolished.

11.4   Mobile Phones

When cell phone technology became available (in the 1980s), no one could understand the real advantage over usual "physical" telephony: basically, a cell phone was just a landline you could carry around with you. Things changed significantly in the 1990s, when 2G (GSM) technology made it possible to send text messages (SMS), and later, 3G technology made it possible to send multimedia messages (MMS) as well, and video calling was also possible. Nowadays, the convenience and flexibility of cellular technology have made it so successful that the use of cell phones is supplanting that of landlines.

The mobile phone networks, a.k.a. cellular networks, are formed by a set of "cells" served by radio base systems (BTSs), that is, antennas equipped with specific transceiver systems. The coverage and activities performed by BTSs can vary depending on the technology used. The most important and appreciated feature of cellular network technology is the ability for users to move from one cell to another (and thus actively move across the territory) while keeping the connection operational.

The newly introduced 5G technology works with decidedly high carrier frequencies, approximately between 30 and 300 GHz. Precisely because of the high operating frequencies of the 5G system, it has come under fire for the risk of causing biological damage. The cause of the concerns raised by 5G lies in the possible risks of high-frequency radio waves, but these are non-ionizing, so the risk should not be real, because non-ionizing radiation is unable to break chemical bonds within molecules of biological interest. The World Health Organization (WHO), in this regard, has concluded that on the basis of extensive research on the effects of electromagnetic radiation, if one stays within the exposure limits recommended by the International Commission on Non-Ionizing Radiation Protection (ICNIRP), in the frequencies between 0 and 300 GHz, no adverse effect on human health should be produced, although there are still some knowledge gaps that need to be filled in order to obtain a better assessment of the risk.

The wave used by 5G are significantly shorter than those used by previous cellular technologies, and this represents an advantage in terms of reliability of communications, and this in practice means that much more devices per surface unit can be supported by the 5G technology.

11.5 Bluetooth

Another widely used transmission system is the Bluetooth (the name in this case seems to have been inspired by King Harald of Denmark, who ruled from 970 to 986 AD, and who was nicknamed precisely "Bluetooth": a King who liked to eat blueberries, to the point that his teeth were stained blue?). Bluetooth technology always uses radio frequencies, between 2.4 GHz and 2.9 GHz; the signal can reach the distance of the order of a hundred meters, with a transmission speed of about 3 Mbps.

The advantages of Bluetooth technology lie mainly in the simplicity of the electtronic circuits used in the design phase, which allows for a low cost of sale to the consumer. Bluetooth technology adapts its transmission frequency by going to one of about 80 transmission frequencies, interspersed with 1 MHz jumps, which prevents its transmission frequency from overlapping with that of similar devices available nearby. The distances covered by a Bluetooth signal range from a few meters to several hundred meters, depending on the class of device. This technology, given its cost-effectiveness (also in terms of energy consumption and transmitted power) and its versatility is particularly suitable for use in wearable biosensors.

The great success both commercially and technologically of wireless systems, such as Wi-Fi and Bluetooth, is demonstrated by the fact that all smartphones and all laptops for several years now have been equipped with these options for communication that reduce the need for wiring: for example, Wi-Fi (at least at home) has replaced the old Ethernet cables to connect to the modem/router, while Bluetooth has made obsolete the use of mouses and keyboards equipped with USB cables to connect to computers. Moreover, it would be unthinkable nowadays not to be able to connect our smartphone to our home and office networks with Wi-Fi.

11.6 Satellite Networks

A satellite orbiting around the earth (in geostationary orbit or otherwise), is a system for repeating the radio signal that is reflected from the satellite, which allows information to be transmitted over great distances between two stations located on the earth's surface. Incidentally, normal consumer Internet services can also be delivered by satellite, just as radiolocation and navigation information is transmitted by satellite. The coverage range of the satellite depends on the height at which the orbit is set. For a geostationary satellite in an equatorial orbit, a rotation synchronous with the earth's rotation (which lasts 86,164.09 s) is required, so an observer on the earth's surface looking at the satellite should see it perfectly still in the sky: from

Kepler's third law, it is derived that the orbital distance from the center of the earth must be 42.164 km, which is slightly greater than the length of the equator. For a geostationary orbit, the latency time exceeds 253 ms; given the orbital distance, the arc of circumference subtended by the satellite on an earth meridian is about 18,000 km.

Communication satellites using Medium Earth Orbit (MEO) rotate at a distance varying between 2,000 km and 35,786 km, thus outside the van Allen belts, but more frequently, they are placed at a distance of about 10,000 km.

In any case, MEO does not allow a single satellite to be used for data transmission, because at that distance the orbital velocity is such that an observer on the Earth's surface would see it move across the sky. It is therefore necessary for communication to "change hands" (handover protocol) between multiple satellites traveling consecutively in the same orbit. To continuously cover the communication, the number of satellites needed is about 15, but this number grows inversely proportional to the orbital distance, and since the distance to the Earth's surface is significantly less than that of a geostationary satellite, the latency time is also less and is reduced to about 130 ms.

One advantage of satellite transmission technology is that it does not depend on any problems on the earth's surface (as long as the integrity of transmitting and receiving stations is safeguarded); a typical disadvantage of satellite communications is the latency time. Another disadvantage of this technology is the high sensitivity to weather events (fog, rain, hail, snow) and solar storms, which cause disturbance and distortion to the transmitted signal. The intensity of the jamming is a function of the frequency of the carrier wave, which can vary between 200 MHz and 40 GHz (in five different transmission bands).

The potential problems of satellite networks mean that their use in telemedicine is quite limited: in particular, latency times and weather-related risks make its use in robotic telesurgery unreliable.

11.7   Infrared

Infrared (IR), also referred to in some cases as thermal radiation, is the part of the spectrum that, in terms of its frequency, lies after that of microwaves and before that of visible red light, thus between 3×10^2 GHz and 4×10^5 GHz, with wavelengths from about 1 mm to about 700 nm.

Infrared radiation is exploited in equipment (viewers, cameras, etc.) for night vision (recall the many military applications of this technology, but also remember their use by fire brigades to search and rescue people during fires), because in the absence of visible light, the thermal radiation emitted by living bodies allows capture by the instrumentation, which transforms the thermal image into a visible monochrome or false-color image, depending on the possible different temperatures.

Other well-known applications of IR technology are remote controls for television and a great many other appliances that can be activated and controlled remotely. The IR frequency emitted by the remote control is picked up by the home appliance, where the receiving sensor converts the received frequency into an instruction. Specifically, the receiving sensor of the home appliance is equipped with a photodiode capable of converting the IR signal into an electric current that implements the conversion between on and off.

From the technological point of view, we can distinguish near infrared (IR-A), generally in use for all night vision applications, and high-frequency infrared, used for wireless applications.

11.8 Blockchains

A blockchain is a form of open digital ledger in which data of various kinds are stored permanently and securely (with encryption). Remarkably, a blockchain is an ever-growing entity. In health care, a blockchain can be used to securely store patient data, but also to transmit it among various authorized healthcare providers in an equally secure manner. Thus, the use of blockchains appears capable of ensuring the accuracy and veracity of transmitted data, also preserving patient privacy from breaches.

Usually, the data in a blockchain are called "transactions." Once the data have been entered, it can no longer be deleted or even modified, unless all the blocks downstream of the block you want to modify are also modified, but such modification would need to obtain permission. Each block contains a pointer targeting the immediately preceding block and a time flag.

When nodes in the network produce together and simultaneously blocks that are connected to the same previous block, but have different contents, a fork is generated. The blocks involved in this situation are called "concurrent," and the protocol will specify the rule by which the protocol to be used will be chosen.

In public and private health care, a blockchain can be one of the most secure ways to store and share patient data among various system operators, so that privacy is ensured through the security of this information storage system.

11.9 Privacy and Cybersecurity Issues

The safeguarding of personal data is defined in the EU Regulation 2016/679 (General Data Protection Regulation, GDPR). A personal data breach is a violation of the security systems of a local network, which occurs due to fraudulent intrusion by a hacker, or due to a virus or other malware that has contaminated the terminals of a network, or due to carelessness, or, again, due to a failure of the network's own protection system, for example, due to outdated antivirus software, or because the protection (hardware and/or software) has weaknesses and allows entry through a communication port, due to a bug in the operating system.

A breach is when one or more of the following events occur to personal data while the data are being processed, stored, or transmitted: (1) destruction; (2)

modification; (3) loss; (4) disclosure; (5) failure to allow access by authorized persons; (6) access allowed to unauthorized persons.

A breach is when the event has occurred unlawfully, but also if it has occurred accidentally and unintentionally. Obviously, the breach is particularly serious when it involves sensitive health data, such as a diagnosis, a treatment pattern, one or more laboratory data.

It is also a violation of personal data to lose or steal or destroy (even by natural disasters) hardware containing it (a laptop, a cell phone, a USB memory stick, a DVD), as well as a paper copy of the data itself, just as it is also a violation to knowingly change the data itself, for example, by altering a diagnosis.

Clearly, in the context of telemedicine, it is imperative that the data be securely protected from hacker intrusion or infection by viruses or malware, and that the servers containing the data be located in non-risk locations (e.g., of flooding), and, finally, that there be constant backups to ensure that the data can be retrieved if needed.

These cases also include problems due to ransomware, in which an entity repository of sensitive data is blackmailed with the threat of divulging the stolen data to, for example, the dark web, where these data are often offered for sale.

From our point of view, it is essential to realize the danger of misappropriation, modification, or deletion of health data or other sensitive data: in telemedicine, not only server-based databases are used but also mobile devices, starting from smartphones, that allow the transmission of the patient's personal data to the hospital and vice versa. Indeed, these are network-connected devices that must provide for security and prevention rules against data theft and hacking. But it is imperative that all biomedical instrumentation equipped with artificial intelligence systems in hospitals be protected.

Therefore, we should be particularly concerned about the security of telemedicine information systems in general, including the various wearable devices, that communicate our health information to a server located in a public and/or private hospital, or care center, and special attention should be paid to smartphone apps and the hardware and software vulnerability of wearable devices.

Clearly, artificial intelligence is not only a passive player in the security process but also an actively engaged player in detecting hidden threats in the data it is examining.

The detection of threats and their elimination can also be done quickly, and even if it is working with big data, generating security protocols that can verify in real time not only threats but also possible vulnerabilities in the software, also carrying out prevention activities and securing the system. The advantage is that these "to serve and protect" attitudes can be automatically updated through self-learning, which must always be of the highest quality right from the training stages of the system.

Self-learning to update security and control activities is indispensable, because in the same way in evolving artificial intelligence techniques, so are evolving threats, which are becoming more and more dangerous and malicious, and because the importance of sensitive data kept in servers continues to increase and become more and more attractive to hackers.

11.10 Computer Virus Infections

A computer virus infection is the worst thing that can happen to a network of interconnected computers, since the infection, if not discovered in time, can spread to all connected machines and cause a form of data breach (one or more of the six types of breaches described in the previous section). It is essential that all machines be equipped with antivirus and antimalware software (which also includes antiransomware features), which must be constantly updated, particularly if the connected machines contain sensitive data, such as individual health data. The possible mechanisms of viral infection (which can represent the spread of a human virus infection, as well as the spread of a computer virus infection) are presented in Fig. 11.3: the arrows explain the transitions from a state to another one. For example, referring to SIRVD model, a computer in the S (susceptible) state can be vaccinated (V) or can be infected by a virus. After infection, the computer may go in the R (recovered) state by means of a suitable antiviral software, or it can be also become definitely unusable, e.g., D (deceased).

There is a wide variety of computer viruses (just as there is a wide variety of viruses that transmit disease in humans), and we do not claim to list them all, but at least highlight certain characteristics of them.

Direct-acting viruses are those that replicate automatically the moment they are activated, physically invading the folder where they are resident or infecting folders linked to batch files.

Another type of viruses are those that overwrite files into which they manage to insert their code, making those files "functionally unrecognizable" by the machine and therefore unusable. They are very harmful because cleaning up the virus, in very many cases can only be done by deleting the infected file.

A related category of computer viruses, and perhaps also the most widespread, is that of files that infect *.exe and *.com files going on to cause a variety of different kinds of damage, depending on what they are programmed to do. Some of these viruses, in order to avoid being intercepted by antivirus software use particularly devious techniques, such as infecting only once every n times they are activated, or infecting only files that have names that begin with a given sequence of letters of the alphabet, or again only files with a predetermined size. We speak, in this case, of slow infector viruses. In other cases, these viruses that attack *.exe and *.com executable files can activate antiviruses, but simultaneously they can move by changing their directory, or more precisely, by changing the path that tells the computer where the infected file is located.

Some viruses are resident in the RAM memory of the computer, from which they can interfere with or even completely erase machine instructions, but the damage, while already very serious, is not limited to this, as they can, for example, also directly corrupt files that are opened. Other types, called boot viruses, on the other

S = susceptible - I = infected - R = recovered - V = vaccinated - D = deceased

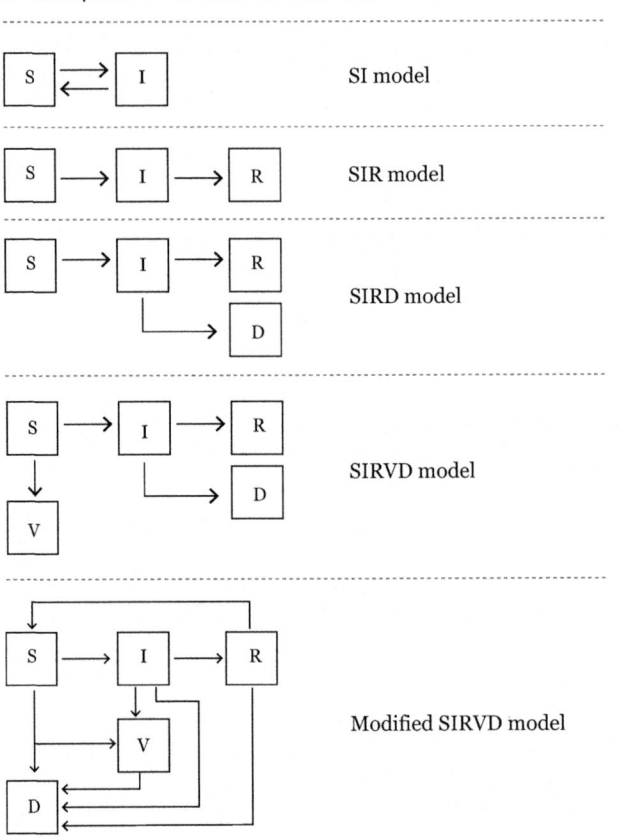

SI model

SIR model

SIRD model

SIRVD model

Modified SIRVD model

Fig. 11.3 Compartmental models for viral infections: some examples. S = susceptible − I = infected − R = recovered − V = vaccinated − D = deceased

hand, go on to infect the boot sector of the hard drive or a USB stick enabled to start the machine.

Particularly insidious are stealth viruses, which are able to hide from the monitoring of antivirus software by intercepting the operating system's communications with the antivirus. Also included among these viruses are the so-called spacefiller viruses that go into hiding inside the empty sectors of certain files so that their length does not change and thus does not make the antivirus software suspicious.

Also worth mentioning are viruses that contaminate the computer's FAT (File Allocation Table), which stores some information about the location of the disk where certain files vital to the machine's operation are located. Damage from infection by these viruses can result in the ultimate loss of this information, so the machine will no longer be able to locate the files. There are also viruses that propagate through macros, which are small files used by some software to automate certain steps of work.

Malicious programs that are not viruses, however, are worms and Trojan horses: the former are able to replicate themselves by occupying physical disk space, while the latter are unable to self-replicate: a Trojan is a malware that is hidden inside a software that is apparently useful, just as the Achaean warriors had hidden inside the wooden horse to enter the besieged city of Troy. In practice, when the user installs the apparently useful software, he also installs the malicious code hidden in it. In some cases, a Trojan can be used to gain remote control of the host computer without the user's knowledge or to pick up data such as credit card numbers or passwords or other login credentials to certain sites (banks, etc.).

Then there are also some specialized network viruses (LAN or WLAN) in this case, the transmission of infection occurs through shared files: after infection of a connected machine, the virus spreads to other machines, one by one, going so far as to infect all of them if not stopped in time.

As we will see, viral infections in computers can be simulated with mathematical models that are conceptually very similar to the compartment models used to analyze infections in human populations: for example, SIS (Susceptible, Infected, Susceptible), SIR (Susceptible, Infected, Recovered), SIRV (Susceptible, Infected, Recovered, Vaccinated), SIRVD (Susceptible, Infected, Recovered, Vaccinated, Deceased).

These will be discussed analytically in the third part of the book, where we will note that the life dynamics (birth, death, etc.) of a population analyzed with these models are analogous to the dynamics of machines in a network, with the addition of new computers and the removal of others (which have become unusable because they are obsolete, or because they have become infected by computer viruses). In turn, we also will see that the use of antivirus software has clear analogies with vaccination campaigns in populations where an epidemic breaks.

References

1. Olifer N, Olifer V. Computer networks: principles, technologies and protocols for network design. New York: John Wiley & Sons; 2015.
2. Newman M. Networks: an introduction. Oxford: Oxford University Press; 2018.
3. Seifert R, Edwards J. The all-new switch book: the complete guide to LAN switching technology. New York: Jahn Wiley & Sons; 2008.
4. Tanenbaum S, Feamster N, Wetherall DJ. Computer networks. Harlow: Pearson Education; 2022.

Communications

12

Communication means transmitting and receiving information, it means being able to share not only information but also emotions and moods; the process of communication has been indispensable for the development of life and to enable cultural evolutionary processes. We think, thousands of years ago, of the need to warn our fellow humans of the presence of a predator so that our ancestors could seek shelter or escape. We think, even nowadays, of the constant, indispensable need to communicate our ideas to each other.

In order to communicate even with voice alone, we need to modulate the signal we convey, using vowels, assembling words, and conveying them to our listeners. Modulation is an indispensable process: in fact, if our voice were just a monotonous, constant buzz, we could not communicate anything.

Our sound wave receivers, which are the ears, are dedicated to processing the verbal signals coming from our interlocutor, but we must remember that communication between human beings does not take place through words alone: indeed, these constitute only about 7% of the information content we receive: this very low percentage amount is generally supported by a small number of words, a vocabulary limited to, say, no more than 200/300 simple words. A much larger percentage of information (about 38%) comes through the expression of words (tone of voice, volume, pauses, accents), while the remaining 55% of the communication we receive comes from body language (posture, attitude, gestures, eye movements, arm movements, hand movements in particular, and leg movements), so the reception of the message is visual and does not use audio channels. For example, we all know how to distinguish between a sincere smile and a false one: it is enough to look at the face of the person smiling: if the smile uncovers the teeth, then the smile is sincere; if, on the other hand, the fold of the mouth widens without uncovering the teeth, then the smile is not sincere, and the person making the smile is lying.

Obviously, the latter type of communication cannot be transmitted or received if a telephone is used, while transmission may be more or less severely restricted during video messages.

© The Author(s), under exclusive license to Springer Nature Switzerland AG 2025   143
M. Nichelatti, *Mathematical Tools for Telemedicine*, TELe-Health,
https://doi.org/10.1007/978-3-031-81709-0_12

Modulation is the production and transmission of a sinusoidal signal, even a complex one (our voice being so); thus, modulation is a process of transmitting information (e.g., radio signals) in which a sinusoidal signal (carrier wave) provides the energy necessary for signal propagation. The carrier wave is superimposed on the modulating wave, which can be modulated in amplitude (AM) or frequency (FM).

12.1   Transmitting and Receiving Signals

Communications and telecommunications consist of the sending and delivery to one or many recipients of a variety of information (from voice messages between one individual to another, to health data files, to songs broadcast on the radio, to television broadcasts). Two people talking to each other is probably the simplest and most immediate example of two-way communication. We can imagine that the information sent from person A (the sender) to person B (the receiver) is a function of time, expressible, for example, as $a(t)$ (a function defined on the interval from 0 to τ, τ being the duration of the signal), which is transmitted in A's voice, conveyed through the air by a series of compressions and rarefactions to reach B's ear, where the compressions and rarefactions will generate a vibration on B's eardrums. In the ideal condition, the message received by B should be the same function $a(t)$, but in reality, things are always different, so the signal received by B will be $b(t) \approx a(t) + c(t)$, so the signal will be received (and the information carried by the signal will be received) with some distortion [1].

A first and immediate cause of distortion is ambient background noise (other people talking, traffic noise, other), defined here as the function $c(t)$ (note that $c(t)$ may well be negative if attenuating the original signal $a(t)$); none of us is capable of filtering out the background noise to derive the initial pure signal, so this will reach the receiver altered and even partly covered by the ambient noise, to which we attribute an additive property with respect to the initial signal $a(t)$.

It is normal when speaking on the telephone or directly by voice to another that the words received are superimposed by background noise, just as the words we say to the other party are superimposed by background noise. In some cases, the noise may be much louder than the signal, so that the latter may almost disappear as it is not perceived. In a sense we can say that $c(t)$ noise becomes part of the original signal, complements it, pollutes it, partially or completely covers it, so in the end, the incoming signal is also made of noise, because the signal contains noise, whether we want it to or not [1].

We are all familiar with a children's game that in English is called the Chinese whispers (in German "stille Post", in French "téléphone arabe", in Italian "telefono senza fili", in Spanish "teléfono descompuesto", and so on), in which players arrange themselves in a row; one player occupying one of the ends of the row, and whispers a sentence into the ear of his immediate neighbor, who repeats the same sentence (or at least as much as he perceives of the sentence) to the next player; the latter will do likewise to the other player next to him, until the other end of the row is reached. The last player will then have to repeat aloud the sentence he heard, and in general, the sentence reported by the last player will be different from the one recited by the first. In practice, the game makes it possible to discover in a very amusing way how much a starting message is "polluted" by the additive effects of many mistakes, resulting in an incoming message that is different from the starting one. The game is an obvious metaphor for gossip that passes from one person to another and is generically modified with each successive passage, but it also has much to do with a possible mechanism by which fake news is also constructed in subsequent passages through the mass media and the social media.

12.2 Signal Transmission Problems

The power of any signal tends to decrease during propagation from the point of departure to the point of arrival. An example of this is sound: the noise of a gunshot is audible up to a certain distance, but then it is no longer audible: this phenomenon is called attenuation. In addition, there is the effect exerted by ambient background noise and noise created by machinery placed near the transmitter, especially if this machinery is also a transmitter.

Noise that "envelops" the signal and covers or modifies or distorts it is capable of making it no longer perceivable properly. Signal distortion is a process that is evident on the shape of the transmitting wave: it is the one that is modified, and it is the one that is received with a different wave shape than the one that is transmitted: the distortion can be at the expense of the frequency, which is modified by the noise, or it can be at the expense of its amplitude. In fact, if a square wave is transformed into a sawtooth wave, or if the amplitude is reduced, the receiver will be left with nothing but receiving a kind of meaningless "buzz."

Added to these problems are those generated by the environment that the signal must traverse (usually the atmosphere) and by obstacles between transmitter and receiver, which contribute to signal attenuation.

If a wave carrying information comes to hit an obstacle such as a mountain, a bell tower, or a multi-story building, problems are generated determined by certain phenomena, that cause a loss of signal strength, generally called "fading," the most important of which are reflection, diffraction, and scattering [1–3].

Reflection is the phenomenon whereby a signal is reflected by an obstacle and transmitted back to its origin, just as a mirror reflects a light signal (a system of transmitting information that was widely used by American Indians). We speak of reflection when the carrier wave of the signal has a much smaller length than the size of the object being hit. The return signal can be easily picked up by a receiving antenna and processed: by knowing the time it takes for the signal to be received by the antenna, and knowing the speed at which the signal is propagated in the air, one can obtain the distance between the object reflecting the signals and the antenna picking up its reflection, so if the object is an airplane, it is easy to calculate its distance D (in kilometers) from the instrument (which is given as $D = vt/2$, in which v is the speed of light in the air in km/s, and t the time in seconds for the signal to return to the transmitter), its height above the ground, and the speed at which it is moving relative to the instrument: this is the principle by which a radar (*ra*dio *d*etection *a*nd *r*anging) works.

When the phenomenon of diffraction occurs, the transmitted signal splits forming secondary waves; it is typically associated with a wave hitting an object that has edges: diffracted waves lose power and are also propagated beyond the obstacle, depending on their wavelength. The effects of diffraction are strongly dependent on the wavelength of the signal: this is why we can hear a person's voice while hiding behind a wall: sound waves easily get around the wall as well as a great many other objects, because the wavelength of sound waves (of speech, but also more generally) is greater than the size of these objects, while if we hide behind a wall, the light rays do not get through, we stay in the shade, because the light rays have an extremely shorter wavelength than the size of a wall or a tree [3].

In the case of diffusion, the signal sent hits an object smaller than the wavelength of the signal, which reflects differently along different trajectories. The case of diffusion typically occurs when light strikes dust moving through the air, or other relatively small particles, or when sunlight strikes the dirty windshield of our car, or again when it strikes porous or rough materials. Diffusion, as mentioned, reflects the signal in multiple directions, and therefore, the signal loss is less than with reflection and diffraction.

It is normal that if a signal is transmitted outdoors, it will find physical obstacles in its path such as mountains, tall buildings, and others. While transmission of a signal may occur along the line of sight (LOS), for radio or electromagnetic signals in general, transmission occurs by following a Fresnel ellipsoid.

The Fresnel ellipsoid is an area of space in which radiation is sent from a transmitting antenna to a receiving one; the effectiveness of the link that therefore guarantees an optimal level for the transmission of information requires the evaluation of the Fresnel zone, because considering the ellipsoid in which the transmission unfolds, the presence of an obstacle that is above or below the LOS can cause the alteration of signals [2].

Power loss during a data transmission is also affected by other factors, such as weather conditions, and thus by fog, rain, or snow; rain can affect heavily the quality of transmission, especially in humid tropical areas, where rain fall can reach more than 10 cm per hour and can last for days. Rain manifests its effects not only according to quantity but also according to the speed of its fall: the heaviest rain results in signal loss proportional to its frequency. The most problematic situations are those with rainfall greater than 20 mm/h and for transmission frequencies greater than 10 MHz. Therefore, communication frequencies below 10 GHz should be preferred in tropical regions or in regions that otherwise have a high rainfall rate.

A telemedicine system cannot ignore this problem of power attenuation, especially operating in weather-critical areas, both because rain reduces the efficiency of transmission systems and because rain itself can be the cause of an accident or a real disaster, which requires to be addressed by organizing relief.

12.3   Radiofrequency Identification

Intuitively, as the name suggests, radio frequency identification (RFID) allows an object or the person wearing it to be identified by means of a radio signal: to be clear, the object has a sort of an electronic label, and the radio frequency reads the tag, identifying the tag, and associating it with the patient wearing it. RFID tags are generally very small and contain a chip in which information is stored and an antenna that allows the information to be sent to the RFID reader. At the production level, it is most important to verify the correct tuning of the tag's antenna: it is necessary to prevent the tag from resonating at the frequency of its reader.

Antenna and chip (which contains the object identification number) are embedded in a small container (a housing made of plastic, fabric, or other material) that mechanically protects them and determines the overall shape and size of the tag. A tag is thus generally composed of a single piece enclosing antenna and chip, although in some cases, it is preferred to keep the antenna separate from the chip.

Tags differ according to frequency of operation, type of power supply, and type of memory. The operating frequencies of RFID tags depend on the function they perform and the structure of the tag itself: more specifically, they can work at low frequency (about 130 kHz, with a rrange of a few centimeters), high frequency (about 14 MHz, with a range of a few tens of centimeters), and very high frequency (about 900 MHz, with a range of a few tens of meters.), denoted as LF, HF, and UHF, respectively. Power depends on whether or not there is a battery built into the tag. In this situation, it is the battery that provides the tag with the necessary power, while other tags do not use batteries, but use the power that comes to them from the reader at the time it transmits the request to read the data: in fact, the signal from the RFID reader contains a certain amount of energy, which reaches the tag's internal antenna producing a small magnetic field that activates the circuit that contains the information: this is called the *inductive coupling*. The memory of an RFID tag can be read-only, or read-write, depending on whether they were programmed at the time they were produced, or whether the chip contains no information and can be programmed at a later time after production.

The RFID tag is a true wireless device, capable of using the incoming energy from the reader, such that this energy is strong enough to let the tag run for the time necessary to transmit the information to the reader, and such that the reader is able to receive it. If a tag is implanted in the body, it will then have to be immediately under the skin to prevent the signal from being scattered and being attenuated by the overlying tissues.

There are some problems that currently prevent intensive use of implantable tags and thus their expanded use in telemedicine: a first problem with RFID tags is the short range of the reader; a second problem is that the tag does not have enough energy to supply to a biosensor anyway; a third problem is the possible interactions between a tag and and an implantable device (a glucometer, or a defibrillator, for example); finally, a fourth problem is UHF tags, which, given their operating frequency, could result in interactions with water absorption frequencies, so they are not suitable for placement on the body.

In the context of telemedicine, there are special requirements for the use of tags. First, a tag must be as small as possible, and it must have adequate transmission capacity. In addition, when a tag is connected through a suitable interface with an implantable biosensor, provision must be made for the tag to store information to be transmitted to the reader for later storage and processing and for the memory to be able to download after reading so as to leave space for subsequent incoming information. This is a job that the interface between sensor and tag must perform: the interface must therefore not only be capable of transmitting the biosensor signals to the tag, but it must also be capable of programming the tag by giving it specific instructions [2].

Despite these problems, which may be permanently solved in the near future, the possibilities for RFID use in the medical field are virtually endless, and so are the possibilities of RFID use in the hospital.

The first type of application of RFID in the hospital setting is in monitoring patients to ensure their appropriate care and safety (especially for in infants).

Patients with a wristband equipped with an RFID tag will be able to be monitored to check their clinical parameters (which can be updated) and to track their location (given the possibility of having RFID real-time location systems, the so-called RFID-RTLS), and this may have advantages in reducing the time of care. In addition, thanks to the wristband, it should become virtually impossible to exchange patient files (and thus, for example, one patient's drug treatment or blood type with another's). With the same security, patients can be prevented from wandering around the hospital's various wards and common parts (bars, cafeterias, etc.) to prevent them from interacting with healthy individuals, perhaps transmitting diseases or causing other accidents.

This system will also prevent unauthorized individuals (relatives or strangers) from taking patients out of their rooms or relatives from doing so outside of visiting hours. The same system will allow employees to gain access to various departments and other various facilities (elevators) by simply placing their badges on an RFID-equipped reader located next to the access door.

In newborns, the application of an RFID-RTLS makes it possible to prevent accidental swapping of newborns, preventing them from being attributable to the wrong parents, as well as preventing other events related to the personal safety of newborns; indeed, whenever an infant's RFID-RTLS device is removed, or whenever an infant with RFID-RTLS is approached at the infant room door, an alarm could be triggered.

Many other applications of RFID systems in hospitals are related to logistics and resource management.

In hospital pharmacy, the use of information acquired with RFIDs at the level of distribution to departments can manage and control inventory, both in the pharmacy (and thus assisting the pharmacist in updating inventory) and in the medicine cabinets of each individual department.

If drug manufacturers use an RFID tag affixed to the drug's label or box, they will be able to provide the pharmacist or warehouseman with encrypted information, such as the production batch number, expiration date, the facility where the drug was manufactured (including the facility of a third party), and any other information to validate the supply. Simply missing the tag will be an evidence of the drug's nonoriginality. Thus, the RFID device will also be an effective tool in verifying the origin of the product, preventing situations of supplying expired drugs with a counterfeit tag or drugs produced by unauthorized companies with a false tag. The same ease of management would be for all the various sterile and nonsterile single-use products: in this case, an RFID tag would be the optimal, low-cost solution for keeping stock up to date and managing the timing for upcoming orders to be placed, so that the hospital never risks a stock shortage for these products, and instead always knows the quantity available in each ward cabinet. To manage these options, it may be sufficient to match staff RFIDs with those associated with parts inventory.

At the management level, the RFID tag can be used for linen cleaning monitoring with a specific tag that can monitor the status within laundry services. Other applications include monitoring the sterilization of surgical instrumentation: the RFID tag will need to be suitable for operation even when applied to a metal object, and most importantly, it will need to be autoclavable, so that to resist to the very high temperatures reached during sterilization: in this way, it will be able to provide the date and time of successful sterilization.

12.4 Chatbots and Medical Chatbots

A chatbot is an application whose purpose is to converse with a human user in a conversational manner, particularly in the course of communication over the Web.

Other chatbots that use artificial intelligence, and are made for more general aims, on the other hand, are much more adaptable, and their response follows paths through neural networks or machine learning; given their flexibility, the responses generated are improvable as time goes on and as the number of times the response is prompted by various customers, to whom they can provide information such as instructions for using a given product.

This type of chatbot is then able to adapt its response style to the patient's question by referring to the very style in which the question was phrased and thus adapt its understanding of the patient's needs, so the chatbot knows what words it will need to say to continue a fluid dialog with the human subject, based on his or her previous requests, so that the general sense of the dialog is obtainable from the context of the conversation, and the system is able to predict with good approximation what the next question might be.

The chatbots may also provide assistance to patients responding to their questions or requests for information and dialoguing with them. Communication takes place through artificial intelligence, or by using natural language processing systems, so that the response to the human interlocutor is hopefully clear and consistent with respect to the questions asked.

There are various types of chatbots. Some work based on simple, predefined rules, being able to answer only precise questions, and giving standard information about the opening hours of an office or instructions for filling out a particular paper or electronic form.

Some others are more able in giving answers to general and clinical questions. Possibly, ChatGPT is the most famous chatbot of this type, whereas Med-PaLM and Med-PaLM[1] 2 (produced by Google) are specifically used for medical and clinical questions. These latter use a completely different approach with respect to ChatGPT: in fact, Med-PaLM is based on some big databases containing real clinical questions and real clinical answers: the answers generated by this chatbot are generally of a good level and sometimes achieve a scientific consensus that can approach that of human clinicians. In general, these chatbots can be a valid interlocutor for medical issues, but they are not completely reliable, may provide answers with some parts insufficient or missing, and still cannot compete with clinical judgment.

Medical chatbots are used by some healthcare providers to converse with patients, and patients often do not notice that they are talking to a system powered by artificial intelligence, especially since some of these systems use algorithms that make the conversation almost identical to what one would have with a real doctor, so these chatbots are able to reduce or at least simplify the workload of human doctors. For patients, there are undeniable practical advantages: a chatbot does not generally require patient registration, nor does it need to be downloaded from a site (since it is contained within the app installed on the patient's smartphone), and it can be accessed 365 days a year and 24 h a day, even at midnight on Christmas (regardless of where the patient is), and it can be a system for raising a health alert.

Chatbots are useful in this regard for making a pre-selection of patients based on the symptoms or problems they tell, so that they can be diverted to the most competent doctor in the field, avoiding wasted time on both sides. Finally, the very dialog with the nonhuman assistant also serves to gather information to be passed on to the designated physician, without the physician having to repeat questions to the patient, and serves to create a waiting list that puts patients in order based on the severity and urgency estimated from the conversation.

For healthcare uses, we can distinguish three main types of chatbots: informational, conversational, and prescriptive.

Informational chatbots are clearly the simplest: they generally handle answers to elementary questions, such as requesting an appointment with a specialist, or information on how to take a medication, or more. They can receive written questions and give written answers, without the need for voice contact, in the form of a text message or popup, or splash window.

---

[1] See https://sites.research.google/med-palm/.

Conversational chatbots are those that provide information or answers by conversing with the patient: they use technologies based on arrtificial intelligence, such as Natural Language Processing.

Prescriptive chatbots are conversational chatbots that have the ability to converse but also suggest medical or rehabilitative therapeutic solutions. It is clear that despite certain excellent performances of chatbots such as MedPaLM 2, these systems with prescriptive suggestions are not on par with the prescriptions and suggestions of a real physician.

More to the point, there may be conditions or concerns in which a chatbot may be prone to manifest racial or sexist biases they are, after all, artificial intelligence systems trained with medical and diagnostic data produced by humans, with all their flaws.

It is likely that someday artificial intelligence-based systems will be able to process health data provided by patients and will enter the diagnostic logic, partly replacing human doctors or helping them. Up to this point, there is nothing negative (of course, it is assumed that the patient's privacy is always respected), indeed: diagnostics and drug therapy could improve if aided by artificial intelligence; however, there will likely be repercussions on the liability aspect. In fact, who will take responsibility for a diagnosis or prescription, or even a single piece of advice to the patient that is incorrect, or openly wrong? It may be a fault of the human doctor who trusted the judgment of artificial intelligence too much, or it may be the fault of the human who trained the system, or, perhaps, it will be a shared blame: certainly, there will be an ethical issue to be settled.

12.5   Networks and Graphs

Here we will assume that we are describing a communication network and using a very simple model to represent it, a table (or more precisely a matrix), that is, a general system by which communications in a railway network, for example, are described.

At the end of this presentation, we will find that the method of representing the network has almost universal value and can be used for numerous other applications, such as studying the transmission of a contagious disease.

Assume that we are analyzing the possibility that 5 people may meet in the place where they live. Let us also assume that the 5 subjects live in 5 different houses that are far enough apart that they cannot meet each other by walking from one house to another. Finally, let us assume that each house is connected to all the others by independent roads, i.e., that from one house to another there is only one direct road, so that to go from a house A to another house B, one does not have to pass through any third house C; in other words, the roads are 10 (but at present, this is just a marginal info).

Let's start from the initial situation where the roads are there and are passable, but none of the inhabitants own a car. The most simpler model for such a network is a table like

House	A	B	C	D	E
A	1	0	0	0	0
B	0	1	0	0	0
C	0	0	1	0	0
D	0	0	0	1	0
E	0	0	0	0	1

where each house is at the intersection of a given row with a given column of the table, e.g., any house occupies a different diagonal element: these are characterized by the value 1, to say that each subject is free to meet himself (in his own home, it's understood); the number 0, on the other hand, means that no meeting is possible between people living in two different houses.

Now, remembering the structure of the table just presented, we can write the table itself in a slightly "more evolved" form, that is, transcribing the table data (the values 1 and 0) into a grid of cells enclosed in parentheses: this new arrangement of our information is called a *matrix*, which we term with the letter $\mathbf{N}$ to remind us that it is a *network matrix*. To make a long story short, we will therefore write:

$$\mathbf{N}_0 = \begin{pmatrix} 1\,0\,0\,0\,0 \\ 0\,1\,0\,0\,0 \\ 0\,0\,1\,0\,0 \\ 0\,0\,0\,1\,0 \\ 0\,0\,0\,0\,1 \end{pmatrix}.$$

We note that in the matrix (and in the table), the numbers are arranged in rows and columns; the position of each number is identified by the intersection of row and column where the number itself is located, and we may generically write n_{11}, n_{24} and n_{51} to denote the numbers that are respectively at the intersection of the first row and first column, between the second row and the fourth column, and between the fifth row and the first column. Going back to our $\mathbf{N}_0$ matrix, we can write $n_{11} = 1$, $n_{24} = 0$ and $n_{51} = 0$.

Now, let us modify the network matrix $\mathbf{N}$ as follows:

$$\mathbf{N}_1 = \begin{pmatrix} 1\,0\,1\,0\,0 \\ 0\,1\,0\,0\,0 \\ 0\,0\,1\,0\,0 \\ 0\,0\,0\,1\,0 \\ 0\,0\,0\,0\,1 \end{pmatrix},$$

to say that now the subject 1 can go to subject 3's house (note that the number n_{13} that is at the intersection of the first row and the third column of the matrix $\mathbf{N}_0$ went from the value 0 to the value 1 in the modified matrix $\mathbf{N}_1$), perhaps because he bought a car, so he can now move around freely. To represent this new situation, we may produce a very simple graph

$$1 \longrightarrow 3$$

telling that among the whole network, we found only one connection between subject 1 and subject 3, in the direction going from 1 to 3.

Again, we now rearrange the network matrix as follows:

$$\mathbf{N}_2 = \begin{pmatrix} 1 & 0 & 1 & 0 & 0 \\ 0 & 1 & 1 & 1 & 0 \\ 1 & 0 & 1 & 0 & 0 \\ 0 & 0 & 0 & 1 & 0 \\ 0 & 0 & 0 & 0 & 1 \end{pmatrix} :$$

where we see that now also $n_{31} = n_{23} = n_{24} = 1$, and therefore, now also subjects 3 and 2 have a car: subject 3 can reciprocate visiting subject 1, while subject 2 can go visit subjects 3 and 4, and the graph representing the network is now

$$1 \rightleftarrows 3 \leftarrow 2$$
$$\swarrow$$
$$4$$

or also

$$\begin{array}{ccc} 1 & & 4 \\ \uparrow\downarrow & & \uparrow \\ 3 & \leftarrow & 2 \end{array}$$

since there are no special requirements in portraying the graph, other than to respect connections between individuals.

Now we are able to describe a somewhat more complicate network with the matrix

$$\mathbf{N}_3 = \begin{pmatrix} 1 & 0 & 1 & 0 & 1 \\ 0 & 1 & 1 & 1 & 1 \\ 1 & 0 & 1 & 0 & 1 \\ 0 & 1 & 0 & 1 & 1 \\ 1 & 0 & 0 & 0 & 1 \end{pmatrix} :$$

where we see that: (a) $n_{13} = n_{31} = 1$; (b) $n_{15} = n_{51} = 1$; (c) $n_{23} = 1$; (d) $n_{24} = n_{42} = 1$; (e) $n_{25} = 1$; (f) $n_{35} = 1$; (g) $n_{45} = 1$. Therefore, the graph can be written as

$$
\begin{array}{c}
3 \;\leftarrow\; 2 \;\rightleftarrows\; 4 \\
\uparrow\downarrow \;\searrow\; \downarrow \;\swarrow \\
1 \;\rightleftarrows\; 5
\end{array} \;\;.
$$

This way to describe a network using the network matrices or their equivalent graphs has general validity and can be used to represent any kind of connections between subjects, objects or events, such as web connections, telephone networks, railway lines between different stations, airline flights between different airports.

It is also evident the utility of the network matrices in studying the disease transmission in a population with known personal relationships. If one is dealing with a number of infected subjects, the network matrices are useful for reconstructing possible subsequent contagions and also to check for the potential presence of individuals who are infected, but who do not yet show symptoms, and who may therefore become dangerous vehicles of disease transmission for other people.

12.6   Ethics in Doctor–Patient Communication

Physician–patient interaction and physician–patient communication in telemedicine have profoundly changed from what happens in face-to-face medicine. It changes the perception of care, now carried out remotely, particularly in elderly and frail individuals, who in the face-to-face fiduciary relationship found the possibility of being refreshed and helped psychologically to cross the "swamp" of illness [4].

A relationship based on video communication may not be sufficient to establish the feeling of trust that one has with the family doctor. All the more so, telemedicine comes not only to replace traditional medicine but also becomes the means on which a new form of treatment is based that had not been initiated before.

It is up to the physician who assists the patient remotely to set up a relationship that can put the patient at ease. The most important tool, initially, is the voice and facial setting. A video link, in fact, cannot always allow one to grasp all the nonverbal conversation patterns that are established between the physician and the patient.

This is something that needs to be given due consideration: verbal communication carries little information, but it is important the modulation of speech, that is, in the tone of voice, its volume, the emphasis on accents put on words, pauses, exclamations, and questions. Just stressing the sentence on one word or another is enough to change the meaning of a sentence, or just moving a word or putting a comma (a pause) is enough to say one thing or say the opposite. The nonverbal communication is contained in the gestures that accompany speech, hand movements, the way one positions the body while standing or sitting, eye gaze setting, frowning, mimic muscle movements, eyebrow twitches, true or false smiles (and anyone can tell a true smile from a false one), and all the small voluntary or involuntary gestures that accompany conversation, in the speaker and the listener. As a result, what you say is important, but how you say it is even more important, and it is necessary for a doctor or nurse to say the things you need to say, but you have to say them in the way the patient would like to hear. And it takes little to figure that out: all it takes is for a doctor or nurse to ask themselves, "If I were the patient, how would I want to be told what I need to say?"

It takes only a little effort to put oneself in the shoes of others, because to behave ethically in dealing with the patient is enough to make sure that we respect the patient and always protect his or her dignity as a person.

The effort to approach the patient has to be made by the doctor and nurse, who are the ones who have to empathize with the patient, have to put themselves in the patient's shoes, have to understand the patient's needs, which are not only health and treatment needs but are also needs for understanding.

When a sick patient is treated, his or her clinical needs are met, but there are all the care needs that are probably still not, and this the healthcare personnel must take in, both in the presence and, especially, remotely, in the condition where the patient has less opportunity to communicate and be understood.

12.7   Mistakes, Slips, Violations

Errors are always possible in all human activities, and medicine is not an exception. In telemedicine, the problem might even be exacerbated by the fact that not prsence in the same place of the physician and patient could potentially delay the discovery of the error.

In any healthcare organization involved in inpatient or remote service delivery, it is essential that clinical risk management (CRM) defines all rules for risk minimization and procedures for their implementation so that patient safety is protected [5].

Moving in this direction, the healthcare company must define a set of risk indicators that are measurable as numbers, and that calculate the probability of the risk: the indicators will be a measure of how possible a risk is and, more importantly, will be indices of its predictability. Hence, the possibility of continuous improvement in the efficiency of service delivery.

Errors can occur for three main reasons: (1) they can occur because of a misconfiguration of the procedures to be used in a given situation, and thus are errors that lie upstream of the execution, which in itself may have been correct (in this case, we speak of *mistakes*); (2) they can occur because of a faulty execution of a procedure that was in itself planned correctly, and thus are attributable to insufficient skill on the part of the operator (in this case, we speak of *slips*); (3) they can occur because operations, or maneuvers, or activities of any kind have been performed (in good or bad faith, or even to remedy a sudden emergency situation) that are instead prohibited by a certain internal regulation (in this case, we speak of *violations*).

Mistakes can be divided into two types: in the first case, they are due to the choice of a wrong procedure, i.e., a procedure that cannot in any way achieve the intended goal (the procedure is in itself right, but it is applied wrongly). In the second case, they are due to the absence or inaccuracy of a given procedure schedule (so the procedure is wrong, no matter how exact the planned activities may have been).

Slips can also be divided into two categories: true slips, which occur due to misapplication of the procedure caused by the operator's lack of skill or inattention, or haste, and memory slips (also called *lapses*), which occur when the operator trusts his or her ability to memorize data in his or her head, only to transcribe it incorrectly. This second type of slips can be very dangerous: as dangerous as the first or even more so.

A generically pessimistic view of the concept of latent error is that of an error that remains hidden in a system until an event causes it to come to the fore: if a miscalculation on a truss is concealed by the other functioning and well-designed trusses, the unleashing of a particularly violent storm (the trigger event) even 20 years after construction can cause the defective truss to fail and cause the roof to collapse. It is a design error then, which does not stand the test of time.

Active errors, on the other hand, are another matter; they occur immediately and are more easily associated with the human factor, but active errors very often originate from latent errors, such as the insufficient training of a physician can cause an injury to a patient (think of the incorrect conducting of an electroencephalogram, causing a misleading result in diagnosi), but it is in turn caused by an organizational error that did not provide for theoretical and practical training or a prolonged series of tests of conducting and reading encephalograms in the presence of a more experienced physician.

The occurrence of an error requires the organization of an investigation that captures all possible causes of the error and removes them from the procedures used at the time the error was observed. If the error was due to a defective sensor, the type or model will be changed to find a more reliable one. This means that the investigation must start from the time the error occurred and proceed backward in time until the origin(s) of the problem is found. The solution to the problem will not only be the eradication of the cause but also a reorganization of the system to prevent that cause (or a similar one) from occurring again. So an error also involves a check of information flows and of procedures.

A deeper and potentially more effective analysis also considers near-misses errors, that is, errors that did not occur only because a series of fortunate situations arose. These are generally small problems that may become more serious in the future and should be reported to the control system. It could be a thermostat applied to an autoclave that appears to be malfunctioning, it could be the door of a washing machine that closes poorly because of a gasket problem, it could be the exchange of a drug between patients that was discovered before administration: in fact, each of these small (or almost small) problems should be reported. The report must be such that it does not cause problems for the reporter or the person who committed the act; it must not generate any kind of company retaliation on the "culprit."

The situation where the possible error is determined by a potential organizational flaw also applies to these near misses. The autoclave thermostat and washing machine porthole gasket are dependent on the fact that regular maintenance is not performed by the company or the third parties to whom maintenance is contracted, and the exchange of a medication between patients may be due to the malfunction of an RFID reader operated by the nurse, or because the nurse has not had sufficient training in the use of the tag reader, or perhaps because the tag's signal has collided with that of other tags. Thus, the response to these near miss events is to improve the organization.

References

1. Dodd AZ. The essential guide to telecommunications, 6th edn. New York: Prentice Hall; 2020.
2. Keers RN, Williams SD, Cooke J, Ashcroft DM. Causes of medication administration errors in hospitals: a systematic review of quantitative and qualitative evidence. Drug Saf. 2013;36:1045–67.
3. Smith DG, Dunlop J. Telecommunication engineering, 3rd edn. Boca Raton: CRC Press; 1994.
4. Veatch RM. Medical ethics. JAMA 1984;252:2296–300.
5. Donaldson L, Ricciardi W, Sheridan S, Tartaglia R, Eds. Textbook of patient safety and clinical risk. Cham: Springer Nature,; 2021.

Wearable Sensors

13

The monitoring of the patient's health parameters in telemedicine practice should be entrusted to appropriate sensors, which are capable of obtaining various information, such as sleep, physical activity, and many other pathophysiological variables. The collection of clinical information in telemedicine is a critical aspect of the whole system. It involves making sure that data collection and transmission is as continuous and accurate as possible. Lacking the ability to keep the patient physically connected to a machine that receives all this information, one must proceed by using sensors that are placed against the patient's body and are capable of storing and transmitting the information [1, 2].

The data arriving from the various body districts are in analog form: the sensors convert them from analog to digital. which are those transmitted to the remote station, where they are memorized and processed.

The role of RFID, which represents, with its ability to detect patient movements and to store and transmit medical chart data, the elementary prototype of all wearable sensors for telemedicine, was discussed earlier.

What might be needed for optimal remote control of the patient is the set of sensors for primary information (heart rate, systolic and diastolic blood pressure, respiratory frequency, a system for checking the correct dosage of a drug, a kind of electronic food diary providing information on the quantity and quality of food, and so on), but sometimes, a small camera might also be needed, consistent with privacy concerns.

All of these sensors should be carried constantly (or nearly so) by the patient and should be wearable (bracelets, necklaces, clocks) or otherwise be very close to the patient's body. Now the sensors, in addition to being wearable, are also invasive or semi-invasive, insertable, or injectable into the body and may also consist of tattoos or patches on the skin, capable of monitoring components of sweat or interstitial fluid.

Sweat is one of the earliest examples of body fluid to be monitored for metabolic and general health status. Sweat, produced by specific glands in the epidermis, can

© The Author(s), under exclusive license to Springer Nature Switzerland AG 2025
M. Nichelatti, *Mathematical Tools for Telemedicine*, TELe-Health,
https://doi.org/10.1007/978-3-031-81709-0_13

convey information not only about the status of electrolytes (sodium, potassium, and others) and some biological metabolites (lactic acid, glucose, cortisol) but also about some metabolites of drugs or toxic substances. Sweat and intestinal fluid also pose a design challenge, as their presence changes skin impedance.

The fundamental problem with sensors is the choice of the material from which they are made and the material with which they are coated, as these can interact with the din information content they need to transmit. In a nutshell, the circuit with which the sensors are equipped must function properly, and the coating must ensure maximum permeability to radio signals transmitted at the output, must protect the circuit from vibration (e.g., in the patient using a motorcycle) and mechanical shocks (falls, etc.), and must prevent the penetration of foreign materials (dust, liquids), which in contact with the circuit could disable it or ruin it completely.

Another fundamental problem with these wearable devices is the possibility of the device moving due to the patient's normal activities. Displacement of the device can be a major determinant of malfunction during data collection, and so it is necessary that the device be fixed stably in the desired location, and if there were more than one device, it is a good idea to ensure that the relative position of the various sensors also remains constant (or is at least checked).

13.1   The Internet of Medical Things

The Internet of Medical Things (IoMT) is the set of all medical devices that are connected through the Internet network, allowing secured transmission, which are transferred to the cloud and then received by doctors or by people, located in hospital or in any other point of care, which must read and elaborate the data to take a clinical decision; it is a connection based on sensors and artificial intelligence. Sensors are bound to the patient's body or are also embedded in clothing (fabrics including electronic devices) or in smartphones (as medical apps) or sport watches or are simply sensors available at home to be used when needed or on demand.

The IoMT extends its competence in controlling drug administration and self-administration by means of electronic drug dispensing so that any time the patient skips a prescription (unintentionally or not), the physician is immediately alerted and can urge the patient to adhere to therapies, as drug treatment is often more likely to be a cocktail than a monotherapy. The problem is quite complex in general: skipping a medication is often an act brought about by a pessimistic perception of therapy ("I have to take ten medications a day"), so monitoring adherence to treatment and contacting the patient at the first signs of error is a mandatory act. A second tool that can be used is the smart bed, which can be tilted as desired and can record the duration and quality of the patient's sleep.

So, all in all, IoMT is a set of technologies that are used in remote patient management and information gathering. We will soon see, without claiming completeness, the most important sensors that contribute to these methods of care.

13.2 Classification of Sensors

Sensors can be classified according to the type of operation: there are pressure and ultrasonic sensors, optical sensors, magnetic sensors, temperature sensors, and chemical sensors.

In all cases, their job is to receive a signal, such as those listed, and to transform it into a radio signal or, if you prefer, into a transmittable electromagnetic type signal, after reading the incoming data and transforming it into direct information to the outside world.

We can briefly describe their operation as follows [1, 2]:

1. Pressure sensors and ultrasonic sensors, both, exploit the piezoelectric effect, that is, the ability of certain materials with crystalline structure to produce an electrical voltage when subjected to compression or deformation or to deform when subjected to an electrical voltage: they are used to measure changes in pressure, density, and electrical conductivity, for blood pressure, heart rate, and many other physiological variables. Pressure sensors have the capacitive effect, which allows to detect changes in electrical capacitance (in addition to biosensors, they are used in touchscreen systems, where they recognize finger contact by the change in electrical capacitance at the screen surface), and the piezoresistive effect, in which the resistive sensor recognizes deformations to which an object is exposed, causing its electrical resistance to change.
2. Optical sensors use photonic signals, in that any change in the concentration of a molecule is measured by a photodetector and transformed into an electrical signal: they are mainly used to measure heart and respiratory rates or oxygen saturation in the blood.
3. Electromagnetic sensors are used to produce signals by means of mechanical energy; the mechanical energy is then transformed into electrical signals or radio signals. They are used in some rehabilitation techniques.
4. Temperature sensors detect changes in body temperature due to the perturbation of the complex metabolic circuits that occur under certain pathological conditions and turn them into signals for external detectors.
5. Chemical sensors are used to measure components of body fluids such as interstitial fluid and saliva.

These sensors must combine durability and reliability; they must be able to adapt to the body's movements without detaching, to remain adherent to the skin while leaving it free to transpire, and must also resist the possible effects of the slightly acidic pH of the skin (which normally ranges between 4.2 and 5.7) and its possible variations. In addition, since various sensors used are basically resting on the skin (and, more importantly, on the skin rests the surface of the sensor that is to read the information), it is also necessary that there be complete biocompatibility between the material used and human tissue. There are various choices in this regard, particularly among hydrogels.

The acquisition of pathophysiological data, and biological data in general, through sensors requires the possession of the necessary engineering know-how (at the design level) and technological know-how (at the data transmission level) and requires great caution regarding privacy issues related to measuring the data and storing them in an appropriate and protected site.

The telemedicine system is able to acquire a wide variety of information about pathophysiological and physiological variables and their dynamics over time, using different data collection techniques, based on the specific properties of different sensors.

13.3   Body Temperature

The measurement of body temperature is one of the first pieces of information that is acquired when there is apparently something "not working right" in our body. In fact, the reaction to many diseases, inflammatory states, or other situations outside of normal physiology is hyperthermia (fever) or hypothermia. The measurement of body temperature can also very well take place within the home. This is done as there is a wide availability of measuring instruments, from the old analog alcohol thermometer to modern thermometers with digital readouts and all the ways to modern temperature detectors that use infrared beams projected onto the patient's forehead and give accurate measurements, without requiring to be physically in contact with the skin.

Using traditional thermometers, temperature is commonly measured with the thermometer in the axillary, groin, mouth, or rectum. As a reference level, the expected temperature in a healthy adult is between 36.0 °C and 37.0 °C, while in children, it can vary between 36.5 °C and 37 °C: anyhow, these are only statistical data that serve only as a rough guideline. There is, however, a fair amount of variability in temperature measurement depending on thermometer placement: an increase to about 0.5 °C is expected if rectal or oral placement is used and a decrease to about 0.5 °C with axillary or groin placement. To be precise, factors that may influence body temperature reading are the age of the patient, environmental temperature, and model of thermometer used: the same temperature reading should be taken with great care without moving the instrument abruptly because vigorous shaking could alter the value reported on the instrument.

A "normal" body temperature does not actually exist, either in the same healthy subject (sitting or while cycling) at various times of the day (which is why we prefer to talk about average temperature) or in the same sick subject (remember that according to a popular tradition, it is said that fever in the morning tends to be lower than in the evening). Temperature also changes according to gender and according to hormonal cycles.

Measuring body temperature is essential in a telemedicine-assisted subject, as hyperthermia could metaphorically "cook" some organs by rendering them no longer functional.

Taking temperature readings by inserting a sensor into the ear seems reliable and very rapid, the ear canal and eardrum being close to the hypothalamus, the endocrine gland that regulates body temperature. The reading can then be transferred from the sensor to the Wi-Fi transmission system and then be stored and processed.

13.4 Blood Pressure

Blood pressure is defined as the force that is exerted on the walls of vessels based on their surface area: it is measured in mmHg (millimeters of mercury), although its International System (SI) unit is the pascal (Pa), which is equal to the pressure exerted by the force of 1 newton on an area of $1\,m^2$. The conversion from mmHg to Pa is such that a systolic pressure of 130 mmHg is equal to 17,330 Pa, thus 17.33 kPa (kilopascal), while a diastolic pressure of 80 mmHg is equal to 10,660 Pa, thus 10.66 kPa.[1]

Measuring blood pressure, systolic (i.e., the pressure exerted on vessel walls by blood being pumped from the heart to various districts) and diastolic (i.e., blood pressure measured while the heart is in relaxation and, by dilating its chambers, is filling with blood.), is one of the first things a physician does when seeing a patient in the clinic. Normal values for the systolic and diastolic pressure are about 120 to 130 mmHg and 70 to 80 mmHg, respectively.

In fact, it is an effective system that can let you know if there is any problem going on, even a serious one; for example, metabolic syndrome also involves an increase in blood pressure, which tends to rise even in obese patients, also because blood is forced to make its way along the fatty tissue and into the panniculus and the heart presumably has to pump the blood more forcefully.

Systolic and diastolic blood pressure can be measured with a traditional mechanical sphygmomanometer or with digital sphygmomanometers, which can be purchased at any store that sells medical supplies or at pharmacies or on the Web. Some mid- to high-end smartwatches are also equipped with a blood pressure monitor.

In the context of telemedicine, the reading and sending of pressure data is done on average once a day: however, in telemedicine, the sending of data is also associated with an analysis of its dynamics (increase or decrease), which can be much more interesting for a physician, in relation to the specific pathology of the monitored subject.

13.5 Heart Rate

Heart rate is measured to assess the efficiency of the circulatory system in delivering oxygen to tissues and to test an individual's ability to work under stress by

---

[1] More specifically, 1 mmHg is equivalent to about 133.3 pascal, while 1 pascal is equivalent to about 0.0075 mmHg.

performing sports activities. Heart rate is measured as the number of beats per minute.

Maximum heart rate (MHR) is, intuitively, the maximum number of pulsations an individual can produce under exertion: it depends on training and a number of other physiological circumstances. In general, it tends to fall with advancing age. The MHR[2] can be derived empirically using the following equation:

$$\text{MHR (beats per minute)} = 207 - 0.7 \times \text{age (yrs)}$$

so that a 20-year-old would have a maximum heart rate given by

$$\text{MHR} = 207 - 0.7 \times 20 = 207 - 14 = 193 \text{ beats per minute}$$

whereas for a 50-year-old, the maximum heart rate is

$$\text{MHR} = 207 - 0.7 \times 50 = 207 - 35 = 172 \text{ beats per minute.}$$

Heart rate is highly dependent on activity and movement, increasing with exertion. The average heart rate can be roughly estimated to be about 70 beats per minute in men and about 80 beats per minute in women. While sleeping, heart rate can drop even more than 20%.

Heart rate in telemedicine is usually taken at least 2 or 3 times a day: the advantage of telemedicine detection is that any emotional factors that may cause beats to rise just because of the restlessness that the subject may feel, feeling evaluated; the same situation may sometimes occur when a patient undergoes blood pressure measurement.

The values and their dynamics over time are sent to the health service provider, and there they are evaluated. However, some situations may occur that are not pathologically determined and that have the potential to change the heart rate, based on the emotions (pleasant and unpleasant, such as seeing the face of a loved one or receiving bad news) that the person feels. Physicians doing the evaluations should therefore be able to take these environmental effects into account, if necessary even contacting the subject directly to ask him or her for any insights. On the other hand, frequent measurement helps quickly detect the appearance of abnormalities in the heartbeat. However, arterial pulse measurement will need to be adjusted according to the subject's age, as mentioned above.

There are many places where the heart rate can be detected: basically anywhere an artery is sufficiently close to the surface so not only the wrist (radial) artery is fine: the ulnar artery, brachial artery, common carotid artery, temporal artery, femoral artery, popliteal artery, and dorsal artery of the foot are also usable.

---

[2] Incidentally, the aerobic threshold is obtained by calculating 75% of the value obtained for MHR, while the anaerobic threshold is obtained by calculating 80% of the value of MHR.

It should be mentioned that all fitness equipment is now provided with heart rate detectors with special transducers found on the knobs of elliptical mats, treadmills, and exercise bikes and that other types of detectors are attached like a small clamp to the earlobe and then are connected to the fitness equipment via a cable.

Obtaining the heart rate is therefore relatively easy, and the arterial pulse gives an easily recognizable signal that is difficult to confuse with other signals. Telemedicine detection is therefore extremely reliable: the use of a sensor applied in close proximity to the artery of interest will be able to record the frequencies and communicate them to the caregiver; alternatively, bands worn on the chest at the level of the heart can be used, which can record the electrical signal produced by the heart muscle contraction.

13.6 Oxygen Saturation

Oxygen saturation (SaO_2) is a measure that tells us how much the hemoglobin in the blood is saturated with oxygen, that is, how much oxygen the blood is carrying relative to its potential capacity. From a certain point of view, oxygen saturation is like the percentage measure of seats occupied by passengers in a train. Lungs, by inhalation, supply the blood with molecular oxygen (O_2) destined for all cells, which is transported through hemoglobin (whose molecules represent the seats where passengers take their seats), and by exhalation, they extract from the blood the carbon dioxide (CO_2) produced by the chemical work of the cells, which basically convert glucose ($C_6H_{12}O_6$) and oxygen into carbon dioxide and water. Metaphorically, then, lungs are the train station where passengers (oxygen) ride the train (blood).

When the lungs are not functioning properly, their ability to send oxygen to the blood is reduced, so the blood becomes depleted of oxygen and carries an insufficient amount [2].

SaO_2 is considered good when its level reaches about 98%, that is, when 98% percent of the hemoglobin molecules are transporting oxygen to the tissues; in contrast, SaO_2 is considered low when it is below 90%, that is, when about 10% of all hemoglobin molecules are not transporting oxygen.

In telemedicine, sensors for measuring SaO_2 use pulse oximetry or blood gas measurement, by means of oximeters that assess the amount of light from an LED that is transmitted from one side of the earlobe to the other (or in the fingers of the hands) as blood passes through. The amount of light not absorbed allows the amount of hemoglobin not saturated by oxygen to be derived.

The detection of SaO_2 is also possible by smartwatches that detect it from the vessels running in the wrist under the bottom of the dial.

13.7   Blood Sugar

Traditionally, the measurement of blood glucose has relied on kits equipped with lancets and test strips to be inserted into a glucometer. This system is very effective, convenient, and widely used by a great many diabetic patients around the world, but it has the shortcoming of taking the measurement at discrete times, which may not be sufficient in some cases.

Today, there are systems available for continuous blood glucose monitoring (CGM), through a patch that sticks to the skin (on the arm but also on the belly, the spot where the patient traditionally injects insulin) and can transmit blood glucose readings to physicians but also allows the patient to read the readings themselves, using a smartphone [1, 2].

The sensor on the arm can then transmit the blood glucose values collected every minute so that information on glucose dynamics is finely tuned. In this way, the system immediately alerts the patient and the doctor as soon as their glucose drops or rises too high.

However, there are highly evolved CGM systems that are able to alert the patient of excessive glucose elevation or lowering before it occurs: based on time-dependent analysis of blood concentration, these CGMs are able to warn of the approach of a value above or below the alert or warning threshold. Thus, these monitoring systems are likewise able to measure the slope of the curve describing blood glucose concentration.

This system is to be implemented with a smartphone on which to install a special app, which is also able to provide real-time suggestions on exercise and food, depending on the circumstances that arise.

13.8   Respiratory Frequency

We breathe autonomously, without realizing it, but we can take control of breathing. Indeed, humans are able to voluntarily change the rate of breathing, as does Astrifiammante (die Königin der Nacht), while singing the marvelous aria "Der Hölle Rache kocht in meinem Herzen," from *Die Zauberflöte* (music by Wolfgang Amadeus Mozart, 1756–1791, *libretto* by Emanuel Schikaneder, 1751–1812).

However, humans can also stop breathing altogether, for example, during skin diving. By the way, before diving, the apneist usually performs hyperventilation, which is a type of forced mouth breathing in which they inhale more air than they normally breathe and at a much higher rate than normal breathing, in order to improve the duration of apnea underwater.

So measuring breathing rate can be complicated, as its variability is quite extensive (a run, a flight of stairs), and is partially governable by the subject. In particular, the respiratory rate is inversely proportional to the length of the breath, i.e., its depth. Actually, a deep breath loads more oxygen into the lungs than a normal breath, so the next breath may follow after a longer time, and thus the respiratory rate will be temporarily slowed.

Respiratory rate varies with physiological state (wakefulness and sleep), and it also varies inversely with age: in the adult, however, respiratory rate is around 20 acts per minute.

Measuring respiratory rate in medicine and telemedicine presents no technical problems whatsoever; it is sufficient for a sensor to pick up the movement of the rib cage to send its rate per minute to the site where it will be recorded and analyzed. Mention should be made of the interaction between heart rate and respiratory rate that is observed in some pathological situations, such as in Cheyne-Stokes breathing, where the patient gradually goes from very deep breathing to less and less deep breathing and then reaches a state of apnea for a few seconds, after which breathing gradually resumes until it becomes very deep again.

It is a periodic pathological breathing that can occur frequently in heart patients but also sometimes appears in terminal cancer patients.

Intuitively, the measurement of respiratory rate is primarily (but not only) intended for individuals with chronic or infectious diseases of the lung or who have problems with dyspnea or sleep apnea.

13.9 Nanomaterials and Nanotechnology

Remembering that a nanometer (nm) is one billionth of a meter, and thus one millionth of a millimeter, the European Union Observatory for Nanomaterials (EUON) provides this definition:[3]

A natural, incidental, or manufactured material containing particles, in an unbound state or as an aggregate or as an agglomerate and where, for 50 % or more of the particles in the number size distribution, one or more external dimensions is in the size range 1 nm–100 nm. In specific cases and where warranted by concerns for the environment, health, safety or competitiveness the number size distribution threshold of 50% may be replaced by a threshold between 1 and 50%. By derogation, fullerenes, graphene flakes and single wall carbon nanotubes with one or more external dimensions below 1 nm should be considered as nanomaterials.

In turn, the European Commission, on June 10, 2022, determined the following:[4]

Nanomaterials consist of differently shaped small particles no larger than one hundred nanometers, or about one thousand times smaller than the thickness of a human hair. As a result, nanomaterials have specific properties and some are exploited by industry and in products. Because of these properties, nanomaterials are subject to specific regulatory scrutiny, both by general chemicals legislation (REACH) and by sectoral legislation addressing their use in certain products, such as biocides, cosmetics or food.

---

[3] See https://euon.echa.europa.eu/definition-of-nanomaterial.

[4] See https://environment.ec.europa.eu/news/chemicals-commission-revises-definition-nanomaterials-2022-06-10_en.

It is well-known that the smaller an object is, the more the ratio of surface area to volume increases: for example, if we consider a cube with faces of $10\,cm^2$ and one with faces of $1\,cm^2$, we see that in the former case, the total surface area is $60\,cm^2$, while in the latter case, it is $6\,cm^2$, while the volume in the first case is $1,000\,cm^3$ and in the second case is $1\,cm^3$ (we recall that $1\,cm^3$ is equivalent to 1 ml). Hence, in the first case, the ratio of surface to volume is $0.06\,cm^{-1}$, while in the second case, the ratio is $6.0\,cm^{-1}$ (i.e., 100 times larger): this is why a small ice cube takes less time to melt than a larger ice cube, and it is also why those who sold ice for old iceboxes transported it in large pieces (after all, melted ice was not saleable and would have been pure loss for the seller).

The increase in the surface-to-volume ratio of nanomaterials (so when we are dealing with objects with size on the order of nanometers) compared to traditional materials is able to make possible quantum effects that alter the electronic properties of molecules, but it is also able to change many other physical properties.

Therefore, nanomaterials can exhibit truly amazing properties compared to their "macro" counterpart, so that gold, which macroscopically, at room temperature is solid and inert, when risen to nanometer size spontaneously melts at room temperature and becomes chemically active (an excellent catalyst), and likewise silicon, which under normal conditions is an insulator, becomes a good electrical conductor when reduced to a nanomaterial.

Nanomaterials are often associated with colloids, which are mixtures of solid in liquid in which there are solid (or semisolid or liquid) particles dispersed but not dissolved: these particles (with diameters in the nanometer to micrometer range) are capable of manifesting Brownian motions, caused by the very large number of random collisions with which solvent molecules, thanks to thermal motions, strike the suspended substances. An example of a colloid is milk, in which an oil phase is dispersed in a liquid phase (the whey), which in turn consists of a solution where proteins, carbohydrates, and mineral salts (including calcium) are dissolved. If particles of a colloid are large enough, the process of sedimentation can occur, which separates the phases, causing the heavier phase to be carried toward the bottom of the vessel.

To the study of these properties of nanomaterials is devoted nanotechnology, which in this situation becomes a meeting point between engineering and the physics of what is small and is the stimulus for the development of new materials suitable for various tasks, including in the case of medicine and telemedicine.

Nanotechnology has an obvious impact on scientific research, but it also has an impact on economic processes and on legislative and ethical aspects. Associated with these are risks commensurate with the possibility of building extremely effective weapons of mass extermination, which may be able to self-replicate, going to increase the dangerousness of some countries that have no scruples in their aims of territorial expansion, or physical elimination of other peoples, perhaps on the basis of racial or religious pretexts.

In medical terms, particularly in the area of telemedicine, nanotechnology is dealing with all the activities that go into the future realm of therapy and pharmacology: there is a lot of potential for nanotechnology to provide effective answers in the therapy of various chronic diseases, including as a possible delivery system or vehicle for new or already proven drugs, allowing specific diseased or infected or mutated (cancer) cells to be reached while minimizing or zeroing the risks of toxicity, because guided by a nanoparticle, the drug could act without attacking healthy cells. Of course, in the field of telemedicine, possible developments of increasingly effective biosensors are of interest.

The development of nanotechnology and the development of artificial intelligence walk hand in hand: making sensors ever smaller and more functional is a task for artificial intelligence and bioengineering, which will pave way for ever more innovative systems, which nanotechnology will put into practice in the form of nanorobots and nano-drugs as they become available. At present, nanomaterials based on graphene and MXenes (two-dimensional biodegradable pressure sensors) are already available to detect information about body movement.

13.10 Desirable Features of Sensors

Sensors must be biocompatible as much as possible, as must all medical devices: this must be clear from the moment the sensor is designed, trying to avoid any risk, even potential risk of harm to the patient. It should be made clear that biocompatibility must be considered even if the contact between sensor or device and patient is only indirect. Moving in this direction is the very popular choice of using materials such as chitin or cellulose, two chemically very similar polymers composed mainly of glucose molecules and known to be biocompatible to a very high degree [2].

When designing a medical device or sensor, characteristics of biocompatibility must be kept in mind, in close connection with the purpose for which the sensor is being designed, so one will immediately have to reason about the nature of the contact between sensor and human and the foreseeable duration of the contact. For it is one thing to design a sensor intended to be in place for a few days and quite another to design a sensor that is to be used for a few months. On this basis, reasoning can be done to identify a priori all possible potential adverse effects at the interaction level, also taking into account their costs in health terms.

We can then distinguish the risk (biohazard) associated with the absence of an actual biocompatibility, as the a priori estimable severity of the damage resulting from the non-biocompatible sensor, multiplied by the probability of the damage occurring, from which we can derive the definition of biosafety, as the absence of unacceptable biological risk due to the use of the sensor.

In addition to this, it should be remembered that all sensors, from the first moment they are worn, are subjected to mechanical wear and tear and can be damaged: for this reason, research has been concerned with finding sensors that can repair themselves. Self-repair can take place through the use of self-healing polymers in case of minor damage from mechanical impact, crushing, excess heat and related temperature rise, and contact with moisture.

In addition to self-healing and biocompatibility, a third possible guideline on the desirable characteristics of a sensor is that of its biodegradability, which should be expected after the sensor has finished performing its task. When a sensor is to be grafted provisionally, for example, to monitor the healing of a bone or deep soft-tissue injury or even to assess the restoration of proper elasticity of a tendon, removal should be planned and done by a surgical technique. But if you have a sensor formed from safe biodegradable materials, the surgery to remove the sensor is no longer essential. There is no longer any need to deal with the cost of the surgery (materials and surgeon's labor cost), nor with the cost of disposing of the sensor, nor to foresee the possible costs resulting from the risks to the patient's health.

In other cases, however, the choice of a biodegradable material may be dictated by the need to keep a patient who lives far away or has limited independent movement capabilities from returning to the hospital. In these circumstances, one sends the patient home with a biodegradable device that will dispose of itself without the need for the patient to return to the hospital. The sensor will degrade on its own without the need for it to be removed by the patient or by a family member.

13.11 Smartglasses

Smartglasses are special glasses used for augmented reality, which use artificial intelligence to ameliorate visual perception. The visual depth and the field of view are both increased. Smartglasses can have multiple fields of use, including the training of medical personnel.

The field of view is equipped with information readable by means of an augmented reality overlay or by a transparent heads-up display (HUD) or, again, by means of other digital interfaces. In all cases, lenses can allow visualization of digital images so that smartglasses are actually a sort of wearable computer, able to work using some specific apps, may access the Internet by means of a Wi-Fi or Bluetooth connection, and can obey voice commands.

13.12 Wrist Sensors

For monitoring some basic physiological parameters such as heart rate, body temperature, oxygen saturation, and physical activity in terms of number of steps and calories burned, wearable devices designed to be worn on the wrist (equipped with accelerometers or pedometers) have been developed, just like a watch: they are called Wrist-Worn Wearables (WWDs).

In fact, intelligent watches (smartwatches) have been on the market for some time: they are available today also at very low prices (although there may be doubts about their reliability) and are capable of performing all these measurements on their own, usually in conjunction with an app that can be downloaded to the smartphone.

Other types of smartwatches are capable of directly measuring daily routes taken on foot, using the Global Positioning System (GPS) technology: thus, from the tracking of the route and its quantification in terms of length (thanks to GPS), it is possible to calculate, albeit indirectly, the amount of energy consumed during walking. For example, a man weighing 80 kg walking for 1 h at normal speed (about 3 km/h) on level ground will consume approximately 200 kcal (which is about one-tenth of his daily caloric requirement). Energy consumption changes with speed and with the type of terrain: by doubling the pace speed and increasing it to 6 km/h, on a slightly uphill stretch, the energy consumption for 1 h of walking rises to about 480 kcal, so it follows that walking is an excellent exercise for keeping fit at all ages.[5]

Although wristbands and smartwatches may appear to be similar devices, smartwatches have had a technological development more related to leisure and non-professional personal fitness monitoring, while wristbands have been designed to monitor the health of patients with the necessary accuracy: in particular, wristbands may be able to measure blood glucose noninvasively, derived from the measurement of glucose in sweat.

To remark on the possible differences between smartwatches and wristbands, it should be added that it is difficult to know exactly how accurately a smartwatch measures oxygen saturation or the number of steps: for the latter, there may be problems with calibration and vibration sensitivity, so that in some cases, the step is not detected or is detected twice.

13.13 Head and Neck Sensors

Medical devices applied to the patient's head have found multiple applications in the field of neuroscience. They can be used in various types of measurements of brain activity and soft tissue activity of the head and neck.

With these devices, it is possible to recognize the emotional responses that humans produce in the presence of external stimuli, particularly in the human-machine relationship.

One monitoring that is likely to have important developments is that of biomarkers in tear fluid, which contains much information that can be used to monitor the development of eyeball disease, diabetes, and other diseases. The measurement can be made through sensors mounted on glasses, which are able to obtain the required data noninvasively.

Measurement of electrical impedance within the head and gas volume dynamics in the airway can monitor respiration not only at the hospital level but also in continuous remote clinical monitoring.

---

[5] The very approximate formula for calculating calories consumed is kcal = weight (kg) × distance (km) × 0.9, if the walking took place on level ground, and kcal = weight (kg) × distance (km), if the walking took place on a slight incline.

13.14 Smart Textiles

Smart textiles have been developed by incorporating biomechanical sensors, based on miniaturized and flexible electronic components, into textiles with technologies that make them integrable and thus wearable within T-shirts, garments, textiles or fibers and are generally called "smart clothing" or "smart T-shirts" or in other ways. These are piezoelectric or resistive, or capacitive sensors, which are generally based on sensitivity to pressure or rubbing or strain.

The factor that makes the use of smart clothes very attractive is their adaptability to body contours and physical skin contact. This virtually unique feature makes skin contact very natural and does not require the sensor to be implanted subcutaneously or be attached in some other way and makes these smart clothes suitable for collecting signals of heartbeat or breathing or muscle contraction.

For an object in contact with a non-negligible surface of the skin, as in the case of a smart T-shirt, the first thing to consider is the presence of sweat, especially when the T-shirt is used in the recording of information gathered during intense physical activity [2].

Sweat is produced by sweat glands (which are eccrine glands because they remain intact after secreting their product), each of which flows onto the skin surface with its own excretory duct; each individual gland is abundantly vascularized (the raw material of sweat, in its initial production is plasma) and surrounded by a nerve network (when you are very stressed you sweat). Sweat is produced for two main purposes: the first is the regulation of body temperature, and the second is the excretion of certain substances (in the latter case, the production of sweat occurs at the apocrine glands, which produce a fatty sweat that flakes into the hair bulbs, and is the probable responsible for the production of pheromones). In cases of psychological changes, stress, sudden emotions, and states of anxiety, sweating occurs at specific body areas and involves vasoconstriction, so this phenomenon is given the name of cold sweating.

Sweat from the eccrine glands during its journey from the glandular body to the outside has a composition similar to that of plasma deprived of its proteins: passing through the excretory duct, there is significant reabsorption of sodium and chloride, along with water (by osmosis), and this reabsorption is inversely proportional to the rate of sweat production by the gland, so when production is intense, less reabsorption occurs. The most conspicuous part of the work of the eccrine sweat glands is that related to the control of body heat, such that in extreme heat situations, sweat production can exceed three or four liters per hour. Equally important is the amount of sweat produced under exertion: a marathoner running the 42.2 km race loses about 4 liters of sweat in the approximately 260 min of running (expected duration for a good marathon runner). There are about three million sweat glands in humans, scattered throughout the body unevenly, and functioning discontinuously, as even under maximum effort about half of the glands do not produce sweat.

Sweat is a solution with an acidic pH (between 4.5 and 6.5) composed of 99% water and the rest of creatinine, ammonia, urea, pyruvate, lactate, amino acids, sodium, potassium, chlorides, and other substances.

The presence of sweat in contact with the skin promotes certain measurements, such as lactate concentration, which can be used to determine the general health status of the body. Measurement can be made by patches or by organometallic substances.

References

1. Reddy DD, Hussain OM, Gopal DVRS, Rao DM, Sastry KS. Biosen- sors and bioelectronics. Delhi: IK Publishing House; 2013.
2. Banica F-G. Chemical sensors and biosensors: fundamentals and applications. New York: John Wiley & Sons; 2012.

Medical Imaging

14

Medical imaging is a virtually indispensable aid in almost every specialty of medicine; therefore, image collection and transmission are high-profile topics in telemedicine. Also for medical imaging, sensors will be responsible for collecting analog information and transmitting it in digital form to the telemedicine service center.

14.1 Ultrasound

Sound is an elastic wave made up of alternating compression and rarefaction of transmission medium (air, water, solid objects). Transmission of sound requires a propagating medium and cannot take place in a vacuum (when in a science fiction movie one hears the sounds of a spaceship swimming in interstellar space, which is known to be empty, this is a serious scientific error).

The speed of sound in air depends on temperature: at $20\,°C$ it is equal to $343.4\,$m/s $(1{,}236.2\,$km/h$)$, while at $0\,°C$ it is equal to $331.2\,$m/s $(1{,}192.3\,$km/h$)$; the speed in water is $1{,}484\,$m/s $(5{,}342\,$km/h$)$, four times the speed in air; the speed in glass is $5{,}770\,$m/s $(20{,}772\,$km/h$)$, and in iron is $5{,}904\,$m/s $(21{,}254\,$km/h$)$.[1]

Audible sound frequencies for humans range between 20 Hz and 20 kHz, but this limit is reduced up to 15 kHz in the elderly (musical instruments are tuned using the frequency of 440 Hz, the note A).

Frequencies audible to animals can be very different; the dog, for example, can hear sounds with frequencies up to 40 kHz (sounds with frequencies higher than that audible to humans are called ultrasound), twice the maximum frequency audible to humans, although much depends on the breed and the configuration of the earcup.

---

[1] To convert the speed from m/s to km/h, it is sufficient to multiply by 3.6 (thus 10 m/s are 36 km/h); therefore, to convert the speed from km/h to m/s, it is sufficient to divide by 3.6 (thus 100 km/h are 27.8 m/s).

M. Nichelatti, *Mathematical Tools for Telemedicine*, TELe-Health, https://doi.org/10.1007/978-3-031-81709-0_14

The ability of bats to produce ultrasounds at 110 kHz, used to detect prey and distinguish obstacles by receiving their echo, is well-known. Other animals, such as the elephant, can produce or hear low-frequency sounds: specifically, elephants hear sounds at low frequencies up to 5 Hz (when the sound frequency is lower than that audible to humans, it is called infrasound).

Ultrasound diagnostics exploits several properties of sound propagation, including speed in fluids and solids, attenuation, and wave phase.

In propagating within tissues, ultrasound waves are able to make, through their echo, a true "acoustic image": the denser the affected tissue, the greater the reflected echo, and the clearer the monochromatic (B/W) image produced on the screen. As a whole, the ultrasound produces a dynamic moving image that follows the movements of the anatomical structures being observed, as happens during ultrasound scans done on pregnant women to check the health of the fetus.

Ultrasound does not require invasive procedures: ultrasounds are produced by the probe, which also receives echoes: it is particularly suitable in the search for clinical problems at the cardiological level, in the search for breast and other neoplasms or kidney stones, and in monitoring the fetal development, as mentioned above. Results of an ultrasound scan are easily transmitted as video files: typically, at the end of an ultrasound check on the fetus, the pregnant woman receives a DVD recorded with the footage.

14.2   X-Rays

A radiography is a photograph in which the image is obtained not with light waves, but with X-ray, an electromagnetic wave characterized by a very high frequency, carrying large amounts of energy, according to Planck's well-known law in which the energy of a photon is $E = h\nu$, where h is Plank's constant (its exact value is $6.62607015 \times 10^{-34}$ J $\times$ Hz^{-1}) and ν is the frequency of the radiation in Hz. The very small wavelength of X-rays, ranging between 0.01 nm (10^{-11} m) and 1 nm (10^{-9} m), allows them to pass through tissue and see things that visible light cannot see. According to a certain vulgate, the name "X-rays" would be derived from the Latin number X (e.g., 10), which would be the sign-changed exponent of the number 10^{-10}, representing an intermediate value of the wavelength between the other sign-changed exponents (9 and 11) that are the upper and lower limits of the X-ray wavelength [1].

X-rays with longer wavelengths carry lower energies and are therefore called "soft X-rays," while those with shorter wavelengths carry higher energies and are called "hard X-rays." Soft X-rays are used for diagnostic imaging, while hard X-rays find use in the therapeutic field for cancer treatment.

High energies of X-rays make them dangerous because they can damage living tissues by breaking certain chemical bonds and causing possible damage to cellular ultrastructures or DNA, so the strictest safety measures must be observed to preserve the health of patients but also that of healthcare workers in charge, who in fact wear small detectors that measure their exposure to radiation.

Radiographic images acquired for their transmission must be converted to digital format, which, however, require very high resolutions that would allow me to visualize even the smallest details, particularly needed to detect small tumor masses when they are still forming.

14.3   Electrocardiogram

Electrocardiograms (ECG), electroencephalograms (EEG), and electromyograms (EMG) are three systems that exploit the properties of electric fields to evaluate the function of the heart, brain, and muscles (together with their associated nerves), respectively.

Electrocardiograms take measurements noninvasively by resting electrodes on the skin, held in situ using painless methods, such as creating a small suction cup effect. Electrodes pick up currents generated by muscle contraction or nerve discharges and record them by means of the electrocardiograph, generating graphs of a periodic function in which the change in current is represented on the ordinate. In these examinations, the patient's body receives no current, nor is it subjected to any potential difference: the current that makes the graph of, say, an ECG is only that produced by the heart as it alternates between systole and diastole.

Abnormalities in the functioning of the heart or any part of it can be read from the irregularities recorded in the graphical trace: it will be the physician who will interpret the nonconforming tracings and attribute them to a specific problem in a ventricle or atrium or other.

The ECG can be used to diagnose many heart diseases, particularly to find coronary artery disease, but the detection system must be as efficient as possible to avoid interference on the signal that will delay diagnosis.

The ECG is performed by the physician who will either keep the graph of the trace, or he will point it out after digitizing it, again taking care to obtain the highest possible resolution in pixels, so that the digital image of the ECG signal is clearly readable, in its eventual black-and-white rendering, making sure that the grid present on the graph strip is clearly distinguishable from the trace.

14.4   Electroencephalogram

The electroencephalogram (EEG) is a device used to record the electrical activity of the encephalon (from the Greek $\varepsilon\gamma\kappa\varepsilon\varphi\alpha\lambda o\sigma$ = that which is contained in the head), which makes a series of wave-shaped tracings. It is performed by noninvasively applying about 20 electrodes to the patient's head and connecting them to the electroencephalograph. An EEG can cover the brain (telencephalon and diencephalon) or the cerebellum or the brainstem.

In the course of recording the tracing, the patient may be asked to perform some simple activities such as reading the page of a book, doing some easy arithmetic calculations, looking at objects, or otherwise answering questions that the doctor asks.

The EEG may be recorded throughout an entire day (we then speak of dynamic EEG): this is a situation that occurs, for example, when the problem of altered brain functioning has not yet been clarified. When encephalography is applied over the 24 h, the patient must perform all activities that occupy his or her day, either at home or at work.

If for various reasons a dynamic EEG is not sufficient, then a recording should also be made over several consecutive days, and in that case, we speak of video EEG, because the EEG recording is accompanied by a video recording made in a specially equipped room in the hospital so that we know what is happening to the patient during the examination, allowing us, for example, to see in what situations a seizure may be triggered, which a pediatric or adult patient perhaps cannot report accurately.

EEG is performed diagnostically to look for the presence of neurological pathology such that the transmission of electrical signals in the brain, cerebellum, and brainstem is altered. The EEG is the most effective system for diagnosing epilepsy, the state of altered functioning of certain neurons, which force the patient to manifest seizures affecting skeletal muscles or to have hallucinations or otherwise sensitive alterations affecting sensory systems. One situation occurs in the case of dementia, where, however, the alteration is to the intellectual functions, language, and memory.

An important use of EEG is in monitoring the status and evolution of a hemorrhagic stroke (from injury to a vessel in the brain that produces bleeding) or ischemic stroke (brought about by failure or insufficient blood supply to an encephalic district)

Use also broadens in cases of mechanical trauma to the head or in cases of inflammation or tumors in the brain, cerebellum, and brainstem, as well as in monitoring patients who are in the state of coma from various causes.

The EEG is also essential for the assessment of brain death, which is defined as the irreversible cessation of electrical activity in the brainstem: when this event occurs, the patient is incapable of responding to stimuli and goes into a definitive state of loss of consciousness. Confirmation of the state of cerebral death is an indispensable step for the removal of those organs that can be transplanted (at the decision of the patient himself or relatives) to other individuals.

14.5   Electromyogram

Electromyography (EMG) is used in the evaluation of the function of skeletal muscles and the peripheral nerve network connected to them. It allows the diagnosis of many diseases and inflammations affecting the muscle and peripheral nerves like muscle afferents, such as in the case of carpal tunnel syndrome, which is quite common in those who, while working at a computer, use the mouse inappropriately or in the case of peripheral neuropathies of diabetics, individuals with renal failure, and alcoholics. Symptoms that should make one suspect the need for electromyography include, among others, constant tingling in a limb, weakness of leg muscles, cramps, and myoclonus.

EMG makes it possible to evaluate situations in which there is involvement of the motor neurons of the brain and spinal cord and thus in cases of poliomyelitis or amyotrophic lateral sclerosis (ALS). It should also be used in cases of herniated disc and crushed spinal nerve emergencies.

EMG is carried out using the appropriate electromyograph and consists of a first phase in which peripheral nerve conduction is studied with electrodes applied to the skin (obviously in the district where there is the innervation you want to study); the second phase, on the other hand, involves the use of needle electrodes with which the electrical activity of the muscle is analyzed. At this stage, the examination can be quite painful, as the skin will be punctured by at least five electro-needles. Prior to EMG, the physician should inquire, among other things, whether the patient has an implantable defibrillator or pacemaker or is possibly using anticoagulants.

14.6 Magnetic Resonance

Magnetic resonance imaging (MRI) uses nuclear magnetic moments to produce high-resolution images of organs [1].

A cylindrical scanner consisting of a ring magnet associated with an electrical coil (a coiled cable) that emits radiofrequencies is used. The patient is inserted into the cylinder [2, 3].

In recent times, the so-called open MRI technique has been introduced, in which the patient is not inserted into the cylinder, and the magnet is placed only near the body district to be analyzed. The condition is more favorable for the patient, who does not suffer from possible claustrophobic effects brought about by being inside the cylinder, nor is not disturbed by the annoying noise produced by the cylindrical scanner. Open MRI is also much more acceptable for pediatric patients.

The very strong magnetic fields generated by the scanner are able to excite the hydrogen nuclei, displacing them from their original position, a position to which they return at the end of the scan, causing a series of radiofrequency signals emitted by the tissues to be generated. These radiofrequency signals are picked up by a spectrometer (the technique is based on the NMR spectroscopes used in chemistry) and translated into high-resolution images, particularly appreciable in details of soft tissues.

NMR can be used in patients with new-generation pacemakers and defibrillators, as well as in subjects with metal prostheses.

14.7   Computed Axial Tomography Scan (CT Scan)

A CT scan is an overlay of X-ray images taken from various positions and angles, which will then be processed by a computer to produce a cross-sectional image of a "slice," which is very useful in seeing if a subject has internal lesions not easily diagnosed by other techniques.

CT scanners are basically made from an X-ray cylinder rotating on its own axis and a series of detectors that analyze how much radiation is being attenuated by the tissues being hit. Patients can be scanned with CT scanners even if they are wearing pacemakers; moreover, CT scanners can analyze in depth almost any part of a patient's body.

The relative disadvantage (probably neutralized by the greater accuracy of the images) is the dose of ionizing radiation the patient must absorb, which is higher than that of an X-ray, although not enough to cause damage.

14.8   Positron Emission Tomography (PET)

Positron emission tomography (PET) is a (quasi) noninvasive diagnostic method that is used in nuclear medicine departments for the diagnosis of diseases affecting certain organs and for the diagnosis of cancer or neurological diseases or in patients with cardiological problems. PET is also used to follow patients in the postoperative course or after radiation treatment.

Positrons, or positive electrons, are elementary particles with mass identical to that of electrons but with positive electrical charge (while electrons have negative charge). Like electrons, neutrons, neutrinos, and quarks, positrons belong to the class of fermions,[2] i.e., the set of elementary particles endowed with a semi-integer spin number (1/2, 3/2, etc.). The other class of particles, namely, bosons[3] (which include the photon, the graviton, the famous Higgs Boson discovered in 2012 at CERN in Geneva, and others), on the other hand, are endowed with an integer spin number (0, 1, 2, etc.).[4]

Positrons are produced in nature during β^+ radioactive decay, or they can also be produced when high-energy photons collide with matter, inducing the production of pairs, in which an electron and a positron are emitted.

PET is performed by intravenously injecting a radiopharmaceutical that selectively binds to certain cells and from a positron-emitting nucleus and highlights

---

[2] To remember the Italian physicist Enrico Fermi (1901–1954).

[3] To remember the Indian physicist Satyendra Nath Bose (1894–1974).

[4] The main difference between fermions and bosons lies in the fact that a quantum state cannot contain two identical Fermions (this is Pauli's exclusion principle, whereby the "no more than one in the same place" rule applies), while two or more identical Bosons can happily coexist (whereby the "the more the merrier" rule applies). If we were made of bosons, then a car could hold several billion passengers, but since we are made of fermions, we must submit to the law of impenetrability of objects.

diseased cells of interest. The intravenous infusion must take place several minutes before the start of the examination so that it can spread to various tissues of the body. A CT scan is also performed before the PET scan to facilitate image reconstruction.

The availability of state-of-the-art tomographs makes the examination quite short and thus also reduces possible risks inherent in the administration of radioactive nuclei.

14.9   Medical Image Transmission

The transmission of images or movies with medical data, collected with the methods previously listed, is not a hard task. We send and receive pictures and videos every day, whether using e-mail or simple smartphone apps such as WhatsApp, and, again, we can easily upload digital images and videos in many Web sites. The only possible problem is an excessive file size, which will take longer and can be blocked by the administrator of the target site. In any case, there are Web sites that allow very large files to be shared among multiple users. Up to 2 GB at a time, the service is free, while to share files without a size limitation, there is a charge.

Obviously, graphic files and movies in the very high resolutions required for telemedicine have very large sizes, so advanced transmission systems are necessary. It is also essential that these systems for transmitting and sharing data respect the necessary privacy and are secure from hacking.

In our daily life, we, if we look at a house, a tree, or a sunset, are dealing with analogic color images that our retina perceives. Visible light, for humans, is an electromagnetic radiation with frequencies ranging from 400 THz[5] of red light (wavelength of 625 nm) to 790 THz of violet light (wavelength of 450 nm): with sunlight, the maximum visual sensitivity is at 540 THz (wavelength of 555 nm), a frequency peculiar to the color green. Thus, there are no limitations in our perception of colors, which in nature are distributed over a continuous spectrum. In addition, our eyes have a constant sensitivity, and this allows our eyesight to observe many more details and to observe them at a much higher resolution than a camera can.

However, such detailed image or video information cannot be transmitted or even stored, so one must resort to digitizing the data, which reduces its size and facilitates its transmission and storage.

Digitizing something means transforming information describable with continuous variables (real numbers) into information describable with discrete variables (natural numbers). Probably the clearest evidence of the difference between analog and digital is seen by looking at the motion of the second hand on an analog mechanical watch and a quartz digital watch. The digitization process is very useful

---

[5] 1 THz is equal to 1000 GHz; thus, 1 THz $= 10^{12}$ Hz.

because it facilitates the transport of information and its storage, but in a sense, it can modify the qualitative content of the same information.[6]

If it is not possible to send an image that is too detailed, digitizing it will require finding the right compromise that preserves its necessary detail resolution but allows for size reduction. A message contained in an image or text that are formed by a series of symbols (a mathematics book contains text and equations, each formed by a sequence of letters, numbers, and mathematical symbols), whereby the entropy H of information is defined as the sum of all the information associated with a symbol (letter, or other), multiplied by the respective probabilities.

Software allows not only file compression but also the merging of several files that are compressed, creating a single new compressed file (in any case, one should never destroy a file after sending it in compressed form: it should be retained, both for archiving purposes and for the eventual need to resend it in case something during the sending was unsuccessful). In addition, it must be remembered that in the last releases of Microsoft Office, files are already compressed, as are music files in mp3 format, so compressing these files can give very poor results.

To define the efficiency of a compression, one uses the compression rate, which is intuitively given as

$$\text{compression rate} = \frac{\text{size of compressed file}}{\text{size of uncompressed file}},$$

provided both sizes are given with the same measure unit. Thus, using this definition, a high compression rate means that the size of the file was significantly reduced. If, for example, the size of uncompressed file was 1,200 MB, and the size of compressed file was 850 MB, then the compression rate is

$$\frac{1,200}{850} \approx 1.412$$

and the space saved on disk with respect to uncompressed file is

$$1 - \frac{850}{1,200} \approx 1 - 0.708 = 0.292 = 29.2\%.$$

Perhaps the most critical part lies in the decompression of the received file. Since compression has reduced the size of the file, restoring the image will mean getting after decompression exactly the same file before compression.

---

[6] A practical test is to listen to a piece of music in the two formats. Take, for example, Keth Jarrett's "The Köln Concert"(ECM Records, Munich): listen first to the concert recorded on CD and then to the one recorded on vinyl. You will notice that these are two different sound experiences, which depend on the frequencies that are differently rendered by a vinyl and by a CD. Of course, vinyl wears out physically because of the friction of the needle in the grooves, while CD is a bit more durable over time.

For this reason, we must first distinguish two main techniques of data compression: (1) lossy (nonsymmetric) compression and (2) loseless (symmetric) compression. In the compression/decompression operations, lossy techniques cause information loss (they are more efficient than accurate), while loseless techniques do not cause information loss (they are more accurate than efficient), so there is a symmetry between original and decompressed files.

The needs of telemedicine call for the use of lossless compression techniques, which allow the decompressed image to retain all original details. In extremely simplified terms, compression of the original details can be achieved by homogeneously marking adjacent (contact) pixels characterized by the same color so that all areas with adjacent pixels of homogeneous color are reduced to a series of monochromatic information requiring less information than the original one.

Giving an extremely simplified example, the information contained in a sequence of pixels labeled as "P," "Q," and "R" (this is obviously a very simplified example), instead of being stored with the string

$$PPPPPPQQQQQQQRRQQQQR$$

can be stored with the string

$$6P7Q2R4Q1R$$

thus saving space. If the data sequence is generally short, as is expected, for example, in text files (ASCII), where sequences (which we call "runs") are limited to two identical characters, the above encoding becomes unnecessary; indeed, it would be harmful because it will produce a sequence longer than the original. For example, coding as "0" (void) the spaces between words, the string "Call me Ishmael" would become "1C1a2l01m1e01I1s1h1m1a1e1l": too long (and, more importantly, lacking that poetic touch).

The zip format (perhaps the most used compression technique) is a lossless compression, so zipped files will return exactly the original file. Of course, a zipped ASCII file will have a very low compression rate. There are other lossless compression techniques, but we are not interested in exploring this topic here.

The substantial thing in medical imaging is the variation in the color of pixels, rather than their color itself: it is the variations that contain the information, and from completely monochromatic images, no one would be able to pick up information, just as from a radio emitting a continuous buzz, one would not be able to understand the information transmitted by a newscast.

In the medical field, however, even slightest changes in color between pixels are important, because they can reveal even very serious situations, such as early stages of tumor growth. The mapping information of various pixels will be entrusted to a set of binary signals included in the file that will judge the reconstruction process of the original image. In this way, the loss of information will be very limited and will not involve critical factors of diagnostic interest: the "cost" of all this necessary image quality is a low compression rate, so compressed images will have a larger size.

14.10 The Excess of Paper Records

Information about the health of patients and the progress of their illness has been recorded practically as long as there has been an activity to treat and heal those who are ill.

Even in the early days of medical care, it was necessary to have a minimal record of the patient's health status yesterday, in order to compare it with the health status today and to understand the evolution of the disease.

After the early stages of the emergence of medicine, patient data began to be recorded on sheets of paper, and later on pre-filled forms, to be filled out by the physician, which—if nothing else—at least tried to give a minimum of uniformity in drawing up reports on patients. Information such as age, sex, body temperature, current drug treatment, and so on were reported. This kind of information was collected until very recently, and only in the last few years, the development of technological resources has made it possible to record medical information on media such as hard drives.

Paper, however, is still widely used today to compile patient records. These paper records have several drawbacks: paper tends to yellow, and over time, it tends to fragment at the touch of the fingers; then in a humid environment, paper deteriorates and tends to make the writing fade, making it illegible. Finally, among other drawbacks is the weight. A 500-sheet ream of A4 paper weighs an average of 2.2 kg, and we have all had the experience of how much books weigh.

References

1. Bushberg JT, Seibert JA. The essential physics of medical imaging. London: Lippincott Williams & Wilkins; 2022.
2. Gurley S. Medical imaging technologies. New York: American Medical Publishers, Inc.; 2023.
3. Holloway M. Optical diagnostics and imaging. New York: American Medical Publishers, Inc.; 2023.

Some Areas of Telemedicine

15

Telemedicine consists of a series of remote implementations of healthcare and can be divided by specialty, just like standard medicine.

Each of the specialties of telemedicine has its own requirements and tools. In some cases, the main needs are related to diagnosis and teleconsultation, while in other cases, there may be different needs, more related to image transmission.

In this brief excursus that follows, an attempt will be made, without claiming to give a complete overview of the various issues involved, to focus on the activities related to the various areas of telemedicine.

In all cases, as an advantage that unites all these techniques, we will observe that the main advantage over the specialty practiced in the presence is for the patient, who will no longer have the need to move and can be cared for in the comfort of his or her own home, with the reassuring presence of family members. The advantage will also be evident for physicians and health facilities, who will not necessarily have to take on the burden of hospitalizations and possible overcrowding in outpatient clinics: thus saving resources and money.

15.1 Telecardiology

Because cardiovascular diseases are among the most common in the population of Western countries, a good deal of medicine is geared toward the prevention and treatment of these diseases. As a result, it is legitimate to emphasize telecardiology as a system for remote diagnosis and treatment of cardiovascular diseases.

The focus on remote treatment of these diseases was brought to the forefront during the last pandemic that affected much of the planet. In many cases, the focus with respect to chronic and degenerative diseases (cardiovascular disease, diabetes, cancers, and others) has been shifted to COVID infection, limiting access to hospitals and drastically restricting elective surgeries to prioritize only emergency surgeries. But the health demand of the population (which, let us remember, is aging

© The Author(s), under exclusive license to Springer Nature Switzerland AG 2025   185
M. Nichelatti, *Mathematical Tools for Telemedicine*, TELe-Health,
https://doi.org/10.1007/978-3-031-81709-0_15

in Western countries) has certainly not decreased: on the contrary, neglecting heart patients (and other chronic patients) in a certain way has had the effect of increasing the care and treatment needs of these individuals.

Indeed, with the pandemic, not only were attention, hospitalizations, and treatment for these diseases diverted to COVID infectiousness, but there was also a reduction in travel, including travel to the doctor's office, because of fears subsumed in patients and generated by the possible risks of leaving home.

The cardiac patient can be assisted at home with all the tools that telemedicine makes available, starting with televisit, which can be managed with one of the many applications available for remote communication using a computer: it is a visit in which there is a lack of physical contact between doctor and patient, and for this very reason, it is not suitable to be the first visit but only to be a follow-up visit, in which the evolution of the patient's health status is recorded, or it can be just a routine visit to renew a prescription and to check for possible side effects. It is pleonastic that in any case, the doctor tries to obtain all the information he can about the evolution of the disease, and, given the importance of the pathology, he makes himself available to receive communication from the patient as often as the patient requests it.

But the quintessential telehealth act with quest patients is telemonitoring, which allows the patient's vital parameters to be monitored and their dynamics to be followed according to ongoing treatment. Sensors and instruments used for this purpose (which are essentially a sphygmomanometer, a saturimeter, a glucometer, and, of course, an electrocardiograph) are able to read the values sought (heart rate, blood pressure, oxygen saturation, etc.), transform them into digital signals, and send them to the remote station for reading and storage. Information can be passed directly to the patient's medical record without the need for additional system-to-system translation, so the physician and caregiver do not have to spend their time to have the patient's data securely saved, and in case of abnormalities, a safety system is activated that contacts the doctor and the patient [1, 2].

In fact, by reading the data transmitted by means of instruments' sensors (e.g., the ECG), the physician is able to decipher any changes in progress and intervene by alerting the patient in a timely manner, to give him or her any transitional arrangements pending a reasoned therapeutic intervention to be made as soon as possible. It is, however, a matter of distinguishing instrumental telemonitoring from the trivial phone call to ask the patient, "how is your health?" The more amenable treatment and management of therapy at home make it easier for patients to accept treatment and rely on the doctor's advice. Greater adherence to therapies means a greater likelihood of staying well and improving quality of life, so telemedicine for cardiac patients yields results that unfold not only in therapy but also in lifestyle.

These are situations that are not limited to the transmission of data over the air but also evolution of algorithms dedicated to the detection of problems such as atrial fibrillation and in the transformation of some technological tools into real diagnostic tools.

So telemonitoring, the real kind, the kind done with biomedical instruments, is a particularly effective system for heart failure and post-infarction patients to prevent consequences such as re-hospitalization.

We had already heard about the heart bands that were worn during some stress tests and sent the signal to a smartphone or smartwatch, but now, some smartwatches are able to perform very sophisticated heart rate analysis using some electrodes added to the crown of the watch, and the patient is able to get an electrocardiogram in less than a minute and have the data recorded, thanks to an app that then gets the results to the doctor.

Among telecardiology, remote assistance for patients with heart failure is emerging, of which telemedicine applications appear very promising as a tool to reduce needs for hospitalization. Hearth failure in these last years has reduced its mortality but has incremented hospitalization and therefore the goal at present to reverse this trend. Diagnostics has been ameliorated with the use of wearable sensors and implantable cardiac devices, making possible remote control of hemodynamic parameters, increasing opportunities for better prevention and therapy and reducing the probability of new hospitalizations. If this result can be limited to patients affected by a mild form of cardiac failure, it is anyway a good result, allowing to divert the physician's attention to more severe situations actually needing a hospital stay.

The use of remote data gathering in hearth failure is an opportunity also because data are collected during time, and this is an excellent way to check the disease dynamics of many patients, so that these data can be used by machine learning algorithms to infer new knowledge about disease, which cannot be reached by using only statistics. AI and ML algorithms are a good system for modelling data: they can be used to find relations between variables and can manage nonlinearity affecting a great part of biological phenomena; therefore, they can also improve our understanding of cardiac failure. Machine learning algorithms in particular can extract information from data practically without the need of programming: these algorithms allow the system to learn by itself and to correct their errors as the knowledge increases [1, 2].

Giving data large enough to the computer and giving also the desired answer (the output one would expect), we are dealing with supervised learning (like students solving an equation of which they already know which will be the result, since the teacher gave it them); this process occurs by means of a training set of data (say, the teacher shows some examples of equation solutions), followed by a test dataset, which are unseen data (the students, after learning the methods of solution to equations, are now challenged with a new equation, never presented by the teacher). With the supervised machine learning, the computer may obtain an output giving a classification (e.g., on the basis of an expected recurrent disease or not), as well as a quantitative model, for example, like a nonlinear multivariate regression.

If one does not know the final outcome, we are dealing with unsupervised learning, which is used for phenogrouping, e.g., to separate patients into different clusters. Unsupervised algorithms are able to reduce the dimensionality of datasets, by using principal component analysis, a statistical technique which condenses variables on the basis of what they actually say: variables with the same meaning or describing similar characteristics are put together to form a new (say, composite or condensed) variable. Unsupervised algorithms do not require labeled data.

A problem that can be considered by supervised and unsupervised algorithms is the time evolution of an event, that is, the time evolution of a disease, in our case. However, if data are continuously transmitted to the hospital and if that data are continuously submitted to AI or ML algorithms, then this new information can be digested and metabolized to be transformed in new knowledge so that a model in function of time can be put at work, and hence it would be possible to know the future of the patients. The statistical instrument to do this was once the time series analysis, where the first requirement was that data are stationary so as to maintain their parameters constant, while new algorithms can manage non-stationary data, where data mean may vary in time.

15.2 Telepathology

Telepathology is the remote study of diseases affecting organs and tissues, diagnosing their causes and possible development, by means of microscope images (optical, electronic, etc.), projected remotely on a monitor, analyzing biopsies or samples of cells or slices of tissue cut with a microtome.

Given the type of activity of telepathology, it is immediate to think that everything or almost everything is based on the ability to obtain high-definition images and transmit them to the remote server where they will be analyzed. Thus, all procedures associated with shipping the biological sample taken and possibly prepared using histochemistry techniques are avoided, and all risks associated with shipping (loss, damage) are avoided. So thanks to telepathology, a physician close to the patient can send images that will be read by a specialized pathologist.

In many other respects, telepathology has the same advantages as all other types of telemedicine, and it allows the same results in terms of teleconsultation, education of junior physicians, and telediagnosis, which is probably the most important aspect inherent in telepathology.

Images can be captured from biological specimens, or they can be recorded as video by robotic systems (and possibly sent in real time): in the latter case, connections must be higher performance and have a sufficiently high speed if the teleconsultation is of an urgent nature. In some situations, given the possibility of losing information by sending still images, hybrid image acquisition systems can be used.

Thus, we have a static-type telepathology that uses the store-and-forward method that allows the remote specialist to see images on the screen when he or she has time availability and a second dynamic-type telepathology that works in real time but requires a large amount of memory, whereas a static image requires less [2].

In its dynamic configuration, although costs are higher than in the static configuration, images are transmitted in real time to the remote specialist, who observes them through a monitor; in this way, the microscope's movements, which can be coordinated using the phone even in its WhatsApp configuration (the signal travels through the Web, and the voice connection is probably more secure), can highlight details of diagnostic interest, such as illumination, zoom, and focus.

Clearly, the quality of transmitted images depends on the bandwidth, processor, and RAM of computers and the quality and capacity of the camera used to capture the static and moving images. The most important functions associated with the operation of the camera will eventually have to be remotely controllable by the pathologist, starting with graphic resolution in pixels and ending with magnification.

In some cases, the transmission of microscope images can be entrusted to a high-performance smartphone, since the necessary, and not only desired, result is for the quality of the original image to be equal to the quality of the received image of the remote pathologist [1–3].

15.3 Teleginecology

In the practice of gynecology, there are situations in which a visit can be made only in presence, as in the case of infection, pregnancy, ultrasound examinations, performance of diagnostic tests, or other types of assessment such as verification of violence. In all other cases, gynecology can take advantage of the availability of technologies that allow tele-medical examination.

Gynecological remote medical examination is able to deliver medical care to patients who cannot or do not wish (for confidentiality or other reasons) to have an in-person medical examination. Remote examination takes place via video and can be either a one-on-one doctor-patient interview or a possible teleconsultation, such as in cases where the patient can manage the health or even psychological problem that arises and—as mentioned above—immediate use of diagnostic techniques to be performed on an outpatient basis is not required. This is the case, for example, of gestational diabetes and gestational hypertension.

Thus, it may be a request for clarification about taking a medication or problems in interpreting a self-administered pregnancy test or for simple monitoring of the patient's or woman's condition (since she does not necessarily have to be sick), who can then undergo a routine examination without traveling to the clinic. In addition, the remote medical examination may include follow-up postoperatively or following the initiation of new treatment [1, 2]. Remote examination may also be done for counseling on contraceptive use or placement of intrauterine devices, if this request does not require the patient's presence, or may be indicated for information on menopause management or physical activity to go along with menopause itself.

Remote medical examination helps understand the patient's real problems and is therefore a method to define which patient will actually need to come to the clinic to solve her problems.

Otherwise, remote examination can be used in all conditions where the patient needs to talk to the doctor, such as in interpreting the results of an examination or laboratory test or when counseling on sexually transmitted infectious diseases is desired.

15.4   Teledermatology

In essence, teledermatology applies to remote diagnosis, in which a camera operated by a physician transmits images or films to a dermatology specialist located at a remote site. Since diagnosis is made through images, a telephone-only consultation makes little sense, so data transfer must take place via a fixed or portable camera.

The camera can be equipped with a single chip to handle three basic colors, or it can have three chips in which one chip handles red, one handles green, and one handles blue: obviously, the camera with three chips is more efficient in color management and is largely preferable to the one with a single chip. With a camera, which can be placed directly on the skin and has its own light source, scans can be made of the affected area, with enlargements on areas to be explored (moles, eruptions, skin infections, or other types of lesion or wound), allowing a detailed view of what is happening; any light reflections can be eliminated by using polarized lenses.

Other types of cameras are available, which instead are capable of performing guided movements in three dimensions, allowing the operator maneuvering it to take images and video footage from multiple angles, which enables them to provide more useful information for diagnosis while minimizing the possible effects of ambient light. Cameras, if equipped with a good resolving power, are able to go so far as to visualize the stratum corneum [1, 2].

Teledermatology can be done in real time, i.e., live, with the remote dermatologist assisting in the acquisition of images and video footage, and can then guide those who capture and transmit the images, asking them to focus their search on a given part of the field or for specific enlargements of certain details, so as to contribute quickly to making the teleconsultation more effective.

In other situations, teledermatology consultation can be done by recording footage and images and sending them to a server where they will be stored for retrieval and viewing by the dermatologist at a later time. While this situation has some possible advantages (e.g., the presence of the dermatologist is not required simultaneously with the acquisition of the images), it can make diagnosis more difficult because the dermatologist has not been able to make any live observations and inquiries to the remote operator, so the collection of information may be incomplete. In order to avoid this particular potentially negative situation, very tight procedures need to be put in place that define the shots, the type of zoom needed, and camera movements depending on the thing to be examined: for example, for a mole, it could be the smooth or jagged edges, the presence of small reliefs within their outer surface, the presence of hairs, the hue of the color, and more.

The software that operates a camera has a very sensitive impact on the result: it must have a very-good-quality freeze frame system, it must be able to filter out ambient light (which must itself be adjusted so that it does not overlap with reflections with that of the images transmitted by the instrument), it must be able to capture images and footage without flickering or blurring, and it must be able to transmit still or moving images to the remote monitor with high fidelity in color and pixel resolution. Only in this way will it be possible for the dermatologist in the remote station to make a reliable and correct diagnosis. The importance of dermatology teleconsultation is very high in the analysis of wounds, to assess their severity and the possibility of infection and to prescribe the most appropriate treatment with antibiotics and drugs that speed or facilitate wound closure and healing.

15.5   Telepediatrics

Standards of care and healthcare for pediatric patients are listed in Article 24 of the "Convention on the Rights of the Child[1]," which was adopted by the United Nations General Assembly on November 20, 1989.

It may be worth quoting part of the article because telepediatrics (as well as traditional pediatrics) must adapt to it. Paragraphs 1 and 2 of the text of Article 24 say verbatim.

> 1. States Parties recognize the right of the child to the enjoyment of the highest attainable standard of health and to facilities for the treatment of illness and rehabilitation of health. States Parties shall strive to ensure that no child is deprived of his or her right of access to such health care services.
> 2. States Parties shall pursue full implementation of this right and, in particular, shall take appropriate measures:
>
> (a) To diminish infant and child mortality;
> (b) To ensure the provision of necessary medical assistance and health care to all children with emphasis on the development of primary health care;
> (c) To combat disease and malnutrition, including within the framework of primary health care, through, inter alia, the application of readily available technology and through the provision of adequate nutritious foods and clean drinking-water, taking into consideration the dangers and risks of environmental pollution;
> (d) To ensure appropriate pre-natal and post-natal health care for mothers;
> (e) To ensure that all segments of society, in particular parents and children, are informed, have access to education and are supported in the use of basic knowledge of child health and nutrition, the advantages of breastfeeding, hygiene and environmental sanitation and the prevention of accidents;
> (f) To develop preventive health care, guidance for parents and family planning education and services.

Premised on the fact that pediatric patients are not small adult patients but rather subjects with specific needs in multiple areas (think, e.g., of nutritional aspects and needs), it must be realized that these specific needs unravel and change throughout the developmental age, from birth to 2 years; then in the second phase, from 2 to 6 years; and then in the third phase, from 6 to about 15 years (or also 18 years), each characterized by its own health needs and specific types of illness. Within the time

---

[1] See https://www.unicef.org/media/52626/file.

spectrum of continuous evolution (continuous, i.e., not in jumps, not in rushes) and characterized by a strong individual imprint (individual, i.e., not all individuals have identical dynamics, even in the same family setting), from infant to child to adult, are included multiple dynamics involving the affective sphere, the cognitive sphere, the psychological sphere, the character sphere, and many other individual and group dynamics.

These "nonphysical" dynamics are juxtaposed with actual physical growth, increased muscle mass, bone growth, and growth in height and weight, with associated changes in metabolism (production of hormones, accentuations of gender differences, and so on) and behavior.

For all these reasons, we can certainly say that the needs of the pediatric subject and those of the adult subject are different, particularly because multidimensional developmental trajectories give the pediatric patient a rapidly changing set of characteristics.

Therefore, traditional and telematic care must also be ready to recognize stages of change and react quickly to the changing conditions not only of health but also of the pediatric subject's whole body and mind.

In general, a telemedicine project designed for adults does not apply to pediatric patients, who also have profoundly different needs. The same is true for the pediatrician who has methods of care that do not always overlap with those of a family physician: moreover, the pediatrician interfaces not only with the little patient but also with his or her family, which interposes itself as a buffer, starting with in-person visits (which a parent always attends) and ending with any televisits in which it is very easy for parents' presence to be necessary for possible interpretation of questions and answers and to put the little one at ease.

Basically, provided that communication in medicine must be justified by an informed consent that the minor's parents will sign (and assuming that all possible privacy issues have been resolved), if a telepediatrics service is to be implemented, certain design arrangements are necessary, starting with the way of interfacing and communicating, which must be congruent with the age of the child or young person, because it is unthinkable that a 7-year-old child will have the same maturity and experience as a 14-year-old boy or girl. If communicating via a computer or tablet, a display with colorful drawings of animals or things will be more effective for a child, while for a young person, one will have to opt for a display with different images, perhaps with animations.

Obviously, the language and paraphrases used for communication will also have a different standard: the goal is to make oneself understood, and so communication strategies will adapt to these needs, just as remote communication tools will use technological devices adapted to the various ages of the patient. Age definitely comes into play when the interaction is based on a question-and-answer sequence, to gather information: the adaptability of the response to the question depends on cultural factors acquired with education and age, so the level of the conversation will have to be adapted to the knowledge and character of the young patient, making sure that the child does not feel looked down upon or questioned or judged for what he or she will say during the remote interview.

Given the special condition of pediatric patients and their variability, there are situations that generally advise against the use of telemedicine. Obviously, the starting context is the bottom-up approach, so if the patient or family does not have adequate connection capabilities (hardware and software), the approach with telemedicine is not possible unless the caregiver is able to make such connection options available.

A possible obstacle to overcome is the family's willingness to accept a telemedicine service for their child: it could be the case of a child not expressing satisfaction, or drawing improvements, that could make the parents reconsider and convince them to desist and turn again to traditional pediatrics.

Given the necessary participation of a family member or guardian, the use of medicine may be excluded where there are histories of family conflict or histories of exploitation or violence or abuse or even situations of social isolation and marginalization.

Telemedicine methods should also be limited when an adverse development can be predicted that might make a condition at the time of non-urgency urgent or when a cognitive or sensory deficit (blindness, deafness) is such that it would impair successful remote communication, unless additional services are guaranteed to supplement.

To summarize, it is necessary to have a computer or tablet connected to the Internet and equipped with antivirus and protection systems capable of ensuring privacy and preventing data theft during communication.

To ensure communication, the computer (or tablet or smartphone) must be equipped with a built-in or external connectable camera and must have adequate RAM memory to handle telecommunication applications, for which a minimal but adequate computer training is also necessary.

Last, but not the least, there needs to be a parent or guardian's signature of informed consent.

15.6 Telenephrology

Telenephrology is the remote delivery (when possible) of nephrology healthcare services, combining advances in engineering technologies with those in clinical nephrology.

Telenephrology is growing substantially as the demand for this type of care is related not only to problems of renal origin but also to problems derived from chronic diseases such as diabetes (diabetic nephropathy). The field of telenephrology is expanding because wherever possible, there is a need to opt for options that provide rapid access to health information and treatment of diseases associated with kidney function.

Telenephrology has some important advantages over classical nephrology, which we could summarize in discussions below.

Improving access to care for patients in rural or geographically distant areas and availability of care for the elderly, frail, or disabled is an advantage inherent in the very idea of telemedicine and therefore does not apply only to telenephrology.

These are coupled with the possibility of organizing nephrology consultations for family physicians; again for physicians but also for caregivers and patients, of receiving video educational information about nephrology therapy (standard or home); self-management of home dialysis by the patient, a simpler and faster management of the transplant patient when sent home; and if the patient is young, for him to receive information and assistance through apps that can be downloaded in the smartphone.

This will be a gap that needs to be overcome quickly, because while it is true that the nephrologist with these remote technologies can treat patients even thousands of kilometers away, scientific demonstration that at least shows equivalence of clinical outcomes for the same disease, stratifying by patient age, and also demonstrating that the cost of treatment is reduced is needed, so that hospitals and nephrology physicians will be convinced to align with telenephrology techniques.

Alongside these possible advantages, however, some potential disadvantages should also be considered. First, the doctor-patient relationship at a distance may be considered worse than the traditional one in presence even if only because of a sense of habit and fear of novelty; on the other hand, a telenephrology approach does not even allow the doctor to perform a complete examination. Finally, the more communication-related part, which is done through apps whose functionality is not fully known, may reduce the quality of service. Added to this are the obvious problems associated with telemedicine in general, namely, the need for the patient to have appropriate hardware and software communication systems and to have the necessary knowledge to use them.

On the other hand, the ability to use new technologies and the confidence with them and hardware and software supports are intuitively inversely proportional to age, so in a few years' time, those who are young today will constitute a generation of older people now adapted to the new availability of technology, which will also have made great strides as time goes on.

With this in mind, it is possible, as well as desirable, that horizons of telenephrology, and telemedicine in general, will grow wider and wider. Smartphone apps make it possible to assist physician and patient for medication and diet management, while wearable or implantable sensors, or smartwatches or even apps, can be used to monitor physiological variables (heart rate, blood glucose, blood pressure, and so on), which, when translated into time-dependent graphs (continuous or discrete), make it very easy to dynamically display parameters kept under observation and share them with the remote nephrologist and the attending physician.

15.7 Teleoncology

Surgical therapies of solid tumors have aimed at total eradication of the tumor using demolitive surgery, with the aim of removing as much of the tumor tissue as possible, but also adjacent topographical areas, so as to minimize the risk of invasion. Chemotherapy, radiotherapy, and hormone therapy have been introduced as an alternative choice to obviate the high likelihood of recurrence among operated patients, succeeding in part to reduce mortality or prolong life expectancy in some cancers.

Today, cancer therapy is based on three fundamentals therapies, medical oncology (drug therapies), surgical oncology (surgical therapies), and radiation therapy (radiation therapy), which in many cases complement each other and alternate so as to optimize outcomes as may be deemed useful by the multidisciplinary clinical staff. This method of encircling the tumor with multidimensional therapy and exchanging views among the clinicians involved is a way of operating that will most likely be the winning method.

In January 2020, WHO officially defined COVID infection a pandemic: this implied a series of limits on the free movement of people to stop the transmission of the infection (whether these limits on free movement were actually effective would be up for debate). What is important, however, is that the movement of patients became a very serious logistical problem: COVID patients were treated mainly in the hospital, and almost only emergency operations were performed. The chronically ill, and especially cancer patients, suffered the most, who were already immunodeficient from treatment, so COVID infection was a risk to be avoided at all costs. The diversion of resources to countering the pandemic thus posed a real risk of lowering the focus on the needs of patients with chronic and degenerative diseases and cancer patients. Treatment of the latter has taken place under risky conditions due to the potential transmissibility of infection.

Priorities for ancology are the cure and the increase of survival with a good quality of life for patients. Basically, in the first row for surgical emergencies were those patients who would be at risk of dying if the surgery was not performed within the immediately following hours; in the second category of urgency were those patients who would be at risk of dying if the surgery was not performed within the immediately following days; and the third priority level was assigned to patients who would be at risk of dying if the surgery was not performed within three months. These provisions were flanked by provisions for staffing and rotation and for disinfection.

Despite the existence of several guidelines for the cancer patient and his or her treatment, problems related to physical isolation, as well as social isolation, such as stigma for the sick patient who also needs psychological support, not only pharmacological or surgical support, are still not solved, since it is certainly possible for the cancer patient to suffer from depression or anxiety, which is multiplied when there is a lack of physical or at least visual contact with attending doctors and nurses. This problem also has obvious repercussions for treatment: if the patient is not followed regularly, there is a lack of confidence in his or her adherence to treatment.

Telemedicine, in these situations, intervenes by facilitating communication so that the patient feels that he or she is being followed, that he or she feels that he or she is the center of attention, and that he or she feels supported by those who are taking care of him or her, so that a word of comfort and help is never missing. Teleoncology therefore assumes a therapeutic dignity equal to that of radiation therapy, medical oncology, and surgical oncology.

Today, if a cancer patient is not suspected to be carrying a viral infection or to have a para-influenza syndrome, he or she can undergo preliminary evaluation before being admitted to the hospital for surgery, chemotherapy, or radiation therapy, while teleoncology can certainly take care of patients undergoing normal follow-up that does not require other investigations or other tests, such as X-rays or blood draws.

As one might guess, teleoncology is very useful in triaging patients to decide how many are or are not suitable for this remote approach. We also need to leverage the psychological profile of patients, as some may benefit from feeling in their own environment, while others may feel more comfortable if they are together with other patients to share their experiences and hopes. Teleoncology is a useful method of prioritization for the patient whose condition requires immediate treatment but who is unable to travel to or stay at the cancer center. Teleoncology consultation can be useful in trying to establish an interim alternative treatment, such as metronomic oral chemotherapy, where possible.

Metronomic therapy (as one might guess, the terminology is derived from the word "metronome") is a method of treatment based on the administration of low-dose chemotherapy, which is taken consistently at short, regular intervals (every day or every few days): of course, it may not necessarily be suitable for all cancers and for all types of patients. The advantage in logistical terms is that metronomic chemotherapy can be managed with the patient at home, while the other advantages lie in a less aggressive treatment than traditional chemotherapy, which is given at high dosages at distant periods. This could mean an improved quality of life, reduction of side effects, reduction of neoformation of tumor-feeding vessels, and reduction of drug resistance of cancer cells.

Prescribing drugs in teleoncology is suitable for all patients who do not have the ability to move or when it is not absolutely necessary for them to do so. Thus, travel in these types of patients becomes necessary only for withdrawals, tests, chemo and radiation therapies, and maneuvers such as insertion of a nasogastric tube, making sure that hospital visits are organized to group non-home activities as much as possible.

Remote communication systems can also be used for normal information exchange, whereas they are probably not the best method for communicating bad news, which should always be made known in a way that preserves privacy and respect for the person. Instead, bad news should be communicated in person, creating the appropriate conditions for communication to be as fair as possible, never, therefore, in the presence of other people, particularly strangers, and never in a depersonalized and aseptic manner, as telematic communication might become or appear to become so. In fact, it seems almost normal that the empathy that should involve the healthcare personnel caring for the patient cannot be easily conveyed through a telematic medium and that person-to-person contact is therefore preferable, with the opportunity to look each other in the eye and concretely express one's participation in the discomfort of those who hear this bad news. However, it is also necessary to communicate hope in cures, even when the situation is difficult, so one may very well express this with phrases such as, "You have cancer in an advanced state, but we will strive to do everything possible and even the impossible to be able to cure you, and to a large extent, the possibility of cure will also depend on you, your strength and courage in facing this disease."

When tumors are in the lungs, head and neck, and breast (both hormone receptor positive and hormone receptor negative), frequent examinations are necessary and should be done at the referring cancer centers. Note that when a breast carcinoma is hormone positive, hormone-based therapy can be used as adjuvant therapy, whereas if the breast carcinoma is hormone negative, OS chemotherapies can be used.

For these tumor types, a transition to teleoncology, using oral drug treatments, is possible in some circumstances [1–3].

For cancer patients, a type of treatment of a multimodal nature is becoming available as a consequence of the effects of the pandemic; through teleoncology, a type of treatment has in fact become available that allows for a remote approach that can be integrated with classic hospital-based oncology and that goes in the direction of optimizing the overall yield of therapy and resource management. This has directed the attitude of general healthcare toward an acceptance of teleoncology practices, which were initially frowned upon. It is now up to the wisdom of health policy measures to make sure that teleoncology is allowed to expand its modes of operation and use.

15.8 Telepsychiatry

To have a psychiatrist at hand is not very simple: most patients cannot have psychiatric help for their mental health problems, and moreover, to go to a psychiatrist can be considered as a luxury medical opportunity for some rare patients. Indeed, some psychiatric diseases are common and may arise from various situation, like depression, bipolar disorders, or attention disorders; again, psychiatric problems may also depend on drug or alcohol addiction, so we are dealing with health problems that are increasing also in the young. Therefore, the demand for psychiatric assistance is also increasing.

The possibility to deliver mental care using telemedicine is now a concrete reality, and the recent pandemic was one of the cause (not the only cause) of telepsychiatry development. Telepsychiatry allows a less formal approach between doctors and patients, which possibly can also make patients feel more comfortable and relaxed at their homes, facilitating comprehension and confidence. As other telemedicine disciplines, telepsychiatry means saving time and saving money for the same reasons we have discussed in preceding sections of this book.

At the moment, telepsychiatry is at an evolutive stage: its future will involve chatbots for requests of information, as well as artificial intelligence and machine learning, but the doctor cannot be excluded; despite possible therapeutic innovations, like virtual reality, some diseases in this field may be dangerous not only for patients but also for other people, including relatives.

One must bear in mind that telepsychiatry is not an alternative to regular psychiatry that is done in the clinic, which may be the preferable approach, like in subjects with strong social anxiety, which could be better resolved by group therapy. Moreover, the psychiatrist would have to look at the nonverbal language of his or her patient, which could be very difficult during a remote visit.

15.9   Teleophthalmology

Image transmission is in essence what characterizes teleophthalmology. Diagnosis, as is the case in dermatology, has as its basis the visualization of anatomical structures of the eye, which may also be small and therefore require detection aided by appropriate magnification. In general, three types of detection are important for the ophthalmologist, involving the anterior chamber (between the cornea and the pupil) and the posterior chamber, which is located in the space that is confined between the iris and the suspensory ligament of the lens (so, it is part of the anterior segment of the eye and not the posterior segment as the name might suggest); the posterior chamber is devoted to the circulation of the aqueous humor, which is produced in the epithelium of the ciliary body, passes into the posterior chamber, and from there, flowing through the pupil, reaches the anterior chamber. Ophthalmologists are of course interested in the outer part of eyes (eyelids, sclera, iris, tear ducts, and so on).

Ophthalmoscopes are used for imaging, and a series of lenses are used to focus on the affected area. Ophthalmologists obtain information about the eye from the images, so if their physical presence next to the patient is not possible, they will have to use remotely transmitted data from an operator.

The posterior chamber is observed with a fundus camera that records and transmits fixed digital images, while video recording and transmissions are generally done by the camera installed on the slit lamp.

As with other telemedicine disciplines, data transmission can be done by a technician ophthalmologist or by a family doctor, who can take advantage of teleconsultation by a trained ophthalmologist who can make diagnoses and prescriptions remotely.

Teleophthalmology uses the store-and-forward method extensively, as still images seem to be much better than moving images that can be transmitted in real time; hence, the mode of sending images to a server is used, so that they are available at the time or at a later time for diagnosis by the ophthalmologist, who can visualize images on a monitor, although in this case the remote specialist is not able to ask for specific shots from the remote operator. Retinal images also appear to be of better quality as obtained with fundus cameras that have higher resolution than the slit lamp and whose contrast and brightness characteristics can be managed. Teleophthalmology is a very practical system for monitoring the progress of diabetic retinopathy, as digital images of the retina are essential for keeping track of one of the most damaging manifestations procured by diabetes. These images can be collected using a non-mydriatic camera. Teleophthalmology is also used to screen diabetic individuals to diagnose the onset of retinopathy, as well as the onset a progression of glaucoma.

Mobile cameras are available that work even in bright light and can be interfaced (directly or via Wi-Fi) with laptops equipped with software that can handle capturing and sending images in high-resolution (on the order of megapixels) compressed, JPEG, or MPEG format that will be associated with patient data.

Images can be shared during teleconsultation, where the specialist can enlarge or manipulate them, adding text or drawings (arrows, or other), which will aid in the understanding of all co-involved healthcare personnel, who can then also use teleconsultation for educational purposes. It is, of course, necessary for the ophthalmic technician to be very knowledgeable and familiar with how to use the camera (the eye is small compared to some other organs) and the transmission system because the collection of images is not a simple operation but, indeed, is quite challenging.

References

1. Gogia SB, Ed. Fundamentals of telemedicine and telehealthh. New York: Academic Press; 2019.
2. Kandpur RS. Telemedicine: technology and applications. New Dehli: PHI Learning; 2017.
3. Sorkin C. Field guide to telehealth and telemedicine. New York: Springer Publishing; 2021.

Telesurgery

16

Telesurgery is based on the robot-assisted surgery and is the result of biomedical engineering and applied mathematics research. To be precise, robot-assisted surgery is a discipline that aims to design and develop automata that enable remote surgical operations, that is, to create automata capable of being maneuvered at a distance, even thousands of kilometers, by a human surgeon.

To begin talking about telesurgery, it is necessary to analyze the various forms through which it can be accomplished: the first of these is remote assistance (e.g., by videoconferencing), where an experienced surgeon is able to assist colleagues who have to operate despite having little specific experience, perhaps because they are constrained by conditions of extreme urgency (floods, earthquakes, rescue of non-transportable wounded patients, etc.) or because of great distance from a surgical center of reference that cannot be covered in a short time, due to the lack of a helicopter or weather conditions that prevent its use.

The activity could take the form in a kind of active live monitoring and mentoring while the operation is in progress, or alternatively, an actual supervisory process could be identified, in which an experienced surgeon is virtually present in the operating room and watches the operation being conducted by the surgeon from whom the supervisor can ask for any clarifications on maneuvers and techniques he or she is using.

Of course, the situation can occur in a mirror-image fashion, in that a newly trained surgeon will be able to watch the operation live from a remote location and will thus be able to increase his or her training by observing live the maneuvers of a more experienced surgeon and possibly asking him or her questions; this type of remote communication is also very useful when a new instrument is introduced or a new device for performing and monitoring a surgical operation.

There are several billion persons in the world who are unable to access adequate health services, either because they live in poverty or because they live in areas far away from large cities with adequate hospitals. This is only a first factor that describes the asymmetry of health services and the demand for care; in fact, the

© The Author(s), under exclusive license to Springer Nature Switzerland AG 2025   201
M. Nichelatti, *Mathematical Tools for Telemedicine*, TELe-Health,
https://doi.org/10.1007/978-3-031-81709-0_16

second factor is the availability of surgeons who can do the job with the appropriate expertise [1, 2].

Obviously, a hospital in a large city cannot always calibrate the number of its staff on the basis of the vastness of the area in which the hospital serves as a referral, but in these situations, surgical tele-mentoring activities can be of fundamental help. Tele-mentoring enables an experienced surgeon to provide active assistance via a video link, guiding execution of appropriate surgical techniques by a novice surgeon where he or she is to operate under emergency conditions as well as under normal conditions. It is obviously desirable that mentoring can take place through audio and video communication, since audio-only communication (via radio or telephone) could not give the inexperienced clinician the ability to effectively show the patient's situation nor enable the mentor to deliver information clearly and consistently [1].

Therefore, visual information sharing appears indispensable for mentoring to be as effective as it should be; in this case, mentoring will be coupled with an increase in safety (due to the guidance of the experienced surgeon), reduction in cost and time (there is no need for the costly physical displacement and loss of time needed to transfer the experienced surgeon or the patient), and training efficiency that shows no difference with the training of the young surgeon in the presence.

Thus, tele-mentoring went on to develop further, dealing with increasingly complex surgeries at greater and greater distances (e.g., between the USA and Europe), for example, remote guidance of laparoscopic nephrectomies and remote control of robotic arms during surgeries to control cutting, hemostasis, and cautery. Parallel development to tele-mentoring has taken place in actual telesurgery, in which the surgeon remotely intervenes directly on the patient, either with biopsies or with actual surgeries (in which real robots such as Da Vinci and Zeus are used), as occurred during a laparoscopic cholecystectomy performed via Zeus robots with the patient in France and the surgeon in New York.

Telesurgery, which has now become reliable enough to rely completely on the technology that supports it, is capable of enabling interventions in areas of oncology, neurology, cardiovascular (remote interventions such as those for coronary stents and aneurysms are now almost routine), and so many other areas of specialization, including that of refractive surgery (which, despite the delicacy of this type of surgery, is based on the use of very advanced laser systems guided remotely by specialists via 5G high-speed connections), having provided, in practice, multiple proofs of efficiency.

16.1   Telesurgery with 5G and 6G Technologies

Telesurgery using 5G enables its application in a variety of areas, including those where short latency time is required and those that required the physical presence and availability of access by personnel with the necessary specialized skills. As we have already seen with telemedicine in general, this new openness of horizon will also enable less experienced surgeons to view and assist in surgeries and learn operating techniques remotely, improving their experience and preparedness.

Improved accessibility to care through these communication systems will make it possible to enhance prognosis of the very many patients unable to have surgery due to factors related to geographic isolation and endemic poverty of certain territories. Of course, it remains essential to perform the necessary clinical, nursing, and care follow-up with remote surgery. But time and cost savings will be two of the additional drivers that will allow for an increasing diffusion of these techniques [1].

As in all things, however, there is a downside, because it is necessary for the same technology to be available in the remote hospital where the patient is physically located, so the success of telesurgery depends on widespread deployment of communication technologies: it is futile to think of using 5G technology to operate remotely if only 2G transmission technology is available in the area where the patient is to be operated on or if 5G connection is unstable due to power supply problems in the electrical grid. In addition, especially at these levels, data protection and shielding of transmission and receiving systems are essential.

It should also be considered that surgical robots are operated by surgeons by means of a remote controller and therefore are not capable of operating on their own (although it is possible that, thanks to artificial intelligence, this truly revolutionary option in the now-distant future may become a reality); the surgeon's gestures are projected and switched through mathematical models into movements of the remote robotic arms, which will thus be able to intervene with very high precision on the patient, always under close visual control (thanks to the endoscope mounted on another surgical arm) of the person performing the surgery.

It is expected that the upcoming availability of the 6G system could significantly improve the already-good latency time and connection stability observed with the current 5G and, most importantly, the improved view of the surgical field in three dimensions, to optimize surgeon's remote viewing. However, 6G technology will unveil its full potential not only for surgery but also for equity in distributing opportunity to everyone to take advantage of this expected improvement.

16.2 Surgical Robots

The word *robot* was first used by Czech dramatist Karel Čapek (1880–1938), who included it in the title of his 1920 play, *Rossumovi Univerzální Roboti* (in English, *Rossum's Universal Robots*[1]). Initially, in the first draft of the drama, Čapek used the term *labori*, derived from Latin labor, but convinced that the word might be too abstruse, he changed it to adopt the term *roboti*, derived from the Slavic word, *robota*, meaning "drudgery" or "forced labor," which originated from medieval terminology defining "serfdom," when house and land rents were paid with the peasants' own labor.

The evolution of surgical techniques began when the need was felt to make operations less risky from the point of view of postoperative management, where

---

[1] See https://en.wikisource.org/wiki/R._U._R._(Rossum%27s_Universal_Robots).

surgical site infections, bleeding, and suture reopening often occurred. Therefore, efforts were made to circumscribe the risk by aiming for less invasive techniques, from which minimally invasive and microinvasive surgery would later emerge, and, if we want, we can say that robotic surgery is the natural technological evolution of laparoscopic surgery.

A surgical robot consists of three parts: a console, a vision cart, and a patient cart [2].

- The control center of the entire robot is the console: it has an ergonomic seat on which the surgeon lays down and a screen for three-dimensional, high-definition viewing.
- The vision cart is the part of the surgical robot where the image processing unit is located, inside which other instrument adjustment systems are also housed.
- The patient cart is a sturdy metal arm, called a boom[2] (like the one on sailboats where the mainsail is connected), where arms branch off onto which cameras and instruments that will be used in the surgery are mounted.

Robotic surgery can be used in thoracic, gynecologic, urologic, andrologic, and pediatric surgeries: it can also be used when trans-oral approaches are used, that is, when the organ to be operated on is reached by passing through the oral cavity.

Robotic surgery is used in the minimally invasive thoracic field for operations involving the lungs and mediastinum (resections) and the esophagus. It is, however, more expensive than video-assisted chest surgery techniques. Minimally invasive robotic surgery adopted in gynecology allows for use in the treatment of fibroids, ovarian tumors, prolapses of the uterus, and other conditions such as endometriosis; it can also be used in hysterectomies and for biopsy retrievals. Use in andrology and urology has seen results in both radical prostatectomy and cystectomy. In the pediatric field, one of the limitations of conventional surgery is the field of view limited by the small size of the abdominal cavity, so some urologic surgeries (nephrectomy, heminephrectomy, pyeloplasty, ureteroureterostomy, etc.) are best conducted in the presence of a surgical robot.

Other areas of use for robotic surgery include kidney transplantation, which is facilitated in obese patients, and abdominal surgery in general. One of the best results is achieved in hernia surgery, where laparoscopic surgery is outperformed particularly with large hernias, allowing reduction of hospital stay and postoperative pain.

The robot is guided by the surgeon, who makes its arms move, on which instruments that will be used during the surgery are mounted. It is not the robot that decides what to do and how to do it. The robot is an extremely advanced interface between surgeon and patient, but it cannot take initiative—it must merely obey the surgeon's commands. Movement of the arms would be impossible even if it occurred completely causally: there are constant controls that prevent even the

---

[2] From the Dutch word "boom" that means "rod".

smallest movement that is not guided by the surgeon. The surgeon stands at the control console with a three-dimensional view of the surgical field (processed by the computer) and uses knobs located under the screen and from the foot pedals at the base of it.

Knobs are used to control instruments and the endoscope, by means of finger and hand movements, which are transformed exactly into movements of arms and surgical instruments attached to them.

Pedals, on the other hand, are connected to instruments involved in the performance of auxiliary complementary maneuvers, such as cautery. There are advantages that arise immediately, as early as the surgery is performed, because robotic surgery eliminates involuntary physiological movements of the surgeon's hand, which are, so to speak, absorbed and buffered by the arms. This is also partly due to the increased comfort of the surgeon, who is in an optimal static position.

This results in increased precision of movements, which are no longer perturbed by small tremors of the hand and thus also in increased speed of performing the surgery, to which high-definition field of view of the display also contributes.

Robotic surgery, where it can be applied, shows several advantages over traditional surgery. In general, by using robotic surgery methods, there is less traumatic impact on internal organs, less persistence of postoperative pain, and a faster follow-up.

There are also disadvantages: the first is the cost of the robot itself and the cost of consumables; the second is the cost to be reserved for training the surgeons and staff. Indeed, one of the goals of telesurgery is the reduction of cost of any single operation.

16.3   Problems with Telesurgery

As can be guessed, the major impediment standing between telesurgery and its future developments lies in the possible technological gaps between the transmitting and receiving stations. Relying on a fast, broadband, and stable connection is essential, as moving images must be transmitted and received and control signals for the robotic arms must be transmitted and received.

In fact, it is necessary that the control of the robotic arms be kept constant by minimizing the latency time between order and execution of the maneuver, and it is also equally important that the control panel be equipped with all the hardware and software updates that allow both to follow the evolution of technology and to improve the translation of the gestures of the surgeon operating remotely.

Reviewing the various information on the possible pros and possible cons of telesurgery, there is an undoubted potential and actual advantage in favor of the widespread use of this technique, which is much less impactful to the patient than in-person surgery. The patient would have no reason to travel to centers of excellence, saving money and time while remaining in his or her local area, in a much more amenable situation. For hospitals of excellence, the reduced influx of patients from remote areas can reduce clogs to the surgical management system by reducing care load requirements.

Projecting these significant benefits to a non-locoregional but rather a global scope, what we have already seen with telemedicine emerges about the possibility of intervening in situations related to territories affected by cataclysms such as earthquakes and floods but also in other situations related to war scenarios or even in cases of surgical problems arising in extreme areas, such as polar scientific bases, oil platforms, or more simply transport ships (oil tankers and others) that cross far from ports. Going even further, telesurgery is expected to become in common use at space stations orbiting Earth and at futuristic lunar space bases.

Obviously, increased human ambitions will drive subsequent developments in telesurgery.

References

1. Costello T. Principles and practice of robotic surgery. Amsterdam: Elsevier; 2023.
2. Giulianotti PC, Benedetti E, Mangano A, (eds.) The foundation and art of robotic surgery. New York: McGraw-Hill; 2024.

Part III

Math Insights

Calculus in One and More Variables

17

This chapter will discuss about differential and integral calculus. Calculus is a tool, possibly the first tool one has to deal with when approaching mathematics. Calculus involves a very wide list of techniques ranging from the set theory to the definition of derivatives and integrals: interconnected topics that need to be understood by a vast audience of researchers with very different educational experiences. However, calculus can be presented as a smooth technique that can be learned by any doctor or biologist.

Given a set $\mathbb{A}$, we say that a is, or is not, an element of $\mathbb{A}$ by writing $a \in \mathbb{A}$ and $a \notin \mathbb{A}$, respectively. If $\mathbb{A}$ is a subset of another set $\mathbb{B}$, we write $\mathbb{A} \subset \mathbb{B}$ to say that any element of $\mathbb{A}$ is also an element of $\mathbb{B}$, but some elements of $\mathbb{B}$ are not elements of $\mathbb{A}$. We should already know the set $\mathbb{N}$ of natural numbers, the set $\mathbb{Z}$ of integer numbers, the set $\mathbb{Q}$ of rational numbers, the set $\mathbb{R}$ of real numbers, and the set $\mathbb{C}$ of complex numbers,[1] where we have $\mathbb{N} \subset \mathbb{Z} \subset \mathbb{Q} \subset \mathbb{R} \subset \mathbb{C}$.

17.1 Functions of One Real Variable

A function f is a law $f : \mathbb{J} \to \mathbb{K}$ connecting two sets $\mathbb{J}$ and $\mathbb{K}$. In other words, the law $f : \mathbb{J} \to \mathbb{K}$ associates with an element $a \in \mathbb{J}$ a unique element $b \in \mathbb{K}$. More intuitively, a function f is a mathematical machine that allows to obtain a specific output from a given input x, chosen among the set containing all acceptable inputs for f (as we will see in the next sections, some functions may also accept a number n of simultaneous inputs $x_1, x_2, ..., x_n$). For example, if $f(x) = x + 1$, we define a function that, for any input x, returns the output $x + 1$, and if $x = 5$, then $f(x) = 6$. We therefore can say that f maps some elements in $\mathbb{J}$ to some elements in $\mathbb{K}$; thus,

---

[1] The term "complex numbers" is not very adequate to describe them: they should more properly be called "lateral numbers."

© The Author(s), under exclusive license to Springer Nature Switzerland AG 2025   209
M. Nichelatti, *Mathematical Tools for Telemedicine*, TELe-Health,
https://doi.org/10.1007/978-3-031-81709-0_17

we may also write $\mathbb{J} \xrightarrow{f} \mathbb{K}$; note that "to map" means "to assign" to a given value of $\mathbb{J}$ a specific value of $\mathbb{K}$; the mapping can be also a composed one, since we may have a situation like $\mathbb{J} \xrightarrow{f} \mathbb{K} \xrightarrow{g} \mathbb{L}$, which can be summarized as $\mathbb{J} \xrightarrow{g \circ f} \mathbb{L}$ or $\mathbb{J} \xrightarrow{g(f)} \mathbb{L}$ to specify that g is applied to the output of f. Thus, if $f(x) = x + 1$ and $g(x) = \frac{1}{3}x$, then $g \circ f(x) = g(f(x)) = \frac{1}{3}f(x)$, and if $x = 5$, then $f(x) = 6$ and $g \circ f(x) = g(f(x)) = \frac{6}{3} = 2$.

The set of all acceptable inputs of a function f is the *domain* of f, Dom(f), and the set containing all possible outputs of the function is the *codomain* (or the *arrival set*, or even the *target set*) Cdm(f), while the range of minimum to maximum values, which actually f may assume, is the *image* of the function Im(f). Note that codomain and image are two different things and that they do not need to define two equivalent sets. Indeed, it is always Im(f) $\subseteq$ Cdm(f); for example, taking $f(x) = x^2$, we have Dom(f) $= \mathbb{R}$, Cdm(f) $= \mathbb{R}$, and Im(f) $= [0, +\infty[$; taking $f(x) = \frac{1}{x+2}$, we have Dom(f) $= \{x \in \mathbb{R} : x \neq -2\}$ (we could also write Dom(f) $= \mathbb{R} \setminus \{-2\}$), Cdm($f$) $= \mathbb{R}$ and Im(f) $= \mathbb{R}$; taking $f(x) = \log(x)$, we have (for x real) Dom(f) $=]0, +\infty[$, Cdm(f) $= \mathbb{R}$, and Im(f) $= \mathbb{R}$; taking $f(x) = \sin(x)$, we have Dom(f) $= \mathbb{R}$, Cdm(f) $= \mathbb{R}$, and Im(f) $= [-1, 1]$. Here, a precisation is needed: we may define a closed interval $[a, b] \in R$ and an open interval $]a, b[\in R$; the difference between closed and open interval is that the closed one contains its endpoints, while the open one does not. In other words, in a closed interval, we have $a, b \in [a, b]$, while in an open interval, we have $a, b \notin]a, b[$. Intuitively, if the interval is defined with $]a, b]$, then $a \notin]a, b]$, and $b \in]a, b]$.

We say that f is *surjective* if any $b \in \mathbb{B}$ is the image of at least one $a \in \mathbb{A}$. We say that f is *injective* if $a_1 \neq a_2$ implies $f(a_1) \neq f(a_2)$. We say that f is *bijective* if f is both surjective and injective; if f is bijective, it is also invertible, e.g., there exists an inverse function $g(x) = f^{-1}(x)$, such that if $f(a)$ is the image of $a \in \mathbb{A}$, then $g(b) = f^{-1}(b)$ is the pre-image of $b \in \mathbb{B}$; moreover, it must be $f^{-1}(f(x)) = x$.

17.2 Limits

A function $f(x)$ defined over a domain Dom(f) is bounded if there is a finite number L such that $|f(x)| \leq L$ over all the domain: in particular, if $f(x) \leq A$, the function is *bounded above* with $A = \sup f(x)$, while if $f(x) \geq B$, the function is *bounded below* with $B = \inf f(x)$.

An *accumulation point* x_0 in a set $\mathbb{X}$ is a neighborhood of x_0 in which one finds at least one point $x_a \neq x_0$. And we may define a *neighborhood* of a point x_0 as an open set where one finds the same x_0 as well as some other points in any direction away from x_0. For example, a neighborhood of x_0 may be given as the open set $]x_0 - \varepsilon, x_0 + \varepsilon[$, ε being a small quantity (say, a small amount at will).

With these premises, we can define the limit of a function as the method to study the behavior of a function $f(x)$ in a neighborhood of a given point x_0 by writing

$$\lim_{x \to x_0} f(x) = \phi,$$ (17.1)

being ϕ a quantity depending on $f(x)$ and on the value of x_0. Note that we calculate the limit for x going to x_0, and not for $x = x_0$; hence, we say that $f(x)$ approaches ϕ as x approaches x_0 and also that $f(x)$ goes arbitrarily close to ϕ as x goes arbitrarily close to x_0 (again, "x going arbitrarily close to x_0" always implies $x \neq x_0$, and thus it does never mean $x = x_0$). Virtually, x_0 may be any point of the real axis: it just needs to be an accumulation point, and so we may take also the limits as x tends to plus or minus infinity.

For what is written above, there are four possible types of limits:

1. Finite limit when x goes to a finite value x_0

$$\lim_{x \to x_0} f(x) = L$$

for example,

$$\lim_{x \to 0} e^{-x^2} = 1;$$

2. Infinite limit when x goes to a finite value x_0

$$\lim_{x \to x_0} f(x) = \pm\infty$$

for example,

$$\lim_{x \to 0} \log(x) = -\infty;$$

3. Finite limit when x goes to an infinite value

$$\lim_{x \to \pm\infty} f(x) = L$$

for example,

$$\lim_{x \to +\infty} e^{-x} = 0;$$

4. Infinite limit when x goes to an infinite value

$$\lim_{x \to \pm\infty} f(x) = \pm\infty$$

for example,

$$\lim_{x \to -\infty} x^2 = +\infty.$$

A special caution must be observed when $\text{Dom}(f) =]x_1, x_2[$ if taking the limit to a boundary point x_1 or x_2; in particular, in these situations, the limit from left $\lim_{x \to x_1^-} f(x)$ and from right $\lim_{x \to x_2^+} f(x)$ should be invoked.

To better understand what the term indeterminate form means, let us focus on equality $\frac{0}{0} = x$: we easily infer that $0 = 0x$, which is true for any value of x, since $0 = 0 \times 1$ is true, but also $0 = 0 \times 2$ is true, and so on, hence any value of x satisfies the equality. Examples of other indeterminate forms are $(+\infty) \mp (\pm\infty)$; $(\pm\infty) \times 0$; $(\pm\infty)^0$; 0^0; $0^{\pm\infty}$; $\frac{\pm\infty}{\pm\infty}$; and $1^{\pm\infty}$. In the case of indeterminate form, the limit must be calculated using the *l'Hôpital rule*.

To explain the l'Hôpital rule , we say that it can be applied in cases

$$\lim_{x \to a} \frac{f(x)}{g(x)} = \frac{0}{0}; \quad \lim_{x \to a} \frac{f(x)}{g(x)} = \frac{\infty}{\infty},$$

assuming that some specific conditions are respected: then, if $f(x)$ and $g(x)$ are continuous and derivable in a neighborhood of a (with $a \in \mathbb{R}$ or $a = \pm\infty$), if $g(x) \neq 0$ in that neighborhood of a, and if the limit $\lim_{x \to a}(f'(x)/g'(x))$ exists, then the limit $\lim_{x \to a}(f(x)/g(x))$ must also exist.

If for a function f at a given point $x_0 \in \text{Dom}(f)$ we have

$$\lim_{x \to x_0^+} f(x) = \lim_{x \to x_0^-} f(x) = f(x_0),$$

then the function is said to be continuous in x_0, and if $f(x)$ is continuous at all the points of the interval $]x_1, x_2[\subseteq \text{Dom}(f)$, then $f(x)$ is said to be continuous over that interval.

A possible example of limit calculus with indeterminate form is

$$\lim_{x \to 2} \frac{x^3 - 2x^2 - x + 2}{x - 2} = \frac{0}{0}$$

where we see that

$$y(2) = \frac{8 - 8 - 2 + 2}{2 - 2};$$

however, if we factor the numerator, we also can see that

$$\frac{x^3 - 2x^2 - x + 2}{x - 2} = \frac{x^2(x - 2) - x + 2}{x - 2} = \frac{(x^2 - 1)(x - 2)}{x - 2} = x^2 - 1$$

so, we get the (only apparently) surprising result

$$\lim_{x \to 2} \frac{x^3 - 2x^2 - x + 2}{x - 2} = \lim_{x \to 2} (x^2 - 1) = 4 - 1 = 3.$$

In some cases, the calculus can be much more difficult and requires some techniques, which are out our scope.

17.3 Derivatives

The derivative $f'(x)$ of a function $f(x)$ is the velocity of instantaneous change of the function; more precisely, it is the angular coefficient of the tangent of the function. It is commonly calculated by means of the well-known equation

$$f'(x) = \lim_{\Delta x \to 0} \frac{f(x + \Delta x) - f(x)}{\Delta x}, \tag{17.2}$$

where Δx is a small (say, small at will) positive amount of x, which becomes arbitrarily small—so small that it can be neglected—when passing to the limit $\Delta x \to 0$. In many textbooks, the value h or even Δ "alone" is used instead of Δx.

For example, if $f(x) = x^2$, then

$$f'(x) = \lim_{\Delta x \to 0} \frac{(x + \Delta x)^2 - x^2}{\Delta x}$$

$$= \lim_{\Delta x \to 0} \frac{x^2 + 2x\Delta x + (\Delta x)^2 - x^2}{\Delta x}$$

$$= \lim_{\Delta x \to 0} \frac{2x\Delta x + (\Delta x)^2}{\Delta x} = \lim_{\Delta x \to 0} (2x + \Delta x)$$

$$= 2x. \tag{17.3}$$

As another example of differentiation, we take $f(x) = e^x$, from which we get

$$f'(x) = \lim_{\Delta x \to 0} \frac{e^{x + \Delta x} - e^x}{\Delta x}$$

$$= \lim_{\Delta x \to 0} \frac{e^x e^{\Delta x} - e^x}{\Delta x}$$

$$= \lim_{\Delta x \to 0} \left(e^x \frac{e^{\Delta x} - 1}{\Delta x} \right)$$

$$= e^x \lim_{\Delta x \to 0} \frac{e^{\Delta x} - 1}{\Delta x}$$

$$= e^x, \tag{17.4}$$

where we used the limit

$$\lim_{\Delta x \to 0} \frac{e^{\Delta x} - 1}{\Delta x} = 1. \tag{17.5}$$

There are various modes to indicate the derivative of a function $y = f(x)$: the simplest are Newton's notation $\dot{f}(x)$(or also $\dot{f}$, often used in physics) and Lagrange's notation $f'(x)$, or even y', which we have used at the beginning of this section. Indeed, in many situations, Leibniz's notation $\frac{df(x)}{dx}$, or even $\frac{dy}{dx}$, is more suitable, while in some other situations, the preferable notation could be $\partial_x y$ or even y_x; thus, one must bear in mind that all of these notations are equivalent. In the next pages, we will use indifferently both Lagrange's and Leibniz's notations, while we will see that notations $\partial_x y$ and y_x will be useful when dealing with partial derivatives.

To avoid confusion, we use $f^2(x)$ (or sometimes f^2 if no ambiguities may arise) as a shortcut for $(f(x))^2$ (bearing in mind that $f^n = (f(x))^n$, whereas $f^{(n)}$ is the n-th derivative of $f(x)$); also, we will use $\sin^2(x)$ as a shortcut to say $\sin(x)\sin(x) = (\sin(x))^2$, which must be not confounded with the functional $\sin(\sin(x))$; a functional (e.g., a compound function) will be always given in the form $f(g(x))$, like $\sin(\sin(x))$. The term $f^{-1}(x)$ will indicate the *inverse function* of $f(x)$, e.g., a function such that $f^{-1}(f(x)) = x$ (assuming that $f(x)$ is invertible); the term $f(x)^{-1}$, as a shortcut for $(f(x))^{-1}$, will therefore be used to mention the multiplicative inverse (the reciprocal) of $f(x)$, hence $f(x)^{-1} = \frac{1}{f(x)}$. To avoid ambiguities, the inverse of trigonometric functions $\sin(x)$ and $\sinh(x)$ will be rendered as $\arcsin(x)$ and arc $\sinh(x)$, respectively.

The differentiation of a function is always possible if $f(x)$ is continuous and differentiable; if also $f'(x)$ is continuous and differentiable, then also $f'(x)$ may be differentiable, obtaining the second derivative of $f(x)$ as

$$f''(x) = \frac{d}{dx} \left(\frac{df(x)}{dx} \right) = \frac{d^2 f(x)}{dx^2},$$

and so on; defining with $f^{(n)}(x)$ the n-th derivative of $f(x)$, we have

$$f^{(n)}(x) = \frac{d}{dx} \left(\frac{d}{dx} \left(\cdots \left(\frac{df(x)}{dx} \right) \right) \right) = \frac{d^n f(x)}{dx^n},$$

of course assuming that also $f^{(n-1)}$ is continuous and differentiable, so that $f(x)$ is differentiable (at least) n times. Note that many functions, like trigonometric ones, the exponential, or the logarithm, are virtually differentiable an infinite number of times over their domains.

If the function f does not depend on x, then $f' = 0$; for example, given $f(y) = 3y^2$, we have $\frac{d(3y^2)}{dx} = 0$, since $f(y)$ is not a function of x. Also, differentiating a constant with respect to x gives a null derivative, since the value of the constant does not depend on x.

The differentiation is linear, thus

$$\frac{d}{dx}[\alpha f(x) \pm \beta g(x)] = \lim_{\Delta x \to 0} \alpha \frac{f(x + \Delta x) - f(x)}{\Delta x} \pm \lim_{\Delta x \to 0} \beta \frac{g(x + \Delta x) - g(x)}{\Delta x}$$

$$= \alpha \lim_{\Delta x \to 0} \frac{f(x + \Delta x) - f(x)}{\Delta x} \pm \beta \lim_{\Delta x \to 0} \frac{g(x + \Delta x) - g(x)}{\Delta x}$$

$$= \alpha \frac{df(x)}{dx} \pm \beta \frac{dg(x)}{dx},$$

being α, β two real constants. For example, if $f(x) = 3x^2 - 4\sin(x)$, then

$$\frac{d}{dx}[3x^2 - 4\sin(x)] = 3\frac{dx^2}{dx} - 4\frac{d\sin(x)}{dx} = 6x - 4\cos(x).$$

As we mentioned at the beginning of this section, the derivative of a function $f(x)$ is the angular coefficient of its tangent line. If the generic point P of coordinates (x_P, y_P) belongs to a planar curve in $\mathbb{R}^2$, then the tangent line in P is given as

$$y - y_P = f'(x_P)(x - x_P)$$
$$= m(x - x_P)$$

or, in other words,

$$y = f(x_P) + f'(x_P)(x - x_P)$$

where

$$f'(x_P) = \frac{df(x)}{dx}\bigg|_{x=x_P}$$

is the derivative calculated at point x_P, e.g., the slope of the tangent line of $f(x)$ at point x_P, assuming that $f(x)$ is continuous and differentiable in x_P. It is evident that if at a given point x_P we have $f'(x_P) > 0$, then $f(x)$ at point x_P is increasing; if $f'(x_P) < 0$, then $f(x)$ at point x_P is decreasing, while if $f'(x_P) = 0$, then we must carry out other evaluations to determine what is actually going to happen at x_P. This cannot be sufficient, and it is a much more convenient complete analysis of the function.

For example, let

$$f(x) = 2x^3 - 3x^2 = x^2(2x - 3); \tag{17.6}$$

we have $\text{Dom}(f) = \mathbb{R}$; thus, $f(x)$ is always defined. We may first search for the intersection points with axes x and y. If $x = 0$, we have $y = f(x) = 0$, and if $y = 0$, we have $x = 0$ and $x = \frac{3}{2}$, so $f(x)$ intercepts both the x axis and the y axis in $P(0, 0)$ and the x axis in $Q(\frac{3}{2}, 0)$; moreover, $f(x)$ is positive for $2x^3 - 3x^2 > 0$, e.g., for $x > \frac{3}{2}$, and is negative for $0 < x < \frac{3}{2}$ and for $x < 0$ (we already saw that at $x = 0$, $f(x) = 0$). Let's now look at limits when $x \to \pm\infty$: we have

$$\lim_{x \to +\infty} (x^2(2x - 3)) = +\infty$$

and

$$\lim_{x \to +\infty} (x^2(2x - 3)) = -\infty$$

then we calculate the first derivative as

$$f'(x) = 6x^2 - 6x = 6x(x - 1)$$

so that

$$\begin{cases} f'(x) > 0 : & \text{for } x < 0 \text{ and } x > 1 \\ f'(x) = 0 : & \text{for } x = 0 \text{ and } x = 1 \\ f'(x) < 0 : & \text{for } 0 < x < 1 \end{cases}$$

Therefore, $f(x)$ has a maximum for $x = 0$ (when $x < 0$, $f'(x) > 0$, and when $x > 0$, $f'(x) < 0$, thus $f(0)$ is a local maximum), while $f(x)$ has a minimum for $x = 1$ (when $0 < x < 1$, $f'(x) < 0$, and when $x > 1$, $f'(x) > 0$, thus $f(1)$ is a local minimum), so that the point of maximum is $(0, 0)$ and the point of the minimum is $(1, -1)$.

The second derivative of $f(x)$ is

$$f''(x) = 12x - 6 = 6(2x - 1)$$

thus

$$\begin{cases} f''(x) > 0 : & \text{for } x > \frac{1}{2} \\ f''(x) = 0 : & \text{for } x = \frac{1}{2} \; ; \\ f''(x) < 0 : & \text{for } x < \frac{1}{2} \end{cases}$$

hence, when $f(x)$ changes its concavity in $x = \frac{1}{2}$, and since $f(\frac{1}{2}) = -\frac{1}{2}$, then the point $R\left(\frac{1}{2}, -\frac{1}{2}\right)$ is an inflection point for $f(x)$.

17.4 Algebraic Properties of the Differential Operator

The differential operator $\frac{d}{dx}$ obeys some algebraic rules. Given the real constants α, β, γ, we may see that the commutative law is obeyed, since

$$\frac{d^\alpha}{dx^\alpha}\left(\frac{d^\beta f(x)}{dx^\beta}\right) = \frac{d^\beta}{dx^\beta}\left(\frac{d^\alpha f(x)}{dx^\alpha}\right)$$

$$= \frac{d^{\alpha+\beta}}{dx^{\alpha+\beta}}f(x)$$

The same is for the associative law

$$\frac{d^\alpha}{dx^\alpha}\left(\frac{d^\beta}{dx^\beta}\left(\frac{d^\gamma f(x)}{dx^\gamma}\right)\right) = \frac{d^\beta}{dx^\beta}\left(\frac{d^\alpha}{dx^\alpha}\left(\frac{d^\gamma f(x)}{dx^\gamma}\right)\right)$$

$$= \frac{d^\gamma}{dx^\gamma}\left(\frac{d^\alpha}{dx^\alpha}\left(\frac{d^\beta f(x)}{dx^\beta}\right)\right)$$

$$= \frac{d^{\alpha+\beta+\gamma}}{dx^{\alpha+\beta+\gamma}}f(x),$$

and for the distributive law

$$\frac{d^\alpha}{dx^\alpha}\left(\frac{d^\beta}{dx^\beta} + \frac{d^\gamma}{dx^\gamma}\right)f(x) = \frac{d^\alpha}{dx^\alpha}\left(\frac{d^\beta f(x)}{dx^\beta}\right) + \frac{d^\alpha}{dx^\alpha}\left(\frac{d^\gamma f(x)}{dx^\gamma}\right)$$

$$= \frac{d^{\alpha+\beta}}{dx^{\alpha+\beta}}f(x) + \frac{d^{\alpha+\gamma}}{dx^{\alpha+\gamma}}f(x).$$

In all cases, we have used also the *index law* , which reads

$$\frac{d^\alpha}{dx^\alpha}\left(\frac{d^\beta f(x)}{dx^\beta}\right) = \frac{d^{\alpha+\beta}f(x)}{dx^{\alpha+\beta}}.$$

In many textbooks, the differential operator is given as

$$\frac{d^\alpha}{dx^\alpha} = D^\alpha,$$

so that, for example, we have

$$2y'''(t) - 3y''(t) + y'(t) + 5y(t) = (2D^3 - 3D^2 + 1D + 5)y(t);$$

this notation is very useful when, for example, one is dealing with a differential equation.

17.5   Main Rules of Differentiation

The differential operator $\frac{d}{dx}$ is linear, that is, given a function $p(x) = \alpha f(x) \pm \beta g(x)$, being α, β two constants, we have

$$\frac{dp(x)}{dx} = \frac{d}{dx}[\alpha f(x) \pm \beta g(x)] = \alpha \frac{df(x)}{dx} \pm \beta \frac{dg(x)}{dx}; \qquad (17.7)$$

since

$$
\begin{aligned}
p'(x) &= \lim_{\Delta x \to 0} \frac{((\alpha f(x + \Delta x)) \pm (\beta g(x + \Delta x)) - (\alpha f(x) \pm \beta g(x))}{\Delta x} \\
&= \lim_{\Delta x \to 0} \frac{\alpha f(x + \Delta x) \pm \beta g(x + \Delta x) - \alpha f(x) \mp \beta g(x)}{\Delta x} \\
&= \lim_{\Delta x \to 0} \frac{(\alpha f(x + \Delta x) - \alpha f(x)) \pm (\beta g(x + \Delta x) - \beta g(x))}{\Delta x} \\
&= \alpha \lim_{\Delta x \to 0} \frac{(f(x) + \Delta x) - f(x)}{\Delta x} \pm \beta \lim_{\Delta x \to 0} \frac{(g(x + \Delta x) - g(x)}{\Delta x} \\
&= \alpha f'(x) \pm \beta g'(x),
\end{aligned}
$$

which can be generalized for an algebraic sum of n functions as

$$\frac{d}{dx} \sum_{k=1}^{n} \alpha_k f_k(x) = \sum_{k=1}^{n} \alpha_k \frac{df_k(x)}{dx},$$

being a_k a positive, negative, or null quantity.

If the function $h(x) = f(x)g(x)$ is a product of two distinct functions, then

$$\frac{dh(x)}{dx} = \frac{d}{dx}[f(x)g(x)] = g(x)\frac{df(x)}{dx} + f(x)\frac{dg(x)}{dx}; \qquad (17.8)$$

in fact, we can write $h(x + \Delta x) = f(x + \Delta x)g(x + \Delta x)$; hence,

$$h'(x) = \lim_{\Delta x \to 0} \frac{f(x + \Delta x)g(x + \Delta x) - f(x)g(x)}{\Delta x}$$

then, adding and subtracting $f(x)g(x + \Delta)$ in the numerator, we have

$h'(x)$

$$
\begin{aligned}
&= \lim_{\Delta x \to 0} \frac{f(x + \Delta x)g(x + \Delta x) + f(x)g(x + \Delta x) - f(x)g(x + \Delta x) - f(x)g(x)}{\Delta x} \\
&= \lim_{\Delta x \to 0} \frac{g(x + \Delta x)(f(x + \Delta x) - f(x)) + f(x)[g(x + \Delta x) - g(x)]}{\Delta x}
\end{aligned}
$$

$$= \lim_{\Delta x \to 0} \frac{[f(x + \Delta x) - f(x)]}{\Delta x} + \lim_{\Delta x \to 0} \frac{f(x)[g(x + \Delta x) - g(x)]}{\Delta x}$$

$$= \lim_{\Delta x \to 0} g(x + \Delta x) \lim_{\Delta x \to 0} \frac{f(x + \Delta x) - f(x)}{\Delta x}$$

$$+ \lim_{\Delta x \to 0} f(x) \lim_{\Delta x \to 0} \frac{g(x + \Delta x) - g(x)}{\Delta x}$$

$$= g(x) \lim_{\Delta x \to 0} \frac{f(x + \Delta x) - f(x)}{\Delta x} + f(x) \lim_{\Delta x \to 0} \frac{g(x + \Delta x) - g(x)}{\Delta x}$$

$$= g(x) f'(x) + f(x) g'(x).$$

The product rule may be extended to an arbitrary number n of functions $p(x) = f_1(x) f_2(x) \cdots f_n(x)$, giving

$$p'(x) = f_1'(x) [f_2(x) \cdots f_n(x)] + f_2'(x) [f_1(x) \cdots f_n(x)]$$

$$+ \cdots + f_n'(x) [f_1(x) \cdots f_{n-1}(x)]$$

$$= \sum_{k=1}^{n} \left(\prod_{i=1, i \neq k} f_i(x) \right) \frac{d f_k(x)}{dx}.$$

It must be pointed out that in most cases, if the product $f(x)g(x)$ is a polynomial, it can be convenient to first expand $f(x)g(x)$ and then to differentiate the product by using the linearity of the $\frac{d}{dx}$ operator. For example, taking $f(x) = 2x - 3$ and $g(x) = x^3 + 2x$, we have

$$f(x)g(x) = (2x - 3)(x^3 + 2x)$$

$$= 2x^4 - 3x^3 + 4x^2 - 6x,$$

then

$$\frac{d(f(x)g(x))}{dx} = \frac{d}{dx} 2x^4 - \frac{d}{dx} 3x^3 + \frac{d}{dx} 4x^2 - \frac{d}{dx} 6x$$

$$= 8x^3 - 9x^2 + 8x - 6$$

which is equivalent to say

$$\frac{d(f(x)g(x))}{dx} = (x^3 + 2x) \frac{d(2x - 3)}{dx} + (2x - 3) \frac{d(x^3 + 2x)}{dx}$$

$$= 2(x^3 + 2x) + (2x - 3)(3x^2 + 2)$$

$$= 2x^3 + 4x + 6x^3 - 9x^2 + 4x - 6$$

$$= 8x^3 - 9x^2 + 8x - 6.$$

Given an arbitrary function $g(x) = \frac{1}{f(x)}$ as the reciprocal, or *multiplicative inverse*, of $f(x)$, we may obtain its derivative as follows:

$$g'(x) = \lim_{\Delta x \to 0} \frac{\dfrac{1}{f(x + \Delta x)} - \dfrac{1}{f(x)}}{\Delta x}$$

$$= \lim_{\Delta x \to 0} \left(\frac{1}{\Delta x} \frac{f(x) - f(x + \Delta x)}{f(x + \Delta x) f(x)} \right)$$

$$= - \lim_{\Delta x \to 0} \left(\frac{1}{\Delta x} \frac{f(x + \Delta x) - f(x)}{f(x + \Delta x) f(x)} \right)$$

$$= - \lim_{\Delta x \to 0} \left(\frac{f(x + \Delta x) - f(x)}{\Delta x} \frac{1}{f(x + \Delta x) f(x)} \right)$$

$$= -f'(x) \lim_{\Delta x \to 0} \frac{1}{f(x + \Delta x) f(x)}$$

$$= -f'(x) \frac{1}{f(x)^2}$$

$$= -\frac{f'(x)}{f(x)^2}. \tag{17.9}$$

provided $f(x)$ is nonzero.

The derivative of the ratio $q(x) = \frac{f(x)}{g(x)}$ of two functions, for any nonzero $g(x)$ is

$$\frac{dq(x)}{dx} = \frac{d}{dx} \frac{f(x)}{g(x)} = \frac{f'(x)g(x) - g'(x)f(x)}{g(x)^2}; \tag{17.10}$$

this can be verified, for example, using the derivation of a product with the substitution $\frac{1}{g(x)} = u(x)$ so as to have

$$\frac{f(x)}{g(x)} = f(x)u(x) = q(x),$$

thus, invoking the derivative of the reciprocal of a function given in Eq. (17.9), we get

$$q'(x) = u(x)f'(x) + f(x)u'(x)$$

$$= \frac{1}{g(x)} f'(x) + f(x) \left(\frac{1}{g(x)} \right)'$$

$$= \frac{f'(x)}{g(x)} - f(x) \frac{g'(x)}{g(x)^2}$$

$$= \frac{g(x)f'(x) - g'(x)f(x)}{g(x)^2}.$$

17.6   The Chain Rule

This is perhaps the most important mathematical tool for anyone dealing with artificial intelligence and with neural networks in particular. For compound functions $f(g(x))$, for example, like $\sin(\exp(x))$, or $\log(\cos(x))$, or $\sin(\cos(x))$, the derivative must be obtained by using the chain rule , that is, first deriving the outer function with respect to the inner function and then multiplying this derivative by the derivative of the inner function, so as to have

$$\frac{\mathrm{d}f(g(x))}{\mathrm{d}x} = \frac{\mathrm{d}f}{\mathrm{d}g}\frac{\mathrm{d}g}{\mathrm{d}x}.$$

For example,

$$\frac{\mathrm{d}}{\mathrm{d}x}\sin(\exp(x)) = \frac{\mathrm{d}[\sin(\exp(x))]}{\mathrm{d}(\exp(x))}\frac{\mathrm{d}(\exp(x))}{\mathrm{d}x}$$

$$= \cos(\exp(x))\ \exp(x)$$

$$= \exp(x)\cos(\exp(x)),$$

or

$$\frac{\mathrm{d}}{\mathrm{d}x}\log(\cos(x)) = \frac{\mathrm{d}[\log(\cos(x))]}{\mathrm{d}(\cos(x))}\frac{\mathrm{d}(\cos(x))}{\mathrm{d}x}$$

$$= \frac{1}{\cos(x)}(-\sin(x))$$

$$= -\tan(x),$$

or, again

$$\frac{\mathrm{d}\sin(\cos(x))}{\mathrm{d}x} = \frac{\mathrm{d}[\sin(\cos(x))]}{\mathrm{d}(\cos(x))}\frac{\mathrm{d}(\cos(x))}{\mathrm{d}x}$$

$$= \cos(\cos(x))(-\sin(x))$$

$$= -\sin(x)\cos(\cos(x)).$$

The chain rule may be repeated for an arbitrary number n of times, so that

$$\frac{\mathrm{d}f_1(f_2(f_3\cdots(f_{n-1}(f_n(x)))))}{\mathrm{d}x} = \frac{\mathrm{d}f_1}{\mathrm{d}f_2}\frac{\mathrm{d}f_2}{\mathrm{d}f_3}\cdots\frac{\mathrm{d}f_{n-1}}{\mathrm{d}f_n}\frac{\mathrm{d}f_n}{\mathrm{d}x}$$

$$= \left(\prod_{k=1}^{n-1}\frac{\mathrm{d}f_k}{\mathrm{d}f_{k+1}}\right)\frac{\mathrm{d}f_n(x)}{\mathrm{d}x}.$$

always starting from the outermost function and arriving to the innermost one.

In some textbooks, the compound function $f(g(x))$ is given as $f \circ g(x)$, to be read as "f after $g(x)$."

17.7 The Power Rule

For a function $h(x) = f(x)^{g(x)}$, the derivative may be calculated recalling that

$$\log(h(x)) = \log\left[f(x)^{g(x)} \right] = g(x) \log(f(x)),$$

thus

$$\frac{\mathrm{d}\log(h(x))}{\mathrm{d}x} = \frac{\mathrm{d}(g(x)\log(f(x)))}{\mathrm{d}x}$$

hence

$$\frac{h'(x)}{h(x)} = \frac{\mathrm{d}(g(x)\log(f(x)))}{\mathrm{d}x}$$

and we define the power rule by writing

$$\frac{\mathrm{d}(f(x)^{g(x)})}{\mathrm{d}x} = h(x)\frac{\mathrm{d}(g(x)\log(f(x)))}{\mathrm{d}x}$$

$$= f(x)^{g(x)}\left(\frac{g(x)f'(x)}{f(x)} + g'(x)\log(f(x)) \right),$$

where we used both the chain rule and the product rule.

A particular case is $g(x) = C$, being C a constant, leading to

$$\frac{\mathrm{d}(f(x)^{C})}{\mathrm{d}x} = \frac{\mathrm{d}(\exp(C\log(f(x))))}{\mathrm{d}x}$$

$$= f(x)^{C}\left(C\frac{f'(x)}{f(x)} \right)$$

$$= Cf(x)^{C-1}f'(x), \qquad\qquad (17.11)$$

where in the case $f(x) = x$, we have

$$\frac{\mathrm{d}(x^{C})}{\mathrm{d}x} = Cx^{C-1},$$

and again having $f(x)^C = f(x)^{-1}$, from Eq. (17.11), we get

$$\frac{d\left(f(x)^{-1}\right)}{dx} = -f(x)^{-2} f'(x)$$

$$= -\frac{f'(x)}{f(x)^2}.$$

A generalization is the derivative of

$$\sqrt[n]{f(x)} = f(x)^{1/n}$$

which may be easily obtained since

$$\frac{d\sqrt[n]{f(x)}}{dx} = \frac{d\sqrt[n]{f(x)}}{df(x)} \frac{df(x)}{dx}$$

$$= \frac{1}{n\sqrt[n]{f(x)^{n-1}}}.$$

17.8 Series Expansion

Assume we may define a given function $f(x)$ in terms of sums of powers of the variable x such that for some coefficients a_k, we may write

$$f(x) = a_0 + a_1 x + a_2 x^2 + a_3 x^3 + a_4 x^4 + a_5 x^5 + \cdots$$

$$= \sum_{k=0}^{+\infty} a_k x^k, \tag{17.12}$$

such that letting $x = 0$, we have $f(0) = a_0$.

The derivative of (17.12) with respect to x will be

$$f'(x) = a_1 + 2a_2 x + 3a_3 x^2 + 4a_4 x^3 + 5a_5 x^4 + \cdots$$

$$= \sum_{k=1}^{+\infty} k a_k x^{k-1}, \tag{17.13}$$

thus, again, letting $x = 0$, we have $f'(0) = a_1$, and deriving (17.13)

$$f''(x) = 2a_2 + 6a_3 x + 12a_4 x^2 + 20a_5 x^3 + \cdots$$

$$= \sum_{k=2}^{+\infty} k(k-1) a_k x^{k-2}, \tag{17.14}$$

in which we have $f''(0) = 2a_2$, and, again, the derivative of (17.14) is

$$f'''(x) = 6a_3 + 24a_4 x + 60a_5 x^2 + \cdots$$

$$= \sum_{k=3}^{+\infty} k(k-1)(k-2)a_k x^{k-3}, \tag{17.15}$$

thus $f'''(0) = 6a_3$, and taking the derivative of (17.15), we get

$$f^{(4)}(x) = 24a_4 + 120a_5 x + \cdots$$

$$= \sum_{k=4}^{+\infty} k(k-1)(k-2)(k-3)a_k x^{k-4}, \tag{17.16}$$

with $f^{(4)}(0) = 24a_4$.

From all what above, since $1! = 1$, $2! = 2$, $3! = 6$, and $4! = 24$, we may deduce that the general form for the n-th derivative of $f(x)$ is

$$f^{(n)}(x) = n!a_n + (n+1)!x + (n+2)!x^2 + \cdots$$

$$= \sum_{k=n}^{+\infty} k(k-1)(k-2)\cdots(k-n+1)a_k x^{k-n}, \tag{17.17}$$

with $f^{(n)}(0) = n!a_n$.

Now, letting $x = 0$, we have seen that

$$a_0 = f(0); \ a_1 = f'(0); \ a_2 = \frac{f''(0)}{2}; \ a_3 = \frac{f'''(0)}{6}; \ a_4 = \frac{f^{(4)}(0)}{6}$$

thus

$$a_n = \frac{f^{(n)}(0)}{n!}.$$

The values a_k are defined the Taylor coefficients of the Taylor series (a.k.a. the *Taylor polynomial* if the series is truncated) of the function $f(x)$; hence, we may write $f(x)$ in its compact form

$$f(x) = \sum_{n=0}^{+\infty} \frac{f^{(n)}(0)}{n!} x^n$$

$$= \sum_{n=0}^{+\infty} \frac{1}{n!} \frac{d^n f(x)}{dx^n}\bigg|_{x=0} x^n, \tag{17.18}$$

where the term

$$\left.\frac{d^n f(x)}{dx^n}\right|_{x=0} = f^{(n)}(0)$$

is the n-th derivative of $f(x)$ calculated at point $x = 0$.

More precisely, we can define the Taylor series expansion in the open interval $]x_0 - \xi, x_0 + \xi[$ around a given point a in the domain of $f(x)$ as follows:

$$f(x) = \sum_{n=0}^{+\infty} \frac{f^{(n)}(x_0)}{n!}(x - x_0)^n$$

$$= \sum_{n=0}^{+\infty} \frac{1}{n!} \left.\frac{d^n f(x)}{dx^n}\right|_{x=x_0} (x - x_0)^n \qquad (17.19)$$

provided $f(x)$ infinitely differentiable in the considered open interval around a.

In the particular case $x_0 = 0$, the expansion is also called the McLaurin series .

The Taylor series can be seen as a generalization of the mean value theorem by Lagrange, stating that if a function $f(x)$ is derivable in an interval $]\lambda, x[$, and $x_0 \in]\lambda, x[$, then $\frac{f(x)-f(\lambda)}{x-\lambda} = f'(x_0)$; thus,

$$f(x) = f(\lambda) + f'(x_0)(x - \lambda)$$

$$= f(\lambda) + \frac{1}{1!} \left.\frac{d f(x)}{dx}\right|_{x=x_0} (x - \lambda).$$

which is a Taylor series expansion at point $x = \lambda$ truncated at first derivative.

Let us now define a remainder function $R_n(x)$ as

$$R_n(x) = \frac{1}{(n+1)!} \left.\frac{d f^{n+1}(x)}{dx^{n+1}}\right|_{x=x_0} (x - \lambda)^{n+1}$$

so that the Taylor series for $f(x)$ can be rewritten

$$f(x) = \sum_{m=0}^{n} \left(\frac{1}{m!} \left.\frac{d^m f(x)}{dx^m}\right|_{x=a} (x - \lambda)^m \right) + R_n(x)$$

$$= \sum_{m=0}^{n} \left(\frac{1}{m!} \left.\frac{d^m f(x)}{dx^m}\right|_{x=x_0} (x - \lambda)^m \right) + \frac{1}{(n+1)!} \left.\frac{d f^{n+1}(x)}{dx^{n+1}}\right|_{x=x_0} (x - \lambda)^{n+1}$$

which is a particular case of Taylor series truncated at n-th derivative with the residual $R_n(x)$ added. Note that the remainder may be given also in the form

$$R_n(x) = o[(x - \lambda)^n]$$

which reads "$R_n(x)$ is small-oh of $(x - \lambda)^n$," meaning that

$$\lim_{n \to +\infty} \frac{R_n(x)}{(x - \lambda)^n} = 0.$$

Let us now take an example calculating the Taylor series of the function

$$y = \frac{1}{1 - x},$$

which is defined for $\forall x \neq 1$. For first we see that

$$f(0) = \left. \frac{1}{1 - x} \right|_{x=0} = 1,$$

thus, calculating the derivatives, and their values at $x = 0$, we have

$$\frac{d}{dx} \left(\frac{1}{1 - x} \right) = \frac{1}{(1 - x)^2} \implies \left. \frac{d}{dx} \left(\frac{1}{1 - x} \right) \right|_{x=0} = 1 = 1!,$$

$$\frac{d^2}{dx^2} \left(\frac{1}{1 - x} \right) = \frac{2}{(1 - x)^3} \implies \left. \frac{d^2}{dx^2} \left(\frac{1}{1 - x} \right) \right|_{x=0} = 2 = 2!,$$

$$\frac{d^3}{dx^3} \left(\frac{1}{1 - x} \right) = \frac{6}{(1 - x)^4} \implies \left. \frac{d^3}{dx^3} \left(\frac{1}{1 - x} \right) \right|_{x=0} = 6 = 3!,$$

$$\frac{d^4}{dx^4} \left(\frac{1}{1 - x} \right) = \frac{24}{(1 - x)^5} \implies \left. \frac{d^4}{dx^4} \left(\frac{1}{1 - x} \right) \right|_{x=0} = 24 = 4!,$$

hence, we may infer the following rule for subsequent differentiation of $\frac{1}{1-x}$:

$$\frac{d^n}{dx^n} \left(\frac{1}{1 - x} \right) = \frac{n!}{(1 - x)^{n+1}} \implies \left. \frac{d^n}{dx^n} \left(\frac{1}{1 - x} \right) \right|_{x=0} = n!,$$

thus, recalling that $0! = 1$, and using the above result, we can write

$$\frac{1}{1 - x} = \sum_{n=0}^{+\infty} \frac{1}{n!} \left. \frac{d^n f(x)}{dx^n} \right|_{x=0} x^n$$

$$= \frac{1}{0!} 0! x^0 + \frac{1}{1!} 1! x^1 + \frac{1}{2!} 2! x^2 + \frac{1}{3!} 3! x^3 + \frac{1}{4!} 4! x^4 + \frac{1}{5!} 5! x^5 + \cdots$$

$$= 1 + x + x^2 + x^3 + x^4 + x^5 + \cdots . \tag{17.20}$$

However, things (as usual) ain't so simple. Let us take $f(x) = \frac{1}{1-x}$ at point $x = 3$: we have $f(3) = \frac{1}{1-3} = -\frac{1}{2}$; hence, using Eq. (17.20), we will find an absurd risultate, like $\frac{1}{1-x} = 1+3+9+27+81+\cdots$, so there should be a criterion to establish at which values of x the Taylor series approximates $f(x)$ in a reasonable way, that is, in which interval of the domain the Taylor series converges to $f(x)$.

In this case, we see that (17.20) is the geometric series

$$\sum_{k=0}^{n} x^k = 1 + x + x^2 + x^3 + x^4 + x^5 + \cdots$$

thus, this series converges if $|x| < 1$, and this may be verified since we can take

$$\sum_{k=0}^{n} x^k = 1 + x + x^2 + x^3 + \cdots + x^n,$$

hence, multiplying both sides by $(1 - x)$

$$(1 - x) \sum_{k=0}^{n} x^k = (1 - x)(1 + x + x^2 + x^3 + \cdots + x^n)$$

$$= 1 - x^{n+1}$$

therefore

$$\sum_{k=0}^{n} x^k = \frac{1 - x^{n+1}}{1 - x}$$

thus, taking the limit in both sides, we get

$$\lim_{n \to +\infty} \sum_{k=0}^{n} x^k = \lim_{n \to +\infty} \frac{1 - x^{n+1}}{1 - x} = \frac{1}{1 - x} \lim_{n \to +\infty} (1 - x^{n+1})$$

hence we see that

$$\sum_{k=0}^{+\infty} x^k = \frac{1}{1 - x}$$

converges only if $|x| < 1$. This means that the Taylor series of Eq. (17.20) converges to $f(x)$ only if $x \in \,] - 1, 1[$. The convergence of the Taylor series to $f(x)$ is of paramount importance and must be always checked.

The Taylor series is a mathematical procedure with great utility: let us take $f(x) = e^x$. Again, we first see that $f(0) = e^0 = 1$, and then we calculate the derivatives at $x = 0$ (in this case, everything is much simpler), to have

$$\frac{de^x}{dx} = e^x \implies \left.\frac{de^x}{dx}\right|_{x=0} = 1,$$

$$\frac{d^2 e^x}{dx^2} = e^x \implies \left.\frac{d^2 e^x}{dx^2}\right|_{x=0} = 1,$$

$$\frac{d^3 e^x}{dx^3} = e^x \implies \left.\frac{d^3 e^x}{dx^3}\right|_{x=0} = 1,$$

and the "rule" is

$$\frac{d^n e^x}{dx^n} = e^x \implies \left.\frac{d^n e^x}{dx^n}\right|_{x=0} = 1,$$

so we once more use Eq. (17.18) to calculate the Taylor series expansion for $f(x) = e^x$ as follows:

$$e^x = \sum_{n=0}^{+\infty} \frac{1}{n!} \left.\frac{d^n f(x)}{dx^n}\right|_{x=0} x^n$$

$$= \frac{1}{0!} 1 x^0 + \frac{1}{1!} 1 x^1 + \frac{1}{2!} 1 x^2 + \frac{1}{3!} 1 x^3 + \frac{1}{4!} 1 x^4 + \frac{1}{5!} 1 x^5 + \cdots$$

$$= 1 + x + \frac{1}{2!} x^2 + \frac{1}{3!} x^3 + \frac{1}{4!} x^4 + \frac{1}{5!} x^5 + \cdots .$$

Using the same procedure with $f(x) = \sin(x)$, we easily obtain

$$\sin(x) = \sum_{n=0}^{+\infty} \frac{1}{n!} \left.\frac{d^n f(x)}{dx^n}\right|_{x=0} x^n$$

$$= \frac{1}{0!} 0 x^0 + \frac{1}{1!} 1 x^1 + \frac{1}{2!} 0 x^2 - \frac{1}{3!} 1 x^3 + \frac{1}{4!} 0 x^4 + \frac{1}{5!} 1 x^5 + \cdots$$

$$= x - \frac{x^3}{3!} + \frac{x^5}{5!} - \frac{x^7}{7!} + \frac{x^9}{9!} + \cdots .$$

Series expansion is very useful, since virtually any function can be treated as the algebraic sum of very simple powers, so that they can be easily derived and integrated. Moreover, they are also useful for the calculus of some limits. For example, we can use this expansion for the calculus of $\lim_{x \to 0} \frac{\sin(x)}{x}$ since we get

$$\lim_{x \to 0} \frac{\sin(x)}{x} = \lim_{x \to 0} \frac{1}{x} \left(x - \frac{x^3}{3!} + \frac{x^5}{5!} - \frac{x^7}{7!} + \frac{x^9}{9!} + \cdots \right)$$

$$= \lim_{x \to 0} \left(1 - \frac{x^2}{3!} + \frac{x^4}{5!} - \frac{x^6}{7!} + \frac{x^8}{9!} + \cdots \right)$$

$$= 1 - \lim_{x \to 0} \left(\frac{x^2}{3!} - \frac{x^4}{5!} + \frac{x^6}{7!} - \frac{x^8}{9!} + \cdots \right)$$

$$= 1.$$

As another example, we may obtain the value of $\lim_{x \to 0} \frac{e^x - 1}{x}$, as

$$\lim_{x \to 0} \frac{e^x - 1}{x} = \lim_{x \to 0} \frac{1}{x} \left[\left(1 + x + \frac{x^2}{2!} + \frac{x^3}{3!} + \frac{x^4}{4!} + \cdots \right) - 1 \right]$$

$$= \lim_{x \to 0} \frac{1}{x} \left(x + \frac{x^2}{2!} + \frac{x^3}{3!} + \frac{x^4}{4!} + \cdots \right)$$

$$= \lim_{x \to 0} \left(1 + \frac{x}{2!} + \frac{x^2}{3!} + \frac{x^3}{4!} + \cdots \right)$$

$$= 1 + \lim_{x \to 0} \left(\frac{x}{2!} + \frac{x^2}{3!} + \frac{x^3}{4!} + \cdots \right)$$

$$= 1.$$

17.9   The Antiderivative (The Indefinite Integral)

The antiderivative , or indefinite integral, of a function $f(x)$, called the integrand , is a function $F(x)$, called the primitive , such that, given an arbitrary constant C,

$$\frac{d}{dx}(F(x) + C) = f(x),$$

which is equivalent to say

$$d(F(x) + C) = f(x)dx,$$

and

$$\int d(F(x) + C) = \int f(x)\, dx,$$

thus

$$F(x) + C = \int f(x)\, dx,$$

so as to have, in general,

$$\int \frac{dy(x)}{dx} \, dx = \int dy(x)$$

$$= \left(\frac{d}{dx}\right)^{-1} \frac{d}{dx} y(x)$$

$$= y(x),$$

hence, the indefinite integration may be interpreted as the inverse of the derivation, and this is the reason why we define $F(x)$ the antiderivative of $f(x)$. Note that the antiderivative is always a function unless $f(x) = 0$ in which case $F(x) = \int 0 \, dx = C$.

The indefinite integration is linear, since given two constants α, β then

$$\int [\alpha f(x) \pm \beta g(x)] \, dx = \int \alpha f(x) \, dx \pm \int \beta g(x) \, dx$$

$$= \alpha \int f(x) \, dx \pm \beta \int g(x) \, dx.$$

Some indefinite integrals can be directly obtained just knowing the derivatives: for example, since

$$\frac{dx^{n+1}}{dx} = (n+1)x^n,$$

then

$$\frac{1}{n+1} \frac{dx^{n+1}}{dx} = x^n$$

therefore

$$\int x^n \, dx = \frac{1}{n+1} x^{n+1} + C;$$

for example,

$$\int \frac{x^4}{3} \, dx = \frac{1}{3} \int x^4 \, dx = \frac{1}{3} \frac{x^5}{5} + C = \frac{x^5}{15} + C.$$

17.10 Integration by Partial Fraction Decomposition

The partial fraction decomposition (p.f.d.) is used to transform a rational function into a polynomial, plus a given number of fractions as follows:

$$R(x) = \frac{N_n(x)}{D_m(x)}$$

$$= Q_{n-m}(x) + \frac{A_1}{x - x_1} + \frac{A_2}{x - x_2} + \cdots + \frac{A_n}{x - x_n}$$

$$= Q_{n-m}(x) + \sum_{k=1}^{n} \frac{A_k}{x - x_k},$$

where $N_n(x)$ is the numerator polynomial of degree n, $D_m(x)$ is the denominator polynomial of degree m, and $Q_{n-m}(x)$ is a polynomial of degree $n - m$, while fractions $\frac{A_k}{x-x_k}$ define at numerator the various roots x_k, and A_k are unknown constants to be found. If $m > n$, the polynomial $Q_{n-m}(x)$ is zero, whereas if $m = n$, the polynomial $Q(x)$ is a constant.

An immediate and very simple case of p.f.d. may be seen, for example, with the function

$$R(x) = \frac{3}{x^2 - 1}$$

$$= \frac{3}{(x - 1)(x + 1)}$$

$$= \frac{A}{x - 1} + \frac{B}{x + 1},$$

where A and B are the unknown constants. Note that the degree of denominator is higher than the degree of numerator, then $Q_{n-m}(x)$ is zero. If we calculate the sum, we get

$$R(x) = \frac{(x + 1)A + (x - 1)B}{(x - 1)(x + 1)}$$

however, we already know that $(x + 1)A + (x - 1)B = 3$, and this is intuitively true if we take $A = \frac{3}{2}$ and $B = -\frac{3}{2}$, since $\frac{3}{2}(x + 1) - \frac{3}{2}(x - 1) = 3$; thus, we obtain the partial fraction decomposition

$$R(x) = \frac{3}{x^2 - 1}$$

$$= \frac{\frac{3}{2}}{x - 1} + \frac{-\frac{3}{2}}{x + 1}$$

$$= \frac{3}{2(x + 1)} - \frac{3}{2(x - 1)}.$$

Indeed, this was only a very simple case: in general, we will deal with more complicate functions, but we can immediately verify the utility of p.f.d. by evaluating the integral

$$\int \frac{3}{x^2 - 1} dx = \int \left(\frac{3}{2(x+1)} - \frac{3}{2(x-1)} \right) dx$$

$$= \frac{3}{2} \left(\int \frac{1}{x-1} dx - \int \frac{1}{x+1} dx \right)$$

$$= \frac{3}{2} \int \frac{1}{x-1} dx - \frac{3}{2} \int \frac{1}{x+1} dx$$

$$= \frac{3}{2} \log(x-1) - \frac{3}{2} \log(x+1) + C.$$

In general, when facing a partial fraction decomposition, the denominator may take one of the following forms (we tacitly assume to have already determined the numerator value):

- Linear

$$\frac{A}{x+a} \rightarrow \int \frac{A}{x+a} dx = A \log |x+a| + C$$

- Linear, raised at n-th power

$$\frac{A}{(x+a)^n} \rightarrow \int \frac{A}{(x+a)^n} dx = \frac{A}{1-n}(x+a)^{1-n} + C$$

- Quadratic

$$\frac{Ax+B}{x^2+ax+b} \rightarrow \int \frac{Ax+B}{x^2+ax+b} dx$$

$$= \frac{A \log |x^2+ax+b|}{2} + \frac{2B-aA}{\sqrt{4b-a^2}} \arctan \left(\frac{2x+a}{\sqrt{4b-a^2}} \right) + C$$

- Quadratic, raised at n-th power

$$\frac{Ax+B}{(x^2+ax+b)^n} \rightarrow \int \frac{Ax+B}{(x^2+ax+b)^n} dx =$$

$$= \frac{1}{2(x^2+ax+b)^n(n-1)(2x+a+\sqrt{a^2-4b})^n} \left(\frac{a+\sqrt{a^2-4b}}{2} \right)^n$$

$$\left[\left(\frac{\sqrt{a^2 - 4b} + a + 2x}{\sqrt{a^2 - 4b}}\right)^n B\left(\sqrt{a^2 - 4b} - a - 2x\right)\right.$$

$$_2F_1\left(1 - n, n; 2 - n; \frac{1}{2} - \frac{2x + a}{2\sqrt{a^2 - 4b}}\right)$$

$$+\left(\frac{\sqrt{a^2 - 4b} + a + 2x}{\sqrt{a^2 - 4b} + a}\right)^n \left(\frac{\sqrt{a^2 - 4b} - a - 2x}{\sqrt{a^2 - 4b} - a}\right)^n 2^n(n - 1)Ax^2$$

$$\left.F_1\left(2; n, n; 3; \frac{-2x}{\sqrt{a^2 - 4b} + a}, \frac{2x}{\sqrt{a^2 - 4b} - a}\right)\right] + C$$

where, in the last equation, $_2F_1$ is the hypergeometric function, while F_1 is the Appell hypergeometric function of first kind.

17.11 Integration by Parts

The integration by parts is based on the well-known product rule for the derivatives:

$$(f(x)g(x))' = f'(x)g(x) + f(x)g'(x),$$

thus

$$f'(x)g(x) = (f(x)g(x))' - f(x)g'(x),$$

and integrating both sides, we get

$$\int f'(x)g(x)dx = \int [(f(x)g(x))' - f(x)g'(x)]dx$$

$$= \int (f(x)g(x))'dx - \int f(x)g'(x)dx$$

$$= f(x)g(x) - \int f(x)g'(x)dx$$

hence the antiderivative of $f'(x)g(x)$ is equal to $f(x)g(x)$ minus the antiderivative of $f(x)g'(x)$. Thus, we have a sort of multiplication rule applied to integration in which one of the functions is a derivative of some other function: to apply this rule, we must bear in mind this concept. Integration by parts can work well if (but not only if), for example, the product is of the type $x^n \log(x)$, say, $f(x)g(x) = 2x^4 \log(x)$.

We know that $2x^4$ is the derivative of $\frac{2}{5}x^5$ and that $\log(x)$ is the antiderivative of $\frac{1}{x}$; hence, we can obtain

$$
\begin{aligned}
\int 2x^4 \log(x)\mathrm{d}x &= \frac{2}{5}x^5 \log(x) - \int \frac{2}{5}x^5 \frac{1}{x}\mathrm{d}x \\
&= \frac{2}{5}x^5 \log(x) - \frac{2}{5}\int x^4 \mathrm{d}x \\
&= \frac{2}{5}x^5 \log(x) - \frac{2}{25}x^5 + C \\
&= \frac{2}{25}x^5(5\log(x) - 1) + C,
\end{aligned}
$$

where C is the constant of integration.

Note that in doing the alternative choice, e.g., considering that $\log(x)$ is the derivative of $x(\log(x) - 1)$ and that $2x^4$ is the antiderivative of $8x^3$, then the integral becomes

$$
\begin{aligned}
\int 2x^4 \log(x)\mathrm{d}x &= 2x^4 x(\log(x) - 1) - \int 8x(\log(x) - 1)x^3 \mathrm{d}x \\
&= 2x^5(\log(x) - 1) - 8\int x^4(\log(x) - 1)\mathrm{d}x \\
&= 2x^5(\log(x) - 1) - 8\left(\frac{1}{5}x^5 \log(x) - \frac{6}{25}x^5 + C_1\right) \\
&= 2x^5(\log(x) - 1) - \left(\frac{8}{25}x^5 (5\log(x) - 6)\right) + C_2 \\
&= \frac{2}{25}x^5(5\log(x) - 1) + C,
\end{aligned}
$$

where $C_2 = -C_1 = C$.

Hence, the result is the same, but in this case, the integration seems a bit more complicated: thus, a crucial issue is the choice of the couple of derivative and antiderivative easier to be managed.

We can take another example by calculating the integral of $x\cos(x)$: since $\cos(x)$ is the derivative of $\sin(x)$ and since x is the antiderivative of 1, then we can write

$$
\begin{aligned}
\int x\cos(x)\mathrm{d}x &= x\sin(x) - \int 1\sin(x)\mathrm{d}x \\
&= x\sin(x) + \cos(x) + C;
\end{aligned}
$$

again, taking the alternative choice (x is the derivative of $\frac{1}{2}x^2$, and $\cos(x)$ is the antiderivative of $-\sin(x)$), we get

$$\int x\cos(x)dx = \frac{1}{2}x^2\cos(x) + \int \frac{1}{2}x^2\sin(x)dx$$

$$= \frac{1}{2}x^2\cos(x) - \frac{1}{2}x^2\cos(x) + \int x\cos(x)dx$$

$$= \int x\cos(x)dx,$$

thus in essence, we have found an identity or—better—a loop, because we were obliged to apply twice the integration by parts and because the first two members on the r.h.s. cancel out. Indeed, this is another example showing the importance of the accurate choice (which is which) of the couple of derivative and antiderivative.

17.12 Integration by Substitution

The integration by substitution is based on the substitution of the variable of integration to get a simpler form to be integrated and then to back substitute the original integration variable in the result. Take the integral

$$\int (x+1)\, dx = \frac{1}{2}x^2 + x + C; \tag{17.21}$$

its result is easy to obtain, but what if we integrate with respect to $x+1$ instead of x? Let us do the substitution $x+1 \rightarrow u$: by virtue of this substitution, we also must impose $du = d(x+1)$, i.e., $du = dx$, thus the integral now reads

$$\int (x+1)\, dx = \int u\, du$$

$$= \frac{1}{2}u^2 + C,$$

and substituting back $u \rightarrow x+1$, we have

$$\frac{1}{2}u^2 + C \rightarrow \frac{1}{2}(x+1)^2 + C$$

and

$$\frac{1}{2}(x+1)^2 + C = \frac{1}{2}x^2 + x + \frac{1}{2} + C$$

$$= \frac{1}{2}x^2 + x + C', \tag{17.22}$$

where $\frac{1}{2} + C = C'$ is the new constant of integration. Note that results in (17.21) and (17.22) coincide.

Assume we want to integrate $f(x) = (2x + 1)^2$: it would not be a difficult task since by the linearity of antiderivative, we obtain

$$\int (2x + 1)^2 dx = \int (4x^2 + 4x + 1)\, dx$$

$$= \int 4x^2\, dx + \int 4x\, dx + \int 1\, dx$$

$$= \frac{4}{3}x^3 + 2x^2 + x + C;$$

however, let us try to see what happens if we put $2x + 1 = u$.

Apparently, the integral would take the form $\int u^2 du$, but

$$du = d(2x + 1),$$

thus

$$du = 2dx,$$

and

$$dx = \frac{1}{2}du$$

hence the integral after the substitution $2x + 1 \to u$ reads

$$\int (2x + 1)^2 dx = \int \frac{u^2}{2} du$$

$$= \frac{1}{2} \int u^2 du$$

and we obtain

$$\frac{1}{2} \int u^2 du = \frac{1}{6}u^3 + C.$$

Now, we can transform this result by substituting u with the original value $2x+1$, obtaining

$$\frac{1}{6}u^3 + C = \frac{1}{6}(2x + 1)^3 + C = \frac{4}{3}x^3 + 2x^2 + x + \frac{1}{6} + C$$

$$= \frac{4}{3}x^3 + 2x^2 + x + C'$$

being $\frac{1}{6} + C = C'$ the new constant of integration.

It is to point out that substitution has effects also on intervals of integration, which may be changed; this will be of great importance when dealing with definite integrals in the next section.

17.13 The Definite Integral (The Area Under a Curve)

A definite integral is a number: thus, despite the apparent similitude, the antiderivative (which is always a function, unless $f(x) = 0$) and the definite integral are two different things.

In general, if

$$\int f(x)dx = F(x) + C,$$

then

$$\int_a^b f(x)dx = F(x)|_a^b = F(b) - F(a),$$

provided the integral converges.

Note that the equation bridging indefinite and definite integral is

$$\int f(x)\,dx = \int_{x_0}^x f(y)\,dy.$$

Let us have $f(x) = \sin(x)$: in this case,

$$\int_a^b \sin(x)dx = -\cos(x)|_a^b = \cos(a) - \cos(b);$$

and if $f(x) = \frac{2}{x^3}$, then

$$\int_a^b \frac{2}{x^3}dx = -\frac{1}{x^2}\Big|_a^b = \frac{1}{a^2} - \frac{1}{b^2};$$

and, again, if $f(x) = \log(x - 1)$, then

$$\int_a^b \log(x - 1)dx = x \log(x - 1) - \log(x - 1) - x|_a^b$$

$$= a - b + (1 - a)\log(a - 1) + (b - 1)\log(b - 1).$$

Assume we are dealing with a function f, defined over the interval $[a, c]$: then the definite integral is additive w.r.t. extremes of integration, that is,

$$\int_a^b f(x)\,\mathrm{d}x + \int_b^c f(x)\,\mathrm{d}x = \int_a^c f(x)\,\mathrm{d}x,$$

provided $b \in [a, c]$; we also have

$$\int_a^b f(x)\,\mathrm{d}x = -\int_b^a f(x)\,\mathrm{d}x$$

and if extremes of integration are coincident

$$\int_a^a f(x)\,\mathrm{d}x = 0.$$

The definite integration maintains the linearity already seen in the indefinite integration as follows:

$$\int_a^b [\alpha f(x) \pm \beta g(x)]\,\mathrm{d}x = \int_a^b \alpha f(x)\,\mathrm{d}x \pm \int_a^b \beta g(x)\,\mathrm{d}x$$

$$= \alpha \int_a^b f(x)\,\mathrm{d}x \pm \beta \int_a^b g(x)\,\mathrm{d}x,$$

of course, assuming that both f and g are continuous and real in $[a, b]$ and with α, β real constants. If a real-valued function f is defined in an interval $[a, b]$ such that $f(x) \geq 0$ over all that interval, then also

$$\int_a^b f(x)\,\mathrm{d}x \geq 0$$

while, if g is also real and defined in the interval $[a, b]$, and if $g(x) \leq 0$ over all $[a, b]$, then

$$\int_a^b g(x)\,\mathrm{d}x \leq 0.$$

In the case f and g continuous and real in $[a, b]$, with $f \geq g$ over all the interval, then

$$\int_a^b f(x)\,\mathrm{d}x \geq \int_a^b g(x)\,\mathrm{d}x$$

which can be verified by taking a function $\phi(x) \geq 0$ over all the interval $[a, b]$ such that $\phi(x) = f(x) - g(x)$; hence,

$$\int_a^b f(x)\,dx = \int_a^b g(x)\,dx + \int_a^b \phi(x)\,dx.$$

The methods used to calculate the indefinite integrals (by partial fractions, by parts, by substitution, and so on) are also applicable to definite integrals; however, one must bear in mind that with the integration by substitution, also the limits of integration may change, depending on the variable substitution. Moreover, in the case of a non-integrable singularity between the range of integration, the integral does not converge, for example, if, for $a < P < b$, we have

$$\int_a^P f(x)\,dx = \pm\infty,$$

and

$$\int_P^b f(x)\,dx = \mp\infty;$$

in this case the Cauchy principal value , defined for a singularity at a finite point $P \in [a, b]$, is

$$\text{p.v.} \int_a^b f(x)dx = \lim_{\xi \to 0^+} \left(\int_a^{P-\xi} f(x)dx + \int_{P+\xi}^b f(x)dx \right)$$

On the other hand, if the singularity is at infinite, then

$$\int_{-\infty}^0 f(x)\,dx = \pm\infty,$$

and

$$\int_0^{+\infty} f(x)\,dx = \mp\infty.$$

so that one must calculate the Cauchy principal value as

$$\text{p.v.} \int_{-\infty}^{+\infty} f(x)dx = \lim_{\xi \to +\infty} \int_{-\xi}^{+\xi} f(x)dx.$$

There can also be the case of both singularities in the same integral: here, a double limit must be taken, in a form like

$$\text{p.v.} \int_{-\infty}^{+\infty} f(x)dx = \lim_{\zeta \to 0^+} \lim_{\xi \to 0^+} \left(\int_{a-\frac{1}{\zeta}}^{P-\xi} f(x)dx + \int_{P+\xi}^{b+\frac{1}{\zeta}} f(x)dx \right);$$

we do not enter more in details for this topic, which is out of our main interest.

As a first example of integration by partial fraction decomposition, we take the following integral:

$$\int_5^{10} \frac{3x^4 + 6x^3 - 9x^2 + 5x + 7}{x^2 + 2x - 3} dx = \int_5^{10} 3x^2 dx + \int_5^{10} \frac{3}{x-1} dx + \int_5^{10} \frac{2}{x+3} dx$$

$$= x^3 \Big|_5^{10} + 3\log(x-1)|_5^{10} + 2\log(x+3)|_5^{10}$$

$$= (1000 - 125) + 3[\log(9) - \log(4)]$$

$$\quad + 2[\ln(13) - \ln(8)]$$

$$= 875 + 6\log(3) - 6\log(2) + 2\log(13)$$

$$\quad - 6\log(2)$$

$$= 875 + 6\log(3) - 12\log(2) + 2\log(13).$$

We observe that the function we are going to integrate is not always defined: since for

$$f(x) = \frac{3x^4 + 6x^3 - 9x^2 + 5x + 7}{x^2 + 2x - 3}$$

we have $\text{Dom}(f) = \{x \in \mathbb{R}; x \neq -3 \text{ and } x \neq 1\}$, with

$$\lim_{x \to -3^-} \frac{3x^4 + 6x^3 - 9x^2 + 5x + 7}{x^2 + 2x - 3} = -\infty;$$

$$\lim_{x \to -3^+} \frac{3x^4 + 6x^3 - 9x^2 + 5x + 7}{x^2 + 2x - 3} = +\infty,$$

and

$$\lim_{x \to 1^-} \frac{3x^4 + 6x^3 - 9x^2 + 5x + 7}{x^2 + 2x - 3} = -\infty;$$

$$\lim_{x \to 1^+} \frac{3x^4 + 6x^3 - 9x^2 + 5x + 7}{x^2 + 2x - 3} = +\infty,$$

thus, for example, we see that within the limits from -2 to $+4$, the integral does not converge (e.g., it is not finite):

$$\int_{-2}^{+4} \frac{3x^4 + 6x^3 - 9x^2 + 5x + 7}{x^2 + 2x - 3}\,\mathrm{d}x \to \text{Does Not Converge}$$

due to a non-integrable singularity at point $x = 1$.

Incidentally, we can obtain the Cauchy Principal Value integral as follows

$$\mathrm{p.v.}\int_{-2}^{+4} \frac{3x^4 + 6x^3 - 9x^2 + 5x + 7}{x^2 + 2x - 3}\,\mathrm{d}x = 72 + \log(49).$$

17.14 Some Integral Functions

Some important functions are given by definite integrals. The most used is possibly the Euler gamma function $\Gamma(m)$, which, given a positive integer m, is defined by

$$\Gamma(m + 1) = m! \tag{17.23}$$

such that

$$\Gamma(m + 1) = m(m - 1)(m - 2) \cdots (m - n + 1)(m - n)!$$
$$= m(m - 1)(m - 2) \cdots (m - n + 1)\Gamma(m - n + 1),$$

We note that $\Gamma(m)$ requires m to be a positive integer. Clearly, $\Gamma(z)$ is a generalization of the factorial: it is defined for positive integers and is not defined for negative integers; however, the gamma function is also defined for possible other values assumed by a real or complex variable z, based on the definition

$$\Gamma(z + 1) = \int_0^{+\infty} t^z e^{-t}\,\mathrm{d}t\,, \tag{17.24}$$

equivalent to

$$\Gamma(z) = \int_0^{+\infty} t^{z-1} e^{-t}\,\mathrm{d}t\,. \tag{17.25}$$

By the way, we see the perfect equivalence of Eqs. (17.23) and (17.24), since, from the integral in (17.24), integrating by parts, taking e^{-t} as the derivative of $-e^{-t}$, also being $z\, t^{z-1}$ the derivative of t^z, one obtains

$$\Gamma(z+1) = \int_0^{+\infty} t^z e^{-t} dt$$

$$= -t^z e^{-t}\big|_0^{+\infty} + z \int_0^{+\infty} t^{z-1} e^{-t}\, dt$$

$$= z\,\Gamma(z)\,.$$

Thus, for the complex variable $z = x + iy$, we can write

$$\Gamma(z) = \int_0^{+\infty} t^{x+iy-1} e^{-t}\, dt$$

$$= \int_0^{+\infty} t^{x-1} t^{iy} e^{-t}\, dt$$

$$= \int_0^{+\infty} t^{x-1} e^{iy\log(t)} e^{-t}\, dt$$

$$= \int_0^{+\infty} [t^{x-1}(\cos(y\log(t)) + i\,\sin(y\log(t))\, e^{-t}]\, dt$$

where we used the known relation $e^{is} = \cos(s) + i\,\sin(s)$.

An important and somewhat unexpected result is

$$\Gamma\left(\frac{1}{2}\right) = \int_0^{+\infty} t^{-1/2} e^{-t}\, dt$$

$$= \int_0^{+\infty} \frac{e^{-t}}{\sqrt{t}}\, dt$$

$$= \int_0^{+\infty} \frac{e^{-\xi^2}}{\sqrt{t}}\, 2\sqrt{t}\, d\xi$$

$$= 2 \int_0^{+\infty} e^{-\xi^2}\, d\xi$$

$$= \int_{-\infty}^{+\infty} e^{-\xi^2}\, d\xi$$

$$= \sqrt{\pi}\,,$$

where we use the substitution $\sqrt{t} \to \xi$, so that $\mathrm{d}t \to 2\sqrt{t}\mathrm{d}\xi$; therefore, $\Gamma(\frac{1}{2})$ is transformed in the Gauss integral.

We note that Eq. (17.25) reads also

$$
\begin{aligned}
\Gamma(z) &= \int_0^{+\infty} t^{z-1} e^{-t}\, \mathrm{d}t \\
&= \int_0^{+\infty} t^{z-1} \left[\lim_{n \to +\infty} \left(1 - \frac{t}{n}\right)^n \right] \mathrm{d}t \\
&= \lim_{n \to +\infty} \int_0^{+\infty} t^{z-1} \left(1 - \frac{t}{n}\right)^n \mathrm{d}t \\
&= \lim_{n \to +\infty} \frac{n^z n!}{z(z+1)(z+2)\cdots(z+n)} \\
&= \lim_{n \to +\infty} \left[n^z n! \left(\prod_{k=0}^{n} (z+k) \right)^{-1} \right].
\end{aligned}
$$

The beta function $B(z_1, z_2)$ is defined for two complex numbers z_1 and z_2 (for which $\mathrm{Re}(z_1)$, $\mathrm{Re}(z_2) > 0$) as follows:

$$
B(z_1, z_2) = \int_0^1 t^{z_1-1}(1-t)^{z_2-1}\, \mathrm{d}t , \tag{17.26}
$$

and since

$$
\Gamma(z_1)\Gamma(z_2) = \int_0^{+\infty} \int_0^{+\infty} p^{z_1-1} q^{z_2-1} e^{-(p+q)}\, \mathrm{d}p\, \mathrm{d}q,
$$

letting $p = \xi\varsigma$ and $q = \xi - \xi\varsigma$, we get

$$
\begin{aligned}
\Gamma(z_1)\Gamma(z_2) &= \int_0^{+\infty} \int_0^1 (\xi\varsigma)^{z_1-1} (\xi - \xi\varsigma)^{z_2-1} e^{-\xi}\, \mathrm{d}\varsigma\, \mathrm{d}\xi \\
&= \int_0^1 \varsigma^{z_1-1}(1-\varsigma)^{z_2-1}\, \mathrm{d}\varsigma \int_0^{+\infty} e^{-\varsigma\xi} \xi^{z_1+z_2-1}\, \mathrm{d}\xi,
\end{aligned}
$$

thus, rearranging and using the definition of the beta function in Eq. (17.26), we obtain

$$
\int_0^1 \varsigma^{z_1-1}(1-\varsigma)^{z_2-1}\, \mathrm{d}\varsigma = \frac{\Gamma(z_1)\Gamma(z_2)}{\displaystyle\int_0^{+\infty} e^{-\varsigma\xi} \xi^{z_1+z_2-1}\, \mathrm{d}\xi} ,
$$

hence we find the important relation between beta and gamma functions as follows:

$$B(z_1, z_2) = \frac{\Gamma(z_1)\Gamma(z_2)}{\Gamma(z_1 + z_2)}.$$

17.15 Partial Derivatives

A function of two or more variables is generally defined as $y = f(x_1, x_2, \ldots, x_n)$ to say that the value of the variable y value depends on the values assumed by n independent variables x_k, such that $f : \mathbb{R}^n \to \mathbb{R}$. A simple example of a function of two independent variables is $w(x, y) = 3xy - y^2$, while a bit more complicated example is $z(x, y) = \log(y \cos(x))$. The number of independent variables is virtually infinite, but for our purposes, we will consider situations in which only few independent variables are involved. In general, given $y = f(x_1, x_2, \ldots, x_n)$, we define

$$\frac{\partial^\alpha y(x_1, x_2, \ldots, x_n)}{\partial x_1^{\beta_1} \partial x_2^{\beta_2} \cdots \partial x_n^{\beta_n}} \tag{17.27}$$

the partial derivative of order α of y taken β_1 times with respect to x_1, β_2 times with respect to x_2,..., and β_n times with respect x_n, provided $\alpha = \beta_1 + \beta_2 + \cdots + \beta_n$.

For a function $f(x, y)$ of two independent variables, we may calculate the derivative with respect to x as

$$f_x(x, y) = \frac{\partial f(x, y)}{\partial x} = \lim_{h \to 0} \frac{f(x + h, y) - f(x, y)}{h}$$

and the derivative with respect to y as

$$f_y(x, y) = \frac{\partial f(x, y)}{\partial y} = \lim_{h \to 0} \frac{f(x, y + h) - f(x, y)}{h},$$

assuming that both limits exist and are finite.

The rules for the differentiation of a function of two or more variables are the same as we already have seen for the function of one variable.

Let us consider the function $w(x, y) = 3xy - y^2$: it can be derived with respect to both x and y as follows: if we derive with respect to x, then y is considered a constant term, and if we derive with respect to y, then x is considered a constant term. This function has six possible partial derivatives as follows:

$$\frac{\partial(3xy - y^2)}{\partial x} = 3y,$$

$$\frac{\partial^2(3xy - y^2)}{\partial x^2} = \frac{\partial}{\partial x}\left(\frac{\partial(3xy - y^2)}{\partial x}\right) = \frac{\partial(3y)}{\partial x} = 0,$$

$$\frac{\partial(3xy - y^2)}{\partial y} = 3x - 2y,$$

$$\frac{\partial^2(3xy - y^2)}{\partial y^2} = \frac{\partial}{\partial y}\left(\frac{\partial(3xy - y^2)}{\partial y}\right) = \frac{\partial(3x - 2y)}{\partial y} = -2,$$

$$\frac{\partial^2(3xy - y^2)}{\partial x \partial y} = \frac{\partial}{\partial y}\left(\frac{\partial(3xy - y^2)}{\partial x}\right) = \frac{\partial(3y)}{\partial y} = 3,$$

$$\frac{\partial^2(3xy - y^2)}{\partial y \partial x} = \frac{\partial}{\partial x}\left(\frac{\partial(3xy - y^2)}{\partial y}\right) = \frac{\partial^2(3x - 2y)}{\partial x} = 3.$$

Note that

$$\frac{\partial^2(3xy - y^2)}{\partial x \partial y} = \frac{\partial^2(3xy - y^2)}{\partial y \partial x},$$

and so when deriving two times, first with respect to x and then with respect to y, we get the same result obtained when deriving first with respect to y and then with respect to x. Of course, deriving a function of y only with respect to x, and vice versa, one obtains zero.

For the other function $z(x, y) = \log(y \cos(x))$, we may use the chain rule to obtain the first two partial derivatives as follows:

$$\begin{aligned}
\frac{\partial}{\partial x} \log(y \cos(x)) &= \frac{\partial \log(v)}{\partial v} \frac{\partial v}{\partial x} \\
&= \frac{1}{y \cos(x)} y \frac{\partial \cos(x)}{\partial x} \\
&= -\frac{1}{\cos(x)} \sin(x) \\
&= -\tan(x)
\end{aligned}$$

and

$$\begin{aligned}
\frac{\partial}{\partial y} \log(y \cos(x)) &= \frac{\partial \log(v)}{\partial v} \frac{\partial v}{\partial y} \\
&= \frac{1}{y \cos(x)} \cos(x) \frac{\partial y}{\partial y} \\
&= \frac{1}{y} 1 \\
&= \frac{1}{y},
\end{aligned}$$

hence (here we stop at fourth partial derivatives even if much more differentiations are possible)

$$\frac{\partial \log(y \cos(x))}{\partial x} = -\tan(x)$$

$$\frac{\partial^2 \log(y \cos(x))}{\partial x^2} = -\frac{1}{\cos^2(x)}$$

$$\frac{\partial^3 \log(y \cos(x))}{\partial x^3} = -2\frac{\tan(x)}{\cos^2(x)}$$

$$\frac{\partial^4 \log(y \cos(x))}{\partial x^4} = 2\frac{\cos(2x) - 2}{\cos^4(x)}$$

while

$$\frac{\partial \log(y \cos(x))}{\partial y} = \frac{1}{y}$$

$$\frac{\partial^2 \log(y \cos(x))}{\partial y^2} = -\frac{1}{y^2}$$

$$\frac{\partial^3 \log(y \cos(x))}{\partial y^3} = \frac{2}{y^3}$$

$$\frac{\partial^4 \log(y \cos(x))}{\partial y^4} = -\frac{6}{y^4}$$

so that other differentiations are simple:

$$\frac{\partial^2 \log(y \cos(x))}{\partial x \partial y} = \frac{\partial^3 \log(y \cos(x))}{\partial x^2 \partial y} = \frac{\partial^4 \log(y \cos(x))}{\partial x^3 \partial y} = 0;$$

$$\frac{\partial^2 \log(y \cos(x))}{\partial y \partial x} = \frac{\partial^3 \log(y \cos(x))}{\partial y^2 \partial x} = \frac{\partial^4 \log(y \cos(x))}{\partial y^3 \partial x} = 0.$$

As a last example, let us consider the function $z = \sin(2xy^2)$: taking into account only the first and second derivatives, this reads

$$\frac{\partial \sin(2xy^2)}{\partial x} = 2y^2 \cos(2xy^2)$$

$$\frac{\partial^2 \sin(2xy^2)}{\partial x^2} = 4y^2 \sin(2xy^2)$$

$$\frac{\partial \sin(2xy^2)}{\partial y} = 4xy \cos(2xy^2)$$

$$\frac{\partial^2 \sin(2xy^2)}{\partial y^2} = 4x\cos(2xy^2) - 16x^2y^2\sin(2xy^2)$$

$$\frac{\partial^2 \sin(2xy^2)}{\partial x \partial y} = \frac{\partial(4y^2\sin(2xy^2))}{\partial y}$$

$$= 4xy\cos(2xy^2) - 8xy^3\sin(2xy^2)$$

$$\frac{\partial^2 \sin(2xy^2)}{\partial y \partial x} = \frac{\partial(4xy\cos(2xy^2))}{\partial x}$$

$$= 4xy\cos(2xy^2) - 8xy^3\sin(2xy^2)$$

where again we see that $\frac{\partial^2 z}{\partial x \partial y} = \frac{\partial^2 z}{\partial y \partial x}$. This last finding, as the previous one, does not occur by chance: indeed, if $f(x, y)$ is a function defined over a given subset of $\mathbb{R}^2$ and both derivatives $\frac{\partial^2 f(x,y)}{\partial x \partial y}$ and $\frac{\partial^2 f(x,y)}{\partial y \partial x}$ are continuous, then it must be always $\frac{\partial^2 f(x,y)}{\partial x \partial y} = \frac{\partial^2 f(x,y)}{\partial y \partial x}$.

Let $f(x, y)$ be a continuous differentiable function on an open set $\mathbb{S}^2 \subset \mathbb{R}^2$, and assume that in any point $P \in \mathbb{S}^2$, the functions $\frac{\partial f}{\partial x}$, $\frac{\partial f}{\partial y}$, $\frac{\partial^2 f}{\partial x \partial y}$, and $\frac{\partial^2 f}{\partial y \partial x}$ are also all defined and continuous. Now, choose a neighborhood $\mathbb{P}(P_0, \varepsilon)$ of a point $P_0 = (x_0, y_0)$, with radius ε, and define

$$u(x, y) = f(x, y) - f(x, y_0);$$

$$v(x, y) = f(x, y) - f(x_0, y),$$

with $x > x_0$, $y > y_0$. Applying the mean value theorem (by Lagrange) twice, after treating $u(x, y)$ first as a function only of x and then only of y, we have

$$u(x, y) - u(x, y_0) = (x - x_0)\left(\frac{\partial f(p, y)}{\partial x} - \frac{\partial f(p, y_0)}{\partial x}\right)$$

$$= (x - x_0)(y - y_0)\frac{\partial^2 f(p, q)}{\partial x \partial y},$$

in which values p and q are, respectively, defined with $x_0 < p < x$ and $y_0 < q < y$ and since $u(x, y)$ is derivable in the interval $[x_0, x]$, as well as $\frac{\partial f(p,y)}{\partial x}$ is derivable in the interval $[y_0, y]$. Using the same procedure for $v(x, y)$, with the same assumptions about derivability, we get

$$v(x, y) - v(x, y_0) = (y - y_0)\left(\frac{\partial f(x, r)}{\partial y} - \frac{\partial f(x_0, r)}{\partial x}\right)$$

$$= (y - y_0)(x - x_0)\frac{\partial^2 f(r, s)}{\partial y \partial x},$$

where r and s are, respectively, defined with $y_0 < r < y$ and $x_0 < s < x$. On the other hand, we see that

$$u(x, y) - u(x, y_0) = v(x, y)$$
$$= f(x, y) - f(x_0, y)$$

thus

$$\frac{\partial^2 f(p, q)}{\partial x \partial y} = \frac{\partial^2 f(r, s)}{\partial y \partial x},$$

but passing to the limits $(x, y) \to (x_0, y_0)$, we have

$$\frac{\partial^2 f(p, q)}{\partial x \partial y} = \frac{\partial^2 f(x_0, y_0)}{\partial x \partial y};$$

$$\frac{\partial^2 f(r, s)}{\partial y \partial x} = \frac{\partial^2 f(x_0, y_0)}{\partial y \partial x},$$

since when $x \to x_0$ then $p, r \to x_0$ and when $y \to y_0$, then $q, s \to y_0$, hence,

$$\frac{\partial^2 f(x_0, y_0)}{\partial x \partial y} = \frac{\partial^2 f(x_0, y_0)}{\partial y \partial x}.$$

The chain rule for partial derivatives is also important: if $z = f(x, y)$ with $x = x(t)$ and $y = y(t)$, then we have

$$\frac{dz}{dt} = \frac{\partial z(x, y)}{\partial x} \frac{dx(t)}{dt} + \frac{\partial z(x, y)}{\partial y} \frac{dy(t)}{dt},$$

and if, instead, $z = f(x, y)$ with $x = x(u, t)$ and $y = y(u, t)$, then

$$\frac{\partial z}{\partial u} = \frac{\partial z}{\partial x} \frac{\partial x}{\partial u} + \frac{\partial z}{\partial y} \frac{\partial y}{\partial u}$$

$$\frac{\partial z}{\partial t} = \frac{\partial z}{\partial x} \frac{\partial x}{\partial t} + \frac{\partial z}{\partial y} \frac{\partial y}{\partial t}.$$

To use a more difficult example, let us take $z = x^2 y \sin(x) + y$ with

$$x = \log(t - 1)$$
$$y = e^{tu - 2t},$$

and then let us first calculate

$$\frac{\partial \log(t-1)}{\partial t} = \frac{1}{t-1}$$

$$\frac{\partial \log(t-1)}{\partial u} = 0$$

and

$$\frac{\partial(e^{tu-2t})}{\partial t} = (u-2)\,e^{t(u-2)}$$

$$\frac{\partial(e^{tu-2t})}{\partial u} = t\,e^{t(u-2)},$$

so that

$$\frac{\partial z(x,y)}{\partial t} = \frac{\partial(x^2 y \sin(x) + y)}{\partial t}$$

$$= \frac{\partial(x^2 y \sin(x) + y)}{\partial x}\frac{\partial \log(t-1)}{\partial t}$$

$$+ \frac{\partial(x^2 y \sin(x) + y)}{\partial y}\frac{\partial(e^{tu-2t})}{\partial t}$$

$$= \frac{\partial(x^2 y \sin(x) + y)}{\partial x}\frac{1}{t-1}$$

$$+ \frac{\partial(x^2 y \sin(x) + y)}{\partial y}\,(u-2)\,e^{t(u-2)}$$

$$= \frac{x^2 y \cos(x) + 2xy \sin x}{t-1}$$

$$+ (x^2 \sin(x) + 1)\,(u-2)\,e^{t(u-2)}$$

and

$$\frac{\partial z(x,y)}{\partial u} = \frac{\partial(x^2 y \sin(x) + y)}{\partial u}$$

$$= \frac{\partial(x^2 y \sin(x) + y)}{\partial x}\frac{\partial \log(t-1)}{\partial u}$$

$$+ \frac{\partial(x^2 y \sin(x) + y)}{\partial y}\frac{\partial(e^{tu-2t})}{\partial u}$$

$$= \frac{\partial(x^2 y \sin(x) + y)}{\partial y}t\,e^{t(u-2)}$$

$$= \left(x^2 \sin(x) + 1\right)t\,e^{t(u-2)}.$$

The search for extreme values when dealing with a function of multiple variables may be represented, without loss of generality, by the following steps evaluated for a function $f(x, y)$ as follows:

- Let

$$\frac{\partial f(x, y)}{\partial x} = 0$$

$$\frac{\partial f(x, y)}{\partial y} = 0$$

- Solve above equations obtaining the critical values x_0 and y_0.
- Calculate the second derivatives

$$\frac{\partial^2 f(x, y)}{\partial x^2} ; \quad \frac{\partial^2 f(x, y)}{\partial x \partial y} ; \quad \frac{\partial^2 f(x, y)}{\partial y \partial x} ; \quad \frac{\partial^2 f(x, y)}{\partial y^2}$$

- Calculate the determinant $\det(\mathbf{M})$ (we will see what a determinant is in the next chapter) at point(s) of coordinates (x_0, y_0)

$$\det(\mathbf{M}) = \begin{vmatrix} \partial_x^2 f(x, y) & \partial_{yx}^2 f(x, y) \\ \partial_{xy}^2 f(x, y) & \partial_y^2 f(x, y) \end{vmatrix}$$

$$= \frac{\partial^2 f(x, y)}{\partial x^2} \frac{\partial^2 f(x, y)}{\partial y^2} - \frac{\partial^2 f(x, y)}{\partial x \partial y} \frac{\partial^2 f(x, y)}{\partial y \partial x}$$

- If $\det(\mathbf{M}) < 0 \Longrightarrow (x_0, y_0)$ is a saddle point
- If $\det(\mathbf{M}) = 0 \Longrightarrow (x_0, y_0)$, more info for classification are needed
- If $\det(\mathbf{M}) > 0$ and $\frac{\partial^2 f(x,y)}{\partial x^2} < 0 \Longrightarrow (x_0, y_0)$ is a local maximum
- If $\det(\mathbf{M}) > 0$ and $\frac{\partial^2 f(x,y)}{\partial x^2} > 0 \Longrightarrow (x_0, y_0)$ is a local minimum

For example, let us consider $f(x, y) = 3x^2 + 2x - y^2$. We have

$$\frac{\partial f(x, y)}{\partial x} = 6x + 2$$

$$\frac{\partial f(x, y)}{\partial y} = -2y$$

then, letting the first derivatives go to zero, we find

$$6x + 2 = 0 \Rightarrow x - \frac{1}{3}$$

$$-2y = 0 \Rightarrow y = 0$$

thus our critical point has coordinates $(-\frac{1}{3}, 0)$.

The second derivatives are

$$\frac{\partial^2 f(x, y)}{\partial x^2} = \frac{\partial}{\partial x}(6x + 2) = 6$$

$$\frac{\partial^2 f(x, y)}{\partial x \partial y} = \frac{\partial}{\partial y}(6x + 2) = 0$$

$$\frac{\partial^2 f(x, y)}{\partial y \partial x} = \frac{\partial}{\partial x}(-2y) = 0$$

$$\frac{\partial^2 f(x, y)}{\partial y^2} = \frac{\partial}{\partial y}(-2y) = -2$$

hence

$$\det(\mathbf{M}) = \frac{\partial^2 f(x, y)}{\partial x^2} \frac{\partial^2 f(x, y)}{\partial y^2} - \frac{\partial^2 f(x, y)}{\partial x \partial y} \frac{\partial^2 f(x, y)}{\partial y \partial x}$$

$$= -12 - 0$$

$$= -12.$$

We see that $\det(\mathbf{M}) = -12$; thus, $\det(\mathbf{M})$ is a constant at any point (x, y), including our critical point $(-\frac{1}{3}, 0)$, and therefore, we may conclude that $(-\frac{1}{3}, 0)$ is a saddle point, being $\det(\mathbf{M}) < 0$.

17.16 Multiple Integrals

Multiple integrals refer to more than one integration, generally evaluated for a function of more than one variable: they can be indefinite or definite as well. For example, if we take the real function of two real variables $f(x, y) = x^2 \sin(y)$, we calculate the indefinite integral as follows:

$$\int \int x^2 \sin(y) dx dy = \int \left(\int x^2 \sin(y) dx \right) dy$$

$$= \int \left(\frac{1}{3} x^3 \sin(y) + C_1 \right) dy$$

$$= C_2 + C_1 y - \frac{1}{3} x^3 \cos(y),$$

thus, the task is to first calculate the innermost integral (in this case, with respect to dx) and then integrate this result in the outermost integral (here, with respect to dy). Caution must be paid to integration constants.

Now, let us take the same function, but switching the order of integration, we have

$$\int\int x^2 \sin(y)\mathrm{d}y\mathrm{d}x = \int\left(\int x^2 \sin(y)\mathrm{d}y\right)\mathrm{d}x$$

$$= \int\left(-x^2 \cos(y) + C_1\right)\mathrm{d}x$$

$$= C_2 + C_1 x - \frac{1}{3}x^3 \cos(y),$$

thus the order of integration is important, since it produces different results.

Now, let us consider the definite multiple integral of $x^2 \sin(y)$ in a given interval, say for x ranging from 1 to 5 and for y ranging from 2 to 3

$$\int_{y=2}^{y=3}\int_{x=1}^{x=5} x^2 \sin(y)\mathrm{d}x\mathrm{d}y = \int_{y=2}^{y=3}\left(\int_{x=1}^{x=5} x^2 \sin(y)\mathrm{d}x\right)\mathrm{d}y$$

$$= \int_{y=2}^{y=3}\frac{124}{3}\sin(y)\mathrm{d}y$$

$$= \frac{124}{3}(\cos(2) - \cos(3)),$$

and, again, switching the integrations, we also have

$$\int_{x=1}^{x=5}\int_{y=2}^{y=3} x^2 \sin(y)\mathrm{d}y\mathrm{d}x = \int_{x=1}^{x=5}\left(\int_{y=2}^{y=3} x^2 \sin(y)\mathrm{d}y\right)\mathrm{d}x$$

$$= \int_{x=1}^{x=5} x^2(\cos(2) - \cos(3))\mathrm{d}y$$

$$= \frac{124}{3}(\cos(2) - \cos(3)),$$

where we see that in this case the definite double integrals get the same result.

Let us now try a function of three variables like $f(x, y, z) = x^2 \sin(y)\log(z)$, and take the integral

$$\int\int\int x^2 \sin(y)\log(z)\mathrm{d}x\mathrm{d}y\mathrm{d}z = \int\left(\int\left(\int x^2 \sin(y)\log(z)\mathrm{d}x\right)\mathrm{d}y\right)\mathrm{d}z$$

$$= \int\left(\int\left(C_1 + \frac{1}{3}x^3 \log(z)\sin(y)\right)\mathrm{d}y\right)\mathrm{d}z$$

$$= \int\left(C_2 + C_1 y - \frac{1}{3}x^3 \cos(y)\log(z)\right)\mathrm{d}z$$

$$= C_3 + C_2 z + C_1 yz + \frac{1}{3} x^3 z \cos(y)$$

$$- \frac{1}{3} x^3 z \cos(y) \log(z).$$

The situation does not appear much simpler in cases like $g(x, y, z) = \alpha x + \beta y + \gamma z$, where we find

$$\int \int \int (\alpha x + \beta y + \gamma z) dx dy dz = \int \left(\int \left(\int (\alpha x + \beta y + \gamma z) dx \right) dy \right) dz$$

$$= \int \left(\int \left(C_1 + \frac{\alpha x^2}{2} + \beta xy + \gamma xz \right) dy \right) dz$$

$$= \int \left(C_2 + Cy + \frac{\alpha x^2 y}{2} + \frac{\beta xy^2}{2} + \gamma xyz \right) dz$$

$$= C_3 + C_2 z + C_1 yz + \frac{\alpha x^2 yz}{2}$$

$$+ \frac{\beta xy^2 z}{2} + \frac{\gamma xyz^2}{2}.$$

Integral Transforms

18

To work with integral transforms, we must recall some concepts regarding complex numbers and complex variables. A complex number $z \in \mathbb{C}$ is given in *Cartesian form* as

$$z = x + iy,$$

where $i = \sqrt{-1}$; any complex number has a real part $\mathrm{Re}(z) = x$ and an imaginary part $\mathrm{Im}(z) = y$, with $x, y \in \mathbb{R}$. Values $\mathrm{Re}(z) = x$ and $\mathrm{Im}(z) = y$ can be considered the coordinates of a point z lying in a Cartesian plane, here more properly called the Gauss plane, so that the point z in that Gauss coordinate system is given as $z(x, y)$ or even $z(\mathrm{Re}(z), \mathrm{Im}(z))$.

We define the module $|z|$ of the complex number z with the equation

$$|z| = \sqrt{(\mathrm{Re}(z))^2 + (\mathrm{Im}(z))^2},$$

thus, for example, if

$$z = 4 + 3i,$$

then

$$|z| = \sqrt{16 + 9} = 5;$$

note that $|z|$ is the distance from the point $z(x, y)$ to the origin $(0, 0)$ of the Gauss plane.

For any number $z \in \mathbb{C}$, we define its complex conjugate number $z^* \in \mathbb{C}$, such that

$$z = x + iy$$
$$z^* = x - iy$$

and

$$zz^* = (x + iy)(x - iy)$$
$$= x^2 + y^2$$
$$= |z|^2,$$

and therefore $zz^* \in \mathbb{R}$. Again, taking $z = 4 + 3i$, we have

$$zz^* = (4 + 3i)(4 - 3i)$$
$$= 16 - 12i + 12i + 9$$
$$= 25,$$

thus the square of the module $|z| = 5$.

In trigonometric form, a complex number is given as

$$z = \rho(\cos(\alpha) + i \sin(\alpha))$$

with

$$\mathrm{Re}(z) = \rho \cos(\alpha)$$
$$\mathrm{Im}(z) = \rho \sin(\alpha)$$

and with

$$z^* = \rho(\cos(\alpha) - i \sin(\alpha))$$
$$= \rho(\cos(\alpha) + i \sin(-\alpha)).$$

In the exponential form, a complex number is

$$z = \rho e^{i\alpha}$$

with

$$|z| = \rho.$$

Taking $z_1, z_2 \in \mathbb{C}$, such that

$$z_1 = \rho_1 e^{i\alpha_1}$$
$$z_2 = \rho_2 e^{i\alpha_2}$$

we have

$$z_1 z_2 = \rho_1 e^{i\alpha_1} \rho_2 e^{i\alpha_2}$$
$$= \rho_1 \rho_2 e^{i(\alpha_1 + \alpha_2)}$$

hence, we evolve

$$|z_1 z_2| = \rho_1 \rho_2$$
$$= |z_1||z_2|$$

as well as

$$\frac{z_1}{z_2} = \frac{\rho_1 e^{i\alpha_1}}{\rho_2 e^{i\alpha_2}}$$
$$= \frac{\rho_1}{\rho_2} e^{i(\alpha_1 - \alpha_2)}$$

from which

$$\left|\frac{z_1}{z_2}\right| = \frac{|z_1|}{|z_2|} = \frac{\rho_1}{\rho_2}.$$

There are complex-valued real functions, real-valued complex functions, and also complex-valued complex variables, which are, respectively, $f : \mathbb{R} \to \mathbb{C}$, $g : \mathbb{C} \to \mathbb{R}$, and $h : \mathbb{C} \to \mathbb{C}$. Possible examples are

$$f(t) = e^{zt}$$
$$g(z) = \text{Re}(z)$$
$$h(z) = z + \sin(z).$$

Among all of these functions, we will deal also with periodic functions, defined as

$$x(t) = x(t \pm T),$$

where T is a time interval called period of $x(t)$. The translation by exactly one period (to the left or to the right) of the graph of a periodic function will give a new graph of $x(t \pm T)$ exactly fitting on top of the original $x(t)$ graph. Moreover, it is evident that

$$x(t \pm T) = x(t \pm nT)$$

hence, if T is a period, then nT is a period, too.

18.1   Fourier Series

A periodic function $g(t)$ with period T_0 may be represented as

$$g(t) = \sum_{k=-\infty}^{+\infty} c_n e^{i 2\pi \nu_0 k t},$$

with $\nu_0 = \frac{1}{T_0}$ [1]. Fourier polynomials (series) are sums of elementary harmonic functions, written as

$$P_n(t) = \sum_{k=-n}^{n} \gamma_k e^{i k \omega t}, \tag{18.1}$$

where $i = \sqrt{-1}$ and where the period is $T = \frac{2\pi}{\omega}$, being ω the angular frequency and

$$\nu = \frac{\omega}{2\pi}$$

the frequency. Note that in Eq. (18.1), we also have $k \in \mathbb{Z}$, $t \in \mathbb{R}$, and $\gamma_k \in \mathbb{C}$.

We may find a Fourier polynomial also in the equivalent forms

$$P_n(t) = \alpha_0 + \sum_{k=1}^{n} (\alpha_k \cos(k\omega t) + \beta_k \sin(k\omega t)); \tag{18.2}$$

$$P_n(t) = \alpha_0 + \sum_{k=1}^{n} \rho_k \sin(k\omega t + \theta_k); \tag{18.3}$$

in fact, given the properties of the sine of a sum, we have

$$\rho_k \sin(k\omega t + \theta_k) = \rho_k (\cos(k\omega t) \sin(\theta_k) + \sin(k\omega t) \cos(\theta_k))$$
$$= (\rho_k \sin(\theta_k) \cos(k\omega t) + (\rho_k \cos(\theta_k) \sin(k\omega t)),$$

where putting

$$\begin{cases} \rho_k \sin(\theta_k) = \alpha_k \\ \rho_k \cos(\theta_k) = \beta_k \end{cases}$$

we obtain the equivalence

$$\rho_k \sin(k\omega t + \theta_k) = \alpha_k \cos(k\omega t) + \beta_k \sin(k\omega t);$$

thus,

$$\alpha_k^2 \beta_k^2 = \rho_k^2 \sin^2(\theta_k) + \rho_k^2 \cos^2(\theta_k)$$
$$= \rho_k^2 (\sin^2(\theta_k) + \cos^2(\theta_k))$$
$$= \rho_k^2$$

since $\sin^2(x) + \cos^2(x) = 1$ by definition.
   Now, since

$$\frac{\alpha_k}{\beta_k} = \frac{\sin(\theta_k)}{\cos(\theta_k)} = \tan(\theta_k),$$

then

$$\theta_k = \begin{cases} \arctan\left(\frac{\alpha_k}{\beta_k}\right); & \beta_k \geq 0 \\ \arctan\left(\frac{\alpha_k}{\beta_k}\right) + \pi; & \beta_k < 0 \end{cases}$$

proves that (18.2) is equivalent to (18.3).
   We see also that

$$x(t) = \gamma_k \exp(ik\omega t) + (\gamma_k \exp(ik\omega t))^*$$
$$= \gamma_k \exp(ik\omega t) + \gamma_k^* \exp(-ik\omega t)$$
$$= \gamma_k (\cos(k\omega t) + i \sin(k\omega t))$$
$$+ \gamma_k^* (\cos(k\omega t) - i \sin(k\omega t))$$
$$= (\gamma_k + \gamma_k^*) \cos(k\omega t) + i (\gamma_k - \gamma_k^*) \sin(k\omega t),$$

where putting

$$\begin{cases} \gamma_k + \gamma_k^* = 2 \operatorname{Re}(\gamma_k) = \alpha_k \\ i(\gamma_k - \gamma_k^*) = -2 \operatorname{Im}(\gamma_k) = \beta_k \end{cases}$$

we have

$$x(t) = \alpha_k \cos(k\omega t) + \beta_k \sin(k\omega t)$$

with

$$\gamma_k = \frac{\alpha_k - i\beta_k}{2}, \tag{18.4}$$

and this proves that (18.1) is equivalent to (18.3) and therefore also equivalent to (18.1).

Any elementary harmonic function $x(t)$ is associated with its *energy*, defined by

$$\|x(t)\|^2 = \int_0^T |x(t)|^2 dt,$$

equivalent to the square of the norm $\|x(t)\|$ and easily evaluable assuming to deal with a complex harmonic, so that

$$\|x_c(t)\|^2 = \int_0^T |\gamma_k \exp(ik\omega t)|^2 dt$$

$$= 1 \int_0^T |\gamma_k|^2 dt$$

$$= |\gamma_k|^2 \int_0^T dt$$

$$= |\gamma_k|^2 T.$$

The energy of a Fourier polynomial reads

$$\|P_n(t)\|^2 = \int_0^T |P_n(t)|^2 dt$$

$$= \int_0^T \left(\sum_{k=-n}^n \gamma_k e^{ik\omega t} \right)^2 dt$$

$$= \int_0^T \left(\sum_{k=-n}^n \gamma_k e^{ik\omega t} \right) \left(\sum_{k=-n}^n \gamma_k^* e^{-ik\omega t} \right) dt$$

$$= \int_0^T \sum_{j=-n}^n \left(\gamma_j e^{ij\omega t} \sum_{k=-n}^n \gamma_k^* e^{-ik\omega t} \right) dt$$

$$= \int_0^T \sum_{j=-n}^n \left(\sum_{k=-n}^n \gamma_j \gamma_k^* e^{-i(j-k)\omega t} \right) dt$$

T being the period. Note that in case $k = j$, then $i(j - k)\omega t = 0$, and $e^{-i0\omega t} = 1$, and so

$$\|P_n(t)\|^2 = \int_0^T \sum_{j=-n}^n \gamma_j \gamma_j^* dt$$

$$= \int_0^T \sum_{j=-n}^n |\gamma_j|^2 dt$$

$$= T \sum_{j=-n}^n |\gamma_j|^2.$$

The Fourier series permit to treat a function $f(t)$ as a sum of sine functions in the form $a_n \sin(\frac{n\pi t}{\ell})$.

The starting point is the orthogonality of the sine function, such that, given two real numbers m and n, with $m \neq n$, and using the *prostapheresis* formula

$$\sin(\alpha) \sin(\beta) = \frac{\cos(\alpha - \beta) - \cos(\alpha + \beta)}{2},$$

we get

$$\int_0^\ell \sin \frac{m\pi t}{\ell} \sin \frac{n\pi t}{\ell} dt = \frac{1}{2} \int_0^\ell \left(\cos \frac{(m-n)\pi t}{\ell} - \cos \frac{(m+n)\pi t}{\ell} \right) dt$$

$$= \frac{1}{2} \left(\int_0^\ell \cos \frac{(m-n)\pi t}{\ell} dt - \int_0^\ell \cos \frac{(m+n)\pi t}{\ell} dt \right)$$

$$= 0.$$

Now, let us write $f(t)$ as a sum of sine functions like

$$f(t) = \sum_{n=1}^{+\infty} a_n \sin\left(\frac{n\pi t}{\ell}\right);$$

hence, multiplying both sides by $\sin(\frac{m\pi t}{\ell})$ and then integrating from 0 to ℓ, we have

$$\int_0^\ell f(t) \sin\left(\frac{m\pi t}{\ell}\right) dt = \sum_{n=1}^{+\infty} a_n \int_0^\ell \sin\left(\frac{m\pi t}{\ell}\right) \sin\left(\frac{n\pi t}{\ell}\right) dt.$$

Note that the integral terms on the r.h.s. of equation are always zero if $m \neq n$ and are nonzero only if $m = n$; thus, we may write

$$\int_0^\ell f(t) \sin\left(\frac{n\pi t}{\ell}\right) dt = a_n \int_0^\ell \sin^2\left(\frac{n\pi t}{\ell}\right) dt$$

$$= a_n \frac{\ell}{2}$$

from which we obtain the a_n term of the Fourier series as

$$a_n = \frac{2}{\ell} \int_0^\ell f(t) \sin\left(\frac{n\pi t}{\ell}\right) dt.$$

In practice, we see that under some conditions, any periodic function can be considered the sum of a number of elementary sine functions. This notion can be virtually extended to any other function, since a nonperiodic function can be seen as a periodic function with an infinite period.

18.2   Convolution

The Dirac delta function $\delta(t)$ can be defined by means of the integral

$$\int_{-\infty}^{+\infty} f(t)\delta(t)dt = f(0),$$

which is a functional, whereas $f(t)$ is a test function, e.g., a function derivable an infinite number of times and equal to zero everywhere in its domain (in particular at $t \to \pm\infty$), except in a small interval. The Dirac delta is a distribution that can be seen as the derivative of a unit step function $u(t)$ defined as

$$u(t) = \begin{cases} 1 \text{ if } t > 0 \\ \frac{1}{2} \text{ if } t = 0 \\ 0 \text{ if } t < 0 \end{cases} \tag{18.5}$$

where the value at $t = 0$ is used only in a formal sense, since at $t = 0$, the step function has a jump discontinuity: however, we may assume that $u'(t)$ is also a functional, and thus, being $u(t) = 0$ in the interval $t \in]-\infty, 0[$, we have

$$\int_{-\infty}^{+\infty} u'(t)f(t)dt = -\int_{-\infty}^{+\infty} u(t)f'(t)dt$$

$$= -\int_0^{+\infty} f'(t)dt$$

$$= -f(t)|_0^{+\infty}$$

$$= -(f(+\infty) - f(0))$$

$$= f(0)$$

since f is always zero out of any limited interval in t.

The Dirac delta can also be defined as a limit

$$\int_a^b f(t)\delta(t)\mathrm{d}t = \lim_{n\to+\infty} \int_a^b \sqrt{\frac{n}{\pi}} f(t)e^{-nt^2}\mathrm{d}t, \tag{18.6}$$

since

$$
\begin{aligned}
\lim_{n\to+\infty} \int_a^b \sqrt{\frac{n}{\pi}} f(t)e^{-nt^2}\mathrm{d}t &= \lim_{n\to+\infty} \frac{1}{\sqrt{\pi}} \int_{a\sqrt{n}}^{b\sqrt{n}} f\left(\frac{\theta}{\sqrt{n}}\right) e^{-\theta^2}\mathrm{d}\theta \\
&= \frac{1}{\sqrt{\pi}} \int_{-\infty}^{+\infty} f(0)e^{-\theta^2}\mathrm{d}\theta \\
&= \frac{1}{\sqrt{\pi}} f(0) \int_{-\infty}^{+\infty} e^{-\theta^2}\mathrm{d}\theta \\
&= f(0) \\
&= \int_a^b f(t)\delta(t)\mathrm{d}t.
\end{aligned}
$$

which is often "translated" in its simpler form

$$\delta(t) = \lim_{n\to+\infty} \sqrt{\frac{n}{\pi}} f(t)e^{-nt^2}.$$

Equation (18.6) is not the only way to give the Dirac delta as a limit (in that case, the limit of a Gaussian): there are several other expressions defining $\delta(t)$ as a limit, for example,

$$\delta(t) = \frac{1}{\pi} \lim_{n\to+\infty} \frac{\sin(nt)}{t}.$$

The integral of the Dirac delta over an interval $[a, b]$ is

$$\int_a^b \delta(t)\mathrm{d}t = 1, \quad 0 \in [a, b]$$

while it is zero if $0 \notin [a, b]$; more precisely, we should write

$$\int_{-\epsilon}^{+\epsilon} \delta(t)\mathrm{d}t = 1, \ \forall \epsilon > 0.$$

Here, a precisation is needed: from a pure mathematical point of view, the above equation has something that is "wrong." Indeed, the integral should have been written just as

$$\int_{-\epsilon}^{+\epsilon} \delta(t) = 1,$$

e.g., without the dt closing the operation, since $\delta(t)$ is already a measure.

A somehow deeper discussion should be done to clarify the sense of the dt used at the end of an integral: its meaning is not just to specify which variable is interested in the integration nor to show where the integral operation stops but rather to tell that we are integrating a function using the Peano measure according to Riemann definition of integral, like a "sum of rectangles." In general, the Riemann integration require strong convergences, and is not always applicable, so new kinds of integration have been developed, like the Lebesgue integration, based on the Lebesgue measure. A measure is a function capable of measuring a set, for example, giving the length of an interval $[a, b]$ of the real line: when working with a measure μ over a given set (e.g., the set $\mathbb{R}$ of real numbers), the integral is given as

$$I = \int_{\mathbb{R}} f \, d\mu.$$

The Dirac delta function freezes the value of the function f (assumed to be continuous) to which it is applied, at the point where the Dirac delta itself is centered. In general, for a Dirac $\delta(t) \equiv \delta(t - 0)$, which is centered at $t = 0$, we will have

$$f(t)\delta(t) = f(0)\delta(t),$$

and for a Dirac delta $\delta(t - a)$, thus centered in $t = a$, we have

$$f(t - a)\delta(t) = f(a)\delta(t - a).$$

From these premises we can take a $\delta(t - \tau)$, thus centered in τ and calculate the integral

$$\int_{-\infty}^{+\infty} f(\tau)\delta(t - \tau)d\tau = \int_{-\infty}^{+\infty} f(t)\delta(t - \tau)d\tau$$

$$= f(t) \int_{-\infty}^{+\infty} \delta(t - \tau)d\tau$$

$$= f(t),$$

and this allows us to define a function (a signal) $f(t)$ in terms of a Dirac delta centered in τ.

What we have seen right above is that

$$f(t) = \int_{-\infty}^{+\infty} f(\tau)\delta(t - \tau)\mathrm{d}\tau \tag{18.7}$$

and the r.s.h. of Eq. (18.7) is called the convolution integral.

The convolution $x(t) * y(t)$ (or also $x * y(t)$) of two functions is the integral

$$x(t) * y(t) = y(t) * x(t) = \int_{-\infty}^{+\infty} x(\tau)y(t - \tau)\mathrm{d}\tau \tag{18.8}$$

which is commutative, as shown in the above equation.

The convolution has a neutral element, which we have already encountered in Eq. (18.7), since it is

$$x(t) * \delta(t) = \int_{-\infty}^{+\infty} x(\tau)\delta(t - \tau)\mathrm{d}\tau$$

$$= \delta(t) * x(t)$$

$$= x(t).$$

The convolution integral always converges if

$$t < 0 \Rightarrow \begin{cases} x(t) = 0 \\ y(t) = 0 \end{cases}$$

or if $x(t) = 0$ when $a > t$ and $b < t$, so as to have

$$x(t) * y(t) = \int_{a}^{b} x(\tau)y(t - \tau)\mathrm{d}\tau.$$

The derivative of a convolution is

$$\frac{\mathrm{d}(x(t) * y(t))}{\mathrm{d}t} = \frac{\mathrm{d}x(t)}{\mathrm{d}t} * y(t)$$

$$= \int_{-\infty}^{+\infty} x'(\tau)y(t - \tau)\mathrm{d}\tau,$$

or even

$$\frac{\mathrm{d}(x(t) * y(t))}{\mathrm{d}t} = \frac{\mathrm{d}y(t)}{\mathrm{d}t} * x(t)$$

$$= \int_{-\infty}^{+\infty} y'(\tau)x(t - \tau)\mathrm{d}\tau.$$

As an example, let us take the function $h(t)$ defined as

$$h(t) = \begin{cases} 0 \text{ if } t \leq -\frac{1}{2} \\ 1 \text{ if } -\frac{1}{2} < t < \frac{1}{2} \; ; \\ 0 \text{ if } t \geq \frac{1}{2} \end{cases}$$

we see that

$$h(t) = u(t + \tfrac{1}{2}) - u(t - \tfrac{1}{2}),$$

where $u(t)$ is the unit step already defined in Eq. (18.5).

Now, let us calculate the convolution $h(t) * h(t)$: we have

$$h(t) * h(t) = \int_{-\infty}^{+\infty} h(\tau)h(t - \tau)d\tau$$

$$= \int_{-1/2}^{+1/2} h(t - \tau)d\tau$$

$$= \int_{-1/2}^{+1/2} (u(t - \tau + \tfrac{1}{2}) - u(t - \tau - \tfrac{1}{2}))d\tau$$

$$= \int_{-1/2}^{+1/2} u(t - \tau + \tfrac{1}{2})d\tau$$

$$- \int_{-1/2}^{+1/2} u(t - \tau - \tfrac{1}{2})d\tau;$$

at this point, we may define

$$\begin{cases} p = t - \tau + \frac{1}{2} \Rightarrow \frac{dp}{d\tau} = -1 \Rightarrow dp = -d\tau \\ q = t - \tau - \frac{1}{2} \Rightarrow \frac{dq}{d\tau} = -1 \Rightarrow dq = -d\tau \end{cases}$$

to get

$$h(t) * h(t) = \int_{t}^{t+1} u(p)dp - \int_{t-1}^{t} u(q)dq$$

$$= pu(p)|_{p=t}^{p=t+1} - qu(q)|_{q=t-1}^{q=t}$$

$$= (t + 1)u(t + 1) - tu(t) - tu(t) + (t - 1)u(t - 1)$$

$$= (t + 1)u(t + 1) + (t - 1)u(t - 1) - 2tu(t)$$

thus

$$h(t) * h(t) = \begin{cases} 0 & \text{if } t \leq -1 \\ t+1 & \text{if } -1 < t \leq 0 \\ -t+1 & \text{if } 0 > t \geq 1 \\ 0 & \text{if } t > 1 \end{cases}.$$

18.3 Fourier Transform

The Fourier series are useful when dealing with periodic functions. Fourier transform can be used to give an alternative representation of several non-periodic functions [1].

We may obtain Fourier transforms from the exponential form of the Fourier series, so that we may also obtain their various properties. Let $x_T(t)$ be a periodic function of period T, such that

$$x_T(t) = \sum_{n=-\infty}^{+\infty} c_n e^{in\omega_0 t}$$

$$= \sum_{n=-\infty}^{+\infty} \left(\frac{\omega_0}{2\pi} \int_{-T/2}^{+T/2} x_T(t) e^{-in\omega_0 t} \, dt \right) e^{in\omega_0 t}$$

$$= \sum_{n=-\infty}^{+\infty} \left(\frac{\omega_0}{2\pi} \int_{-T/2}^{+T/2} x_T(t) e^{-itn_0 2\pi/T} \, dt \right) e^{itn_0 2\pi/T},$$

with $n_0 = 0, \pm 1, \pm 2, \pm 3, \ldots$

Now, letting $T \to \infty$, and using an integration to represent all the frequencies ω, instead of the discrete ones, we obtain that for a generic nonperiodic $x(t)$, it must be

$$x(t) = \int_{-\infty}^{+\infty} \left(\frac{1}{2\pi} \int_{-\infty}^{+\infty} x(t) e^{-i\omega t} \, dt \right) e^{i\omega t} \, d\omega,$$

where $x(t)$ is represented as the Fourier anti-transform $\mathcal{F}^{-1}$ of its Fourier transform $X(\omega) = \mathcal{F}[x(t)]$; hence,

$$x(t) = \int_{-\infty}^{+\infty} \left(\frac{1}{2\pi} \int_{-\infty}^{+\infty} x(t) e^{-i\omega t} \, dt \right) e^{i\omega t} \, d\omega$$

$$= \frac{1}{2\pi} \int_{-\infty}^{+\infty} \left(\int_{-\infty}^{+\infty} x(t) e^{-i\omega t} \, dt \right) e^{i\omega t} \, d\omega$$

$$= \frac{1}{2\pi} \int_{-\infty}^{+\infty} X(\omega)e^{i\omega t}\, d\omega$$

$$= \mathcal{F}^{-1}[\mathcal{F}[x(t)]]$$

Thus, given a function $x(t)$, we *here* define its Fourier transform the integral

$$\mathcal{F}[x(t)] = \int_{-\infty}^{+\infty} x(t)e^{-i\omega t}\, dt \qquad (18.9)$$

$$= X(\omega),$$

and its Fourier antitransform (the inverse Fourier transform) the integral

$$\mathcal{F}^{-1}[X(\omega)] = \frac{1}{2\pi} \int_{-\infty}^{+\infty} X(\omega)e^{i\omega t}\, d\omega \qquad (18.10)$$

$$= x(t),$$

obviously, with $i = \sqrt{-1}$ (note that the expression $e^{-i\omega t}$ is a bunch of circumferences).

Note that we used the term "here": indeed, for pure mathematics, the couple transform/antitransform is often rendered as

$$F(y) = \frac{1}{\sqrt{2\pi}} \int_{-\infty}^{+\infty} f(x)e^{-iyx}\, dx; \qquad (18.11)$$

$$f(x) = \frac{1}{\sqrt{2\pi}} \int_{-\infty}^{+\infty} F(y)e^{ixy}\, dy, \qquad (18.12)$$

while in the probability theory the couple transform/antitransform is often given by

$$F(y) = \int_{-\infty}^{+\infty} f(x)e^{iyx}\, dx;$$

$$f(x) = \int_{-\infty}^{+\infty} F(y)e^{-ixy}\, dy,$$

but a transform/antitransform couple may be given in the more general form

$$F(y) = a \int_{-\infty}^{+\infty} f(x)e^{-iryx}\, dx;$$

$$f(x) = b \int_{-\infty}^{+\infty} F(y)e^{irxy}\, dy,$$

where r is a nonzero real number, with a, b real positive numbers (they could also be complex numbers, but it is preferable to set them as real), such that

$$|r| = 2\pi ab \tag{18.13}$$

and therefore, in Eqs. (18.9) and (18.10), we use $r = \pm1$, $a = 1$, and $b = \frac{1}{2\pi}$, whereas in Eqs. (18.11) and (18.12), we use $r = \pm1$, $a = \frac{1}{\sqrt{2\pi}}$, and $b = \frac{1}{\sqrt{2\pi}}$. However, from Eq. (18.13), we may understand that also a transform/antitransform couple given by

$$F(y) = \int_{-\infty}^{+\infty} f(x)e^{-i6yx}dx;$$

$$f(x) = \frac{3}{\pi} \int_{-\infty}^{+\infty} F(y)e^{i6xy}dy,$$

could potentially make sense, since the relationship $|r| = 2\pi ab$ is obeyed, given $2\pi \times 1 \times \frac{3}{\pi} = |6|$, despite the lack of an evident mathematical meaning.

The Fourier transform, as we defined above in Eqs. (18.9) and (18.10), allows to shift from the time domain to frequency domain (and vice versa; it's understood). However, depending on what we are dealing with, other domain changes are possible: for example, in quantum mechanics and in statistical thermodynamics, the Fourier transform is used to shift from position p to momentum q domains (again and vice versa), so as to have

$$y(p) = \frac{1}{2\pi} \int_{-\infty}^{+\infty} Y(q)e^{iqp}dq$$

$$Y(q) = \int_{-\infty}^{+\infty} y(p)e^{-iqp}dp.$$

Coming back to Eqs. (18.9) and (18.10), from the trigonometry, we recall that

$$e^{\pm i\omega t} = \cos(\omega t) \pm i \sin(\omega t)$$

$$= \frac{e^{i\omega t} + e^{-i\omega t}}{2} \pm i \frac{e^{i\omega t} - e^{-i\omega t}}{2i},$$

thus, the Fourier transform $\mathcal{F}[x(t)]$ of the function $x(t)$ is also

$$\mathcal{F}[x(t)] = X(\omega)$$

$$= \int_{-\infty}^{+\infty} x(t)e^{-i\omega t}dt$$

$$= \int_{-\infty}^{+\infty} x(t)[\cos(\omega t) - i\sin(\omega t)]dt$$

$$= \int_{-\infty}^{+\infty} x(t)\cos(\omega t)dt - i\int_{-\infty}^{+\infty} x(t)\sin(\omega t)dt.$$

We define $x(t)$ the inverse Fourier transform of $X(\omega)$ by means of the integral

$$x(t) = \mathcal{F}^{-1}[x(t)]$$

$$= \frac{1}{2\pi}\int_{-\infty}^{+\infty} X(\omega)e^{i\omega t}d\omega,$$

and the definition of the inverse transform may be immediately verified by writing

$$\frac{1}{2\pi}\int_{-\infty}^{+\infty} X(\omega)e^{i\omega t}d\omega = \frac{1}{2\pi}\int_{-\infty}^{+\infty}\left(\int_{-\infty}^{+\infty} x(t)e^{-i\omega t}dt\right)e^{i\omega t}d\omega$$

$$= \frac{1}{2\pi}\int_{-\infty}^{+\infty}\left(\int_{-\infty}^{+\infty} x(\theta)e^{-i\omega\theta}d\theta\right)e^{i\omega t}d\omega$$

$$= \frac{1}{2\pi}\int_{-\infty}^{+\infty} x(\theta)\left(\int_{-\infty}^{+\infty} e^{i\omega(t-\theta)}d\omega\right)d\theta$$

$$= \frac{1}{2\pi}\int_{-\infty}^{+\infty} x(\theta)\left(\int_{-\infty}^{+\infty} e^{-i\omega(\theta-t)}d\omega\right)d\theta$$

$$= \frac{1}{2\pi}\int_{-\infty}^{+\infty} x(\theta)\left(\int_{-\infty}^{+\infty} 1e^{-i\omega(\theta-t)}d\omega\right)d\theta$$

$$= \frac{1}{2\pi}2\pi\int_{-\infty}^{+\infty} x(\theta)\delta(\theta - t)d\theta$$

$$= \int_{-\infty}^{+\infty} x(\theta)\delta(t - \theta)d\theta$$

$$= x(t) * \delta(t)$$

$$= x(t).$$

Note that the function to be transformed must be square integrable: this means (in the more generalized definition), that, being f a complex-valued function, $\int_{-\infty}^{+\infty}|f(x)|^2dx$ must be finite, and this implies that also the integrals of the positive and negative parts of $\mathrm{Re}(f)$ and $\mathrm{Im}(f)$ must be finite, too.

Surely, the simplest Fourier transform is the Dirac delta one: from the definition, we have

$$\mathcal{F}[\delta(t)] = \int_{-\infty}^{+\infty} \delta(t - t_0) e^{-i\omega t} \, dt$$

$$= e^{-i\omega 0}$$

$$= 1,$$

so, we see that the transform of the infinitely thin impulse produces an infinite number of frequencies; in general, the thinner the impulse, the larger its set of frequencies.

In the case of a Dirac comb $C_\delta(t)$, e.g., a repeated sequence of impulses with period T, we have

$$C_\delta(t) = \sum_{n=-\infty}^{+\infty} \delta(t - nT)$$

thus

$$\mathcal{F}[C_\delta(t)] = \mathcal{F}\left[\sum_{n=-\infty}^{+\infty} \delta(t - nT) \right]$$

$$= e^{-i\omega(nT)} \mathcal{F}[\delta(t)]$$

$$= e^{-i\omega(nT)}.$$

A notable transform is $\mathcal{F}[\sin(t)]$, for which it is convenient to use $\sin(t)$ expressed as exponential as follows:

$$\sin(t) = \frac{e^{it} - e^{-it}}{2i}$$

so that

$$\mathcal{F}[\sin(t)] = \int_{-\infty}^{+\infty} \frac{e^{it} - e^{-it}}{2i} e^{-i\omega t} \, dt$$

$$= \frac{1}{2i} \int_{-\infty}^{+\infty} (e^{it} - e^{-it}) e^{-i\omega t} \, dt$$

$$= \frac{1}{2i} \int_{-\infty}^{+\infty} e^{it} e^{-i\omega t} \, dt - \frac{1}{2i} \int_{-\infty}^{+\infty} e^{-it} e^{-i\omega t} \, dt$$

$$= i\pi \delta(\omega + 1) - i\pi \delta(\omega - 1),$$

while if the sine wave has an angular frequency ω_0, then

$$\mathcal{F}[\sin(\omega_0 t)] = \int_{-\infty}^{+\infty} \frac{e^{i\omega_0 t} - e^{-i\omega_0 t}}{2i} e^{-i\omega t} dt$$

$$= \frac{1}{2i} \int_{-\infty}^{+\infty} (e^{i\omega_0 t} - e^{-i\omega_0 t}) e^{-i\omega t} dt$$

$$= \frac{1}{2i} \int_{-\infty}^{+\infty} e^{i\omega_0 t} e^{-i\omega t} dt - \frac{1}{2i} \int_{-\infty}^{+\infty} e^{-i\omega_0 t} e^{-i\omega t} dt$$

$$= i\pi \delta(\omega + \omega_0) - i\pi \delta(\omega - \omega_0).$$

The Fourier transform of the function

$$f(t) = \frac{1}{\sigma\sqrt{2\pi}} \exp\left(\frac{-t^2}{2\sigma^2}\right)$$

is another Gaussian function, since

$$\mathcal{F}\left[\frac{1}{\sigma\sqrt{2\pi}} \exp\left(\frac{-t^2}{2\sigma^2}\right)\right] = \frac{1}{\sigma\sqrt{2\pi}} \int_{-\infty}^{+\infty} \frac{1}{\sigma\sqrt{2\pi}} \exp\left(\frac{-t^2}{2\sigma^2}\right) \exp(-i\omega t) dt$$

$$= \frac{1}{\sigma\sqrt{2\pi}} \int_{-\infty}^{+\infty} \exp\left(\frac{-t^2 - 2\sigma^2 i\omega t}{2\sigma^2}\right) dt$$

$$= \frac{1}{\sigma\sqrt{2\pi}}$$

$$\times \int_{-\infty}^{+\infty} \exp\left(\frac{-t^2 + 2\sigma^2 i\omega t + \sigma^4 \omega^2 - \sigma^4 \omega^2}{2\sigma^2}\right) dt$$

$$= \frac{e^{-\sigma^2\omega^2/2}}{\sigma\sqrt{2\pi}} \int_{-\infty}^{+\infty} \exp\left(-\frac{(t + \sigma^2 i\omega)^2}{2\sigma^2}\right) dt$$

$$= \frac{\sigma\sqrt{2\pi}}{\sigma\sqrt{2\pi}} \exp\left(\frac{-\sigma^2\omega^2}{2}\right)$$

$$= \exp\left(\frac{-\sigma^2\omega^2}{2}\right),$$

which reads

$$\exp\left(\frac{-\sigma^2\omega^2}{2}\right) = \exp\left(\frac{-\omega^2}{2\varsigma^2}\right)$$

if one uses the variance $\varsigma = \frac{1}{\sigma}$ in the frequency domain.

The Fourier transform has some important properties: first, it is linear; hence,

$$\mathcal{F}[af(t) \pm bg(t)] = \int_{-\infty}^{+\infty} [af(t)e^{-i\omega t} \pm bg(t)e^{-i\omega t}]\mathrm{d}t$$

$$= a \int_{-\infty}^{+\infty} f(t)e^{-i\omega t}\,\mathrm{d}t \pm b \int_{-\infty}^{+\infty} g(t)e^{-i\omega t}\,\mathrm{d}t$$

$$= a\mathcal{F}[f(t)] \pm b\mathcal{F}[g(t)],$$

moreover, the Fourier transform is symmetric: since $\mathcal{F}[f(t)] = F(\omega)$ we also may search for $F(t)$; in this case, we can put

$$f(t) = \frac{1}{2\pi} \int_{-\infty}^{+\infty} f(t)e^{-i\omega(-t)}\,\mathrm{d}\omega,$$

to have

$$2\pi f(-t) = \int_{-\infty}^{+\infty} f(t)e^{-i\omega t}\,\mathrm{d}\omega,$$

and if we exchange the name of the variables

$$2\pi f(-\omega) = \int_{-\infty}^{+\infty} f(t)e^{-i\omega t}\,\mathrm{d}t$$

$$= \mathcal{F}[F(t)].$$

Notably, the Fourier transform of a convolution product of two functions $f(t)$ and $g(t)$ is equal to the algebraic product of the respective Fourier transforms, since

$$\mathcal{F}[f(t) * g(t)] = \mathcal{F}\left[\int_{\infty}^{+\infty} f(\tau)g(t - \tau)\mathrm{d}\tau\right]$$

$$= \int_{\infty}^{+\infty} \left(\int_{\infty}^{+\infty} f(\tau)g(t - \tau)\mathrm{d}\tau\right) e^{-i\omega t}\,\mathrm{d}t$$

$$= \int_{\infty}^{+\infty} f(\tau)\mathrm{d}\tau \int_{\infty}^{+\infty} g(t - \tau)e^{-i\omega(t-\tau)}e^{-i\omega\tau}\,\mathrm{d}(t - \tau)$$

$$= e^{-i\omega\tau} \int_{\infty}^{+\infty} f(\tau)\mathrm{d}\tau \int_{\infty}^{+\infty} g(t - \tau)e^{-i\omega(t-\tau)}\mathrm{d}(t - \tau)$$

$$= e^{-i\omega\tau} \int_{\infty}^{+\infty} f(\tau)\mathrm{d}\tau\, G(\omega)$$

$$= \int_{\infty}^{+\infty} f(\tau)e^{-i\omega\tau}\,\mathrm{d}\tau\, G(\omega)$$

$$= F(\omega)G(\omega).$$

The Fourier transform can be derived w.r.t. time t, since we see that

$$\frac{\mathrm{d}f(t)}{\mathrm{d}t} = \frac{\mathrm{d}}{\mathrm{d}t}\left(\frac{1}{2\pi}\int_{-\infty}^{+\infty} F(\omega)e^{i\omega t}\,\mathrm{d}\omega\right)$$

$$= \frac{1}{2\pi}\int_{-\infty}^{+\infty} F(\omega)\left(\frac{\mathrm{d}}{\mathrm{d}t}e^{i\omega t}\right)\mathrm{d}\omega$$

$$= \frac{1}{2\pi}\int_{-\infty}^{+\infty} F(\omega)i\omega e^{i\omega t}\,\mathrm{d}\omega$$

$$= \frac{1}{2\pi}\int_{-\infty}^{+\infty} i\omega F(\omega)e^{i\omega t}\,\mathrm{d}\omega$$

$$= \mathcal{F}^{-1}[i\omega F(\omega)]$$

hence

$$\mathcal{F}\left[\frac{\mathrm{d}f(t)}{\mathrm{d}t}\right] = i\omega F(\omega),$$

whereas the derivative w.r.t. the frequency ω is

$$\frac{\mathrm{d}F(\omega)}{\mathrm{d}t} = \frac{\mathrm{d}}{\mathrm{d}t}\left(\int_{-\infty}^{+\infty} f(t)e^{-i\omega t}\,\mathrm{d}t\right)$$

$$= \int_{-\infty}^{+\infty} f(t)\left(\frac{\mathrm{d}}{\mathrm{d}t}e^{-i\omega t}\right)\mathrm{d}t$$

$$= \int_{-\infty}^{+\infty} (-i\omega)f(t)\left(\frac{\mathrm{d}}{\mathrm{d}t}\right)e^{-i\omega t}\,\mathrm{d}t$$

$$= \mathcal{F}[-itf(t)].$$

If we have a signal with a time scaling λ, the Fourier transform reads

$$\mathcal{F}[f(\lambda t)] = \int_{-\infty}^{+\infty} f(\lambda t)e^{-i\omega t}\,\mathrm{d}t$$

thus, changing the variable from λt to θ, such that $\mathrm{d}t = \frac{\mathrm{d}\theta}{\lambda}$, the integral becomes

$$\mathcal{F}[f(\lambda t)] = \int_{-\infty}^{+\infty} f(\theta)e^{-i\omega\theta/\lambda}\,\mathrm{d}\theta$$

$$= \begin{cases} \dfrac{1}{\lambda}\displaystyle\int_{-\infty}^{+\infty} f(\theta)e^{-i\omega\theta/\lambda}\,\mathrm{d}\theta, & \text{if } \lambda > 0 \\ -\dfrac{1}{\lambda}\int_{-\infty}^{+\infty} f(\theta)e^{-i\omega\theta/\lambda}\,\mathrm{d}\theta, & \text{if } \lambda > 0 \end{cases}$$

$$= \frac{1}{|\lambda|} \int_{-\infty}^{+\infty} f(\theta) e^{-i\omega\theta/\lambda} d\theta$$

$$= \frac{1}{|\lambda|} \int_{-\infty}^{+\infty} f(\theta) \exp\left(-i\frac{\omega}{\lambda}\theta\right) d\theta$$

$$= \frac{1}{|\lambda|} F\left(\frac{\omega}{\lambda}\right).$$

18.4   The Laplace Transform

For a function $f(t)$, we may define its Laplace transform $\mathcal{L}[f(t)]$ as the integral

$$\mathcal{L}[f(t)] = \int_{-\infty}^{+\infty} f(t) e^{-st} dt$$

$$= F(s),$$

assuming that the integral converges: here we have two functions that must behave in two different manners, since as t increases, then $f(t)$ increases and e^{-st} decreases; therefore, the criterion for convergence of the integral states that the rate at which $f(t)$ grows must be less than the rate at which e^{-st} decreases.

The variable s is the complex number $s = \sigma + i\omega$; thus, we see that

$$\mathcal{L}[f(t)] = \int_{-\infty}^{+\infty} f(t) e^{-st} dt$$

$$= \int_{-\infty}^{+\infty} f(t) e^{-\sigma t} e^{-i\omega t} dt$$

$$= \mathcal{F}[f(t) e^{-\sigma t}]$$

$$= F_\sigma(\omega),$$

representing the connection between Laplace and Fourier transforms. In other words, we find

$$f(t) e^{-\sigma t} = \mathcal{F}^{-1}[F_\sigma(\omega)],$$

so that, under some conditions applied to the domain of $\mathcal{L}[f(t)]$, and considering that $F_\sigma(\omega)$ is the Fourier transform calculated if $\text{Re}(s) = \sigma$, we get

$$f(t) = e^{\sigma t} \mathcal{F}^{-1}[F_\sigma(\omega)]$$

$$= e^{\sigma t} \frac{1}{2\pi} \int_{-\infty}^{+\infty} F_\sigma(\omega) e^{i\omega t} d\omega$$

$$= \frac{1}{2\pi} \int_{-\infty}^{+\infty} F_\sigma(\omega) e^{\sigma t} e^{i\omega t} \, d\omega$$

$$= \frac{1}{2\pi} \int_{-\infty}^{+\infty} F(s) e^{\sigma t + i\omega t} \, d\omega$$

$$= \frac{1}{2\pi i} \int_{-\infty}^{+\infty} i F(s) e^{\sigma t + i\omega t} \, d\omega$$

$$= \frac{1}{2\pi i} \int_{-\infty}^{+\infty} F(s) e^{(\sigma + i\omega) t} \, d(\sigma + i\omega)$$

$$= \frac{1}{2\pi i} \int_{-\infty}^{+\infty} F(s) e^{st} \, ds$$

thus, being the integral evaluated on a vertical axis parallel to imaginary axis and passing by σ, we define the inverse Laplace transform $\mathcal{L}^{-1}[F(s)]$ in the form

$$\mathcal{L}^{-1}[F(s)] = \frac{1}{2\pi i} \int_{\sigma - i\infty}^{\sigma + j\infty} F_\sigma(\omega) e^{i\omega t} \, ds$$

$$= f(t),$$

assuming that integral converges.

The Laplace transform is used in many fields of mathematical and physical sciences; in general, it can be very useful when solving a differential equation: the Laplace transform changes the domain of a function, transforming it in a more easily solvable expression. Once we find a solution in this new domain, we can take this solution and calculate its inverse transform, so that we may translate that solution in the original domain.

The Laplace transform is linear, since

$$\mathcal{L}[af(t) + bg(t)] = aF(s) + bG(s),$$

and its linearity depends on the linearity of the integral, being

$$\mathcal{L}[af(t) + bg(t)] = \int_{-\infty}^{+\infty} [af(t) + bg(t)] e^{-st} \, dt$$

$$= a \int_{-\infty}^{+\infty} f(t) e^{-st} \, dt + b \int_{-\infty}^{+\infty} g(t) e^{-st} \, dt$$

$$= aF(s) + bG(s),$$

and in the case of translation of its domain $\text{Dom}_{\mathcal{L}}(F(s))$ by a term t_a, we have

$$\mathcal{L}[f(t - t_a)] = \int_{-\infty}^{+\infty} f(t - t_a)e^{-st}\,\mathrm{d}t$$

$$= e^{-t_a s} \int_{-\infty}^{+\infty} f(t - t_a)e^{-s(t-t_a)}\mathrm{d}(t - t_a)$$

$$= e^{-t_a s} F(s).$$

Here we introduce the derivatives (w.r.t. s and t) of a Laplace transform. The derivative with respect to s is

$$\mathcal{L}[f'(t)] = \int_{-\infty}^{+\infty} f'(t)e^{-st}\,\mathrm{d}t$$

$$= f(t)e^{st}\,\Big|_{-\infty}^{+\infty} - \int_{-\infty}^{+\infty} -sf(t)e^{-st}\,\mathrm{d}t$$

$$= -\int_{-\infty}^{+\infty} -sf(t)e^{-st}\,\mathrm{d}t,$$

where we hypothesized $f(t)e^{-st}$ to be always integrable, for all s.

Regarding the derivative with respect to t, assuming that $F'(s)$ is the derivative of $F(s)$, we have

$$F'(s) = \frac{\mathrm{d}}{\mathrm{d}s}\left(\int_{-\infty}^{+\infty} f(t)e^{-st}\,\mathrm{d}t\right)$$

$$= -\int_{-\infty}^{+\infty} tf(t)e^{-st}\,\mathrm{d}t$$

$$= \mathcal{L}[-tf(t)],$$

where we also assumed that we may exchange derivation and integration. Note also that it is

$$\mathcal{L}[f^{(n)}(t)] = s^n F(s) - \sum_{k=0}^{n-1} s^{n-k-1} \frac{\mathrm{d}^k f(t)}{\mathrm{d}t^k}\bigg|_{t=0} = s^n F(s) - \sum_{k=0}^{n-1} s^k \frac{\mathrm{d}^{n-k-1} f(t)}{\mathrm{d}t^{n-k-1}}\bigg|_{t=0}.$$

The last very important property of the Laplace transform is given by its effect on the convolution integral: we may see that the Laplace transform of a convolution product of two functions is equal to the algebraic product of the Laplace transforms of the functions, as we saw also for the Fourier transform. Indeed, we define the convolution $f(t) * g(t)$ of two functions $f(t)$ and $g(t)$ as the integral

$$f(t) * g(t) = \int_{-\infty}^{+\infty} f(\tau)g(t - \tau)\,\mathrm{d}\tau = g(t) * f(t),$$

since convolution commutes. The Laplace transform of a convolution is therefore

$$\mathcal{L}[f(t) * g(t)] = \int_{-\infty}^{+\infty} \left(\int_{-\infty}^{+\infty} f(\tau)g(t - \tau)d\tau \right) e^{-st} dt$$

$$= \int_{-\infty}^{+\infty} f(\tau)d\tau \int_{-\infty}^{+\infty} g(t - \tau)e^{-s(t-\tau)}e^{-st}d(t - \tau)$$

$$= \int_{-\infty}^{+\infty} f(\tau)e^{-st}d\tau \, \widehat{g}(s)$$

$$= F(s)F(s).$$

We have seen the Laplace transform of a function defined over all the time domain; however, there are situations in which the function is defined only if t is nonnegative. In this last case, we may define a unilateral Laplace transform as follows:

$$\mathcal{L}_u[f(t)] = F_u(s)$$

and using the unit step function

$$u(t) = \begin{cases} 0 \text{ if } t < 0 \\ 1 \text{ if } t \geq 0 \end{cases},$$

we get

$$F_u(s) = \mathcal{L}_u[f(t)]$$

$$= \int_0^{+\infty} f(t)e^{-st}dt,$$

and the convolution becomes

$$(u(t)f(t)) * (u(t)g(t)) = \int_{-\infty}^{+\infty} u(t)f(\tau)u(t - \tau)g(t - \tau)d\tau$$

$$= \int_0^t f(\tau)g(t - \tau)d\tau,$$

since here the convolution integral is defined only for $t \geq 0$.

Reference

1. Sneddon IN. Fourier transforms. New York: McGraw-Hill; 1951.

A Primer of Fractional Calculus

19

The derivative of a function $f(x) = x^m$, assuming $m > 0$, is

$$f'(x) = \frac{\mathrm{d}\, x^m}{\mathrm{d}\, x} = m x^{m-1},$$

and the second derivative is

$$f''(x) = \frac{\mathrm{d}^2 x^m}{\mathrm{d}x^2} = m(m-1)x^{m-2},$$

and so on, such that, for $m > n$, with $m, n > 0$, we write

$$\frac{\mathrm{d}^n x^m}{\mathrm{d}x^n} = m(m-1)(m-2)\cdots(m-n+1)x^{m-n}$$

$$= \frac{m!}{(m-n)!}x^{m-n}, \tag{19.1}$$

and if we use the Euler Gamma function, Eq. (19.1) reads

$$\frac{\mathrm{d}^n x^m}{\mathrm{d}x^n} = \frac{\Gamma(m+1)}{\Gamma(m-n+1)} x^{m-n} \tag{19.2}$$

Leonhard Euler, in 1730, observed a very interesting fact: the definition of the derivative in terms of $\Gamma(m)$ in Eq. (19.2), permits also the definition of a non-integer derivation. The same Euler, letting $n = \frac{1}{2}$, calculated the $\frac{1}{2}$-th order derivative of $y = x$ as follows:

$$\frac{\mathrm{d}^{1/2} x}{\mathrm{d}x^{1/2}} = \frac{\Gamma(1+1)}{\Gamma\left(1 - \frac{1}{2} + 1\right)} x^{1-1/2}$$

$$= \frac{\Gamma(2)}{\Gamma\left(\frac{3}{2}\right)} \sqrt{x}$$

$$= \frac{1}{\frac{\sqrt{\pi}}{2}} \sqrt{x}$$

$$= 2\frac{\sqrt{x}}{\sqrt{\pi}}. \tag{19.3}$$

If we go ahead deriving again the result with respect to $x^{1/2}$, we obtain

$$\frac{\mathrm{d}^{1/2}\left(2\frac{\sqrt{x}}{\sqrt{\pi}}\right)}{\mathrm{d}x^{1/2}} = \frac{2}{\sqrt{\pi}}\frac{\mathrm{d}^{1/2}x^{1/2}}{\mathrm{d}x^{1/2}} = \frac{2}{\sqrt{\pi}}\frac{\Gamma(\frac{1}{2}+1)}{\Gamma\left(\frac{1}{2}-\frac{1}{2}+1\right)}x^{(1-1)/2}$$

$$= \frac{2}{\sqrt{\pi}}\frac{\Gamma(\frac{3}{2})}{\Gamma(1)}x^0 = \frac{2}{\sqrt{\pi}}\frac{\sqrt{\pi}}{2} = 1;$$

in other words, we have found that

$$\frac{\mathrm{d}^{1/2}}{\mathrm{d}x^{1/2}}\left(\frac{\mathrm{d}^{1/2}x}{\mathrm{d}x^{1/2}}\right) = \frac{\mathrm{d}x}{\mathrm{d}x} = 1$$

so that, the equivalence of operators

$$\frac{\mathrm{d}^{1/2}}{\mathrm{d}x^{1/2}}\left(\frac{\mathrm{d}^{1/2}}{\mathrm{d}x^{1/2}}\right) \equiv \frac{\mathrm{d}}{\mathrm{d}x}$$

is verified.

Let us now see what is going to happen when calculating the derivatives of x^2, respectively, of order 3/4, 1/2, 1/4, and 0. Bearing in mind that $\frac{\mathrm{d}x^2}{\mathrm{d}x} = 2x$, we obtain

$$\frac{\mathrm{d}^{3/4}x^2}{\mathrm{d}x^{3/4}} = \frac{\Gamma(2+1)}{\Gamma\left(2-\frac{3}{4}+1\right)}x^{2-3/4} = \frac{\Gamma(3)}{\Gamma\left(\frac{9}{4}\right)}x^{5/4} \approx 1.765\sqrt[4]{x^5};$$

$$\frac{\mathrm{d}^{1/2}x^2}{\mathrm{d}x^{1/2}} = \frac{\Gamma(2+1)}{\Gamma\left(2-\frac{1}{2}+1\right)}x^{2-1/2} = \frac{\Gamma(3)}{\Gamma\left(\frac{5}{2}\right)}x^{6/4} \approx 1.505\sqrt[4]{x^6};$$

$$\frac{d^{1/4} x^2}{dx^{1/4}} = \frac{\Gamma(2+1)}{\Gamma\left(2 - \frac{1}{4} + 1\right)} x^{2-1/4} = \frac{\Gamma(3)}{\Gamma\left(\frac{11}{4}\right)} x^{7/4} \approx 1.244 \sqrt[4]{x^7} \, ;$$

$$\frac{d^0 x^2}{dx^0} = \frac{\Gamma(2+1)}{\Gamma(2-0+1)} x^{2-0} = \frac{\Gamma(3)}{\Gamma(3)} x^2 = x^2 \, ,$$

where the last result is trivial.

To deal with fractional derivatives of a function $f(x)$, it could be generally more convenient to use the so-called integrodifferential operator D, instead of $\frac{d}{dx}$, so that we write

$$D(f(x)) = \frac{df(x)}{dx},$$

and

$$D^n(f(x)) = \frac{d^n f(x)}{dx^n},$$

where we recall that superscript does not define a power, since it is just an index; the integrodifferential operator could well be used also for antidifferentiation, putting

$$D^{-1}(f(x)) = \int f(x) \, dx,$$

and

$$D^{-n}(f(x)) = \underbrace{\int\!\int \cdots \int}_{n \text{ times}} f(x) \, dx.$$

The linearity of the operator may be verified observing that, for a scalar λ, it is

$$D^m(D^n(\lambda f(x))) = \lambda D^{m+n}(f(x)) = \lambda \frac{d^{m+n} f(x)}{dx^{m+n}},$$

but the operator D^m can also be "decomposed," for example, by writing

$$D^m(f(x)) = D^{m-n}(D^n(f(x))),$$

and the power rule reads

$$D^m(f(x)^n) = \frac{\Gamma(n+1)}{\Gamma(n-m+1)} x^{n-m}$$

$$= \frac{n!}{(n-m)!} x^{n-m}.$$

19.1   Introduction to Fractional Derivatives and Integrals

Fractional calculus can be used when we are dealing with two or more events producing two or more different mathematical (or physical, or biological) effects [1]. Examples can be taken from physics like a cooling down of a hot object, which also radiates heat (note that here we have the first event governed by an exponential law, while the second event is governed by a power law).

Despite the large number of physical phenomena that may be studied with fractional calculus, there are also notable applications to medicine and biology, like transmission and spread of an infective disease, where many effects are simultaneously exerted on the system by even a single individual.

Since the first and second derivatives of $f(x)$ can be written as

$$f'(x) = \lim_{h \to 0} \frac{f(x) - f(x-h)}{h}; \quad f''(x) = \lim_{h \to 0} \frac{f(x) - 2f(x-h) + f(x-2h)}{h^2}$$

then, by induction,

$$f^{(n)}(x) = \lim_{h \to 0} \frac{1}{h^n} \sum_{k=0}^{n} (-1)^k \binom{n}{k} f(x-hk),$$

where $\binom{n}{k}$ is the binomial coefficient

$$\binom{n}{k} = \frac{n!}{k!(n-k)!} = \frac{n(n-1)(n-2)\cdots(n-k+1)}{k!}.$$

Let us now define the integral and the double integral of $f(x)$ as a limit

$$f^{(-1)}(x) = \lim_{h \to 0} h \sum_{k=0}^{n} f(x-hk); \quad f^{(-2)}(x) = \lim_{h \to 0} h^2 \sum_{k=0}^{n} (k+1)f(x-hk),$$

thus, again by induction, we obtain

$$f^{(-n)}(x) = \lim_{h \to 0} h^n \sum_{k=0}^{n} \binom{n+k-1}{k} f(x-hk),$$

so that we gain a unique equation for n-fold integration and differentiation as follows:

$$f^{(n)}(x) = \lim_{h \to 0} \frac{1}{h^n} \sum_{k=0}^{n} \binom{k-n-1}{k} f(x-hk) \tag{19.4}$$

corresponding to a n-fold integration if $n < 0$ and $|n| \in \mathbb{N}$ and to a n-fold differentiation if $n > 0$ and $n \in \mathbb{N}$. Note that letting $n = 0$, Eq. (19.4) reads

$$f^{(0)}(x) = \lim_{h \to 0} \frac{1}{h^0} \sum_{k=0}^{0} \binom{k - 0 - 1}{k} f(x - 0k) = \frac{1}{1} f(x) = f(x),$$

as expected; moreover, taking Eq. (19.4) and inserting $\alpha \in \mathbb{R}$ instead of $n \in \mathbb{N}$, we have

$$f^{(\alpha)}(x) = \lim_{h \to 0} \frac{1}{h^n} \sum_{k=0}^{n} \binom{k - \alpha - 1}{k} f(x - hk). \tag{19.5}$$

Another concept to bear in mind is the Cauchy formula for an n-fold integral, e.g., the operator

$$(J^n f)(x) = \frac{1}{(n - 1)!} \int_a^x (x - t)^{n-1} f(t) dt,$$

where, again, substituting $n \in \mathbb{N}$ with $\alpha \in \mathbb{R}$, we get

$$(J^\alpha f)(x) = \frac{1}{\Gamma(\alpha)} \int_0^x (x - t)^{n-1} f(t) dt,$$

so that we can see that the semigroup property of fractional operators

$$(J^\alpha)(J^\beta f)(x) = (J^\beta)(J^\alpha f)(x) = (J^{\beta+\alpha} f)(x) = (J^{\alpha+\beta} f)(x)$$

holds.

Thus, we can take into account the general form for derivation given in the formula

$$\frac{d^a x^{-n}}{dx^a} = (-1)^a \frac{\Gamma(n + a)}{\Gamma(n)} x^{-(n+a)}, \quad n \geq 0$$

which is not useful only for real powers. Indeed, letting $a < 0$, the formula leads to integrals.

19.2   The Mittag-Leffler Function

The Mittag-Leffler (M-L) function is an important tool for the development and the working capability in the area of fractional calculus [1]. It can be considered a natural extension of the exponential function e^x. The two-parameter M-L function

$E_{\alpha,\beta}(z)$ is defined as

$$E_{\alpha,\beta}(z) = \sum_{k=0}^{+\infty} \frac{z^k}{\Gamma(\alpha k + \beta)},$$

for $\mathrm{Re}(\alpha), \mathrm{Re}(\beta) > 0$, and we immediately realize that when $\alpha = \beta = 1$, then $E_{1,1}(z) = e^z$, since

$$E_{1,1}(z) = \sum_{k=1}^{+\infty} \frac{z^k}{\Gamma(k+1)} = \sum_{k=1}^{+\infty} \frac{z^k}{k!} = e^z$$

is exactly the Taylor series expansion corresponding to e^x; therefore, we can say that M-L function can be seen as a generalization of the exponential.

In the more general form, the M-L function reads

$$E_{\alpha,\beta}(\lambda(z-z_0)^\alpha) = \sum_{k=1}^{+\infty} \frac{(\lambda(z-z_0)^\alpha)^k}{\Gamma(\alpha k + \beta)},$$

again, for $\mathrm{Re}(\alpha), \mathrm{Re}(\beta) > 0$.

19.3   The Riemann-Liouville and Caputo Fractional Derivatives

We define the *Riemann-Liouville (RL) fractional derivative* of non-integer order α, with the relation

$$
{}^{RL}_{0}\mathrm{D}^\alpha_t f(t) =
\begin{cases}
\dfrac{1}{\Gamma(m-\alpha)} \dfrac{\mathrm{d}^m}{\mathrm{d}t^m} \displaystyle\int_0^t \dfrac{f(\theta)}{(t-\theta)^{\alpha+1-m}}\mathrm{d}\theta, & m-1 < \alpha < m \\[4mm]
\dfrac{\mathrm{d}^m}{\mathrm{d}t^m} f(t), & \alpha = m
\end{cases}
\tag{19.6}
$$

where $m \in \mathbb{N}$ and $\alpha \in \mathbb{R}$.

We also define the *Caputo (C) fractional derivative* of non-integer order α as

$$
{}^{C}_{0}\mathrm{D}^\alpha_t f(t) =
\begin{cases}
\dfrac{1}{\Gamma(m-\alpha)} \displaystyle\int_0^t \dfrac{\mathrm{d}^m f(\theta)}{\mathrm{d}\theta^m} \dfrac{1}{(t-\theta)^{\alpha+1-m}}\mathrm{d}\theta, & m-1 < \alpha < m \\[4mm]
\dfrac{\mathrm{d}^m f(\theta)}{\mathrm{d}\theta^m}, & \alpha = m
\end{cases}
$$

$$\tag{19.7}$$

again, with $m \in \mathbb{N}$ and $\alpha \in \mathbb{R}$.

The RL and the C fractional derivatives intuitively differ for the order of operators; the first differentiates an integral; the latter integrates a differential, and we may expect some changes in the results. Let's take a very simple example with

$f(t) = K$ (K being a constant), and with $\alpha = 0.5 = \frac{1}{2}$, such that $m - 1 = 0 < \alpha < m = 1$: with the Riemann-Liouville differentiation, using a suitable a as the lower limit of integration, we have

$$
{}^{RL}_{a}D^{1/2}_{t}K = \frac{1}{\Gamma(1 - \frac{1}{2})} \frac{d}{dt} \int_{a}^{t} \frac{K}{(t - \theta)^{\frac{1}{2} - 1 + 1}} d\theta
$$

$$
= \frac{1}{\Gamma(\frac{1}{2})} \frac{d}{dt} \int_{a}^{t} \frac{K}{(t - \theta)^{\frac{1}{2}}} d\theta
$$

$$
= \frac{1}{\sqrt{\pi}} \frac{d}{dt} \int_{a}^{t} \frac{K}{\sqrt{(t - \theta)}} d\theta
$$

$$
= \frac{K}{\sqrt{\pi} \sqrt{(t - a)}},
$$

which is not zero, as we would expect with the usual differentiation rules.

With the Caputo differentiation we get, instead

$$
{}^{C}_{a}D^{1/2}_{t}K = \frac{1}{\Gamma(\frac{1}{2} - 1)} \int_{a}^{t} \frac{dK}{dt} \frac{1}{(t - \theta)^{\frac{1}{2} - 1 + 1}} d\theta
$$

$$
= \frac{1}{\Gamma(-\frac{1}{2})} \int_{a}^{t} \frac{0}{(t - \theta)^{\frac{1}{2}}} d\theta
$$

$$
= -\frac{1}{2\sqrt{\pi}} 0
$$

$$
= 0,
$$

where the differentiation of a constant is zero, like with the integer differentiation.

Using the same $\alpha = \frac{1}{2}$ and $n = 1$, we now apply the two fractional derivatives at the very simple function $f(t) = t$: with the Riemann-Liouville differentiation, we have

$$
{}^{RL}_{a}D^{1/2}_{t}t = \frac{1}{\Gamma(1 - \frac{1}{2})} \frac{d}{dt} \int_{a}^{t} \frac{t}{(t - \theta)^{\frac{1}{2} - 1 + 1}} d\theta
$$

$$
= \frac{1}{\Gamma(\frac{1}{2})} \left(\frac{a}{2\sqrt{t - a}} - \sqrt{t - a} \right)
$$

$$
= \frac{1}{\sqrt{\pi}} \left(\frac{a}{2\sqrt{t - a}} - \sqrt{t - a} \right)
$$

and with the Caputo differentiation, we have

$$
\begin{aligned}
{}_a^C \mathrm{D}_t^{1/2} t &= \frac{1}{\Gamma(\frac{1}{2} - 1)} \int_a^t \frac{\mathrm{d}t}{\mathrm{d}t} \frac{1}{(t - \theta)^{\frac{1}{2} - 1 + 1}} \mathrm{d}\theta \\
&= \frac{1}{\Gamma(-\frac{1}{2})} \int_a^t \frac{1}{(t - \theta)^{\frac{1}{2}}} \mathrm{d}\theta \\
&= -\frac{\sqrt{t - a}}{\sqrt{\pi}},
\end{aligned}
$$

such that, in both cases, we don't obtain the usual result $\frac{\mathrm{d}}{\mathrm{d}t} t = 1$ of the integer-valued differentiation.

Of course, the two definitions (19.6) and (19.7), which in essence have the form of a convolution, do not come out of the blue. We first must consider the causal function $f(t)$, e.g., a function vanishing if $t < 0$; note that $f(t)$ can be either a real or complex valued function of real variable t. The Cauchy-Dirichlet formula for the n-fold ($n \in \mathbb{N}$) primitive of $f(t)$ is given by the convolution integral

$$
{}_0 I_t^n f(t) = \frac{1}{(n - 1)!} \int_0^t (t - \theta)^{n-1} f(\theta) \mathrm{d}(\theta),
$$

where we see that $f(t)$, as well as all its derivatives until the $(n - 1)$-th order, vanishes at $t = 0$. Now, simply taking the Gamma function and $\alpha \in \mathbb{R}^+$, the Cauchy-Dirichlet formula becomes

$$
{}_0^{RL} I_t^\alpha f(t) = \frac{1}{\Gamma(\alpha)} \int_0^t (t - \theta)^{\alpha-1} f(\theta) \mathrm{d}(\theta), \quad t > 0, \alpha \in \mathbb{R}^+ \tag{19.8}
$$

which is the RL fractional integral. Note that, since ${}_0^{RL} I_t^0 f(t) = f(t)$, we may define ${}_0^{RL} I_t^0$ the identity operator.

Considering the operator composition

$$
{}_0^{RL} I_t^\alpha \circ {}_0^{RL} I_t^\beta f(t) = {}_0^{RL} I_t^\alpha \left({}_0^{RL} I_t^\beta f(t) \right) = {}_0^{RL} I_t^{\alpha+\beta} f(t),
$$

with $\alpha, \beta \geq 0$, we verify the semigroup property. Indeed, given the definition of RL integral, and using the equality

$$
\int_a^p \int_a^q f(r) \mathrm{d}q \mathrm{d}r = \int_a^p \int_r^p f(x) \mathrm{d}q \mathrm{d}r
$$

we find that, for $\alpha, \beta > 0$,

$$
{}^{RL}_{a}I^{\alpha}_{t}{}^{RL}_{a}I^{\beta}_{t}f(t) = \frac{1}{\Gamma(\alpha)\Gamma(\beta)} \int_{a}^{t}(t-\theta)^{\alpha-1}\int_{0}^{t}(\theta-\tau)^{\beta-1}f(\tau)\mathrm{d}\tau\mathrm{d}\theta
$$

$$
= \frac{1}{\Gamma(\alpha)\Gamma(\beta)} \int_{a}^{t}\int_{\tau}^{t}(t-\theta)^{\alpha-1}(\theta-\tau)^{\beta-1}f(\tau)\mathrm{d}\tau\mathrm{d}\theta
$$

$$
= \frac{1}{\Gamma(\alpha)\Gamma(\beta)} \int_{a}^{t}(t-\tau)^{\alpha+\beta-1}f(\tau)\left(\int_{0}^{1}(1-y)^{\alpha-1}y^{\beta-1}\mathrm{d}y\right)\mathrm{d}\tau
$$

where we see that the second integral in the r.h.s. is a Beta distribution with arguments α and β, since

$$
\mathrm{B}(\alpha, \beta) = \int_{0}^{1}(1-y)^{\alpha-1}y^{\beta-1}\mathrm{d}y
$$

$$
= \frac{\Gamma(\alpha)\Gamma(\beta)}{\Gamma(\alpha+\beta)}, \quad \mathrm{Re}(\alpha, \beta) > 0.
$$

therefore

$$
{}^{RL}_{a}I^{\alpha}_{t}{}^{RL}_{a}I^{\beta}_{t}f(t) = \frac{1}{\Gamma(\alpha)\Gamma(\beta)}\frac{\Gamma(\alpha)\Gamma(\beta)}{\Gamma(\alpha+\beta)}\int_{a}^{t}(t-\tau)^{\alpha+\beta-1}f(\tau)\mathrm{d}\tau
$$

$$
= \frac{1}{\Gamma(\alpha+\beta)}\int_{a}^{t}(t-\tau)^{\alpha+\beta-1}f(\tau)\mathrm{d}\tau
$$

$$
= {}^{RL}_{a}I^{\alpha+\beta}_{t}f(t).
$$

which also implies

$$
{}^{RL}_{0}I^{\alpha}_{t}\circ{}^{RL}_{0}I^{\beta}_{t}f(t) = {}^{RL}_{0}I^{\beta}_{t}\circ{}^{RL}_{0}I^{\alpha}_{t}f(t),
$$

thus RL fractional integrals commute. Note that for $\alpha \geq 0, t > 0$, dealing with a power function t^k, with $k > -1$, the RL fractional integral becomes

$$
{}^{RL}_{0}I^{\alpha}_{t}t^{k} = \frac{\Gamma(k+1)}{\Gamma(k+1+\alpha)}t^{k+\alpha},
$$

which is a generalization of the results we get when working with integer order.

The RL integral is linear like the usual Riemann integral, since

$$\begin{aligned}
{}_a^{RL}I_t^\alpha(pf(t) + qg(t)) &= p\frac{1}{\Gamma(\alpha)}\int_a^t (t - \theta)^{\alpha-1}f(\theta)d\theta \\
&\quad + q\frac{1}{\Gamma(\alpha)}\int_a^t (t - \theta)^{\alpha-1}g(\theta)d\theta \\
&= p{}_a^{RL}I_t^\alpha f(t) + q{}_a^{RL}I_t^\alpha g(t).
\end{aligned}$$

Now we can define the *Gel'fand-Shilov function* of order α as

$$\Phi_\alpha(t) = \frac{t^{\alpha-1}}{\Gamma(\alpha)}, \quad \alpha > 0,$$

which is absolutely integrable in the $\mathbb{R}^+$ support and vanishes if $t < 0$. Here we may easily verify that

$$\begin{aligned}
\Phi_\alpha(t) * f(t) &= \frac{1}{\Gamma(\alpha)}\int_0^t (t - \theta)^{\alpha-1}f(\theta)d(\theta) \\
&= {}_0^{RL}I_t^\alpha f(t).
\end{aligned}$$

Since the Laplace transform of $f(t)$ is

$$\mathcal{L}[f(t)] = F(s) = \int_0^{+\infty} f(t)e^{-st}dt, \; s \in \mathbb{C}$$

and since given the convolution product of two functions $f(t) * g(t)$, we have

$$\mathcal{L}[f(t) * g(t)] = \int_{-\infty}^{+\infty} \left(\int_{-\infty}^{+\infty} f(\tau)g(t - \tau)d\tau\right) e^{st}dt = F(s)G(s),$$

thus we get also

$$\mathcal{L}[\Phi_\alpha(t)] = \frac{1}{s^\alpha}$$

$$\mathcal{L}[{}_0^{RL}I_t^\alpha f(t)] = \frac{F(s)}{s^\alpha}$$

in both cases with $\alpha > 0$.

Now we can observe that defining the derivative of order n (with $n \in \mathbb{N}$) of a given $f(t)$ as

$$D_t^n f(t) = \frac{d^n}{dt^n}f(t), \tag{19.9}$$

then, for $t > a$, it is

$$D_t^n \circ {}_a^{RL} I_t^n f(t) = f(t)$$

and therefore we may say that $_0 D_t^n$ is the left inverse operator of $_0^{RL} I_t^n$, and we get the definition of the RL fractional derivative of non-integer order α given in Eq. (19.6), and again invoking the semigroup property, and looking at effects on the power function, we have

$$_0 D_t^\alpha t^k = \frac{\Gamma(k+1)}{\Gamma(k+1-\alpha)} t^{k-\alpha}, \quad \alpha, t > 0, k > -1$$

where $k + 1 - \alpha$ can be negative.

At this point, we can define the Caputo fractional derivative $_a^C D_t^\alpha f(t)$ as

$$_a^C D_t^\alpha f(t) = {}_0 I_t^{m-\alpha} \circ D_t^m f(t), \quad m - 1 < \alpha \le m,$$

with $m \in \mathbb{N}$ and $\alpha \in \mathbb{R}$, to get Eq. (19.7).

Note that since

$$_a^C D_t^\alpha = \frac{1}{\Gamma(n-\alpha)} \int_a^t \frac{d^n f(\theta)}{d\theta^n} \frac{1}{(t-\theta)^{1+\alpha-n}} d\theta,$$

then

$$_a^C I_t^{n-\alpha} f(t) = {}_a^C D_t^\alpha f(t),$$

thus, integrating by parts

$$_a^C D_t^\alpha y(t) = \frac{(t-a)^{n-a}}{\Gamma(n-\alpha+1)} \frac{d^n y(a)}{da^n}$$

$$+ \frac{1}{\Gamma(n-\alpha+1)} \int_a^t \frac{1}{(t-\theta)^{\alpha-n}} \frac{d^{n+1} y(\theta)}{d\theta^{n+1}} d\theta$$

where $t > \alpha$, with $n - 1 < \alpha \le n$.

The Caputo operator differs from the Riemann-Liouville operator because it represents the integration of a derivative of f, which must be differentiable at least n times. If we pass to the limit $\alpha \to n - 1$, we get $n - \alpha = 1$, and therefore, $\Gamma(n-\alpha) = \Gamma(1) = 1$; thus, $\frac{1}{\Gamma(1)} = 1$, and $\alpha - n + 1 = 1$, hence

$$_0^C D_t^\alpha y(t) = \int_0^t \frac{1}{(t-\theta)} \frac{d^n y(\theta)}{d\theta^n} d\theta = \frac{d^{n-1} y(t)}{dt^{n-1}},$$

thus the Caputo operator becomes the regular differential operator, provided y is differentiable n times.

Reference

1. Anastassiou GA. Generalized fractional calculus. Cham: Springer Nature; 2021.

Vectors

In a n-dimensional vector space, $\mathbb{V}$, we define a n-dimensional vector $\mathbf{v}$, as well as its transposed vector $\mathbf{v}^\top$, respectively, as

$$
\mathbf{v} = \begin{pmatrix} v_1 \\ v_2 \\ \vdots \\ v_n \end{pmatrix}; \qquad \mathbf{v}^\top = \begin{pmatrix} v_1 \\ v_2 \\ \vdots \\ v_n \end{pmatrix}^\top = \begin{pmatrix} v_1 & v_2 & \cdots & v_n \end{pmatrix}, \tag{20.1}
$$

where v_1, v_2, and v_n are components (or the *elements*) of the vector; these elements are generally scalars and can be, for example, real or complex numbers. In most cases, there is no need to specify the number of components of a vector, e.g., its dimensions; however, if dimensions must be given, this may be done by placing the number of dimensions as a subscript, for example, writing $\mathbf{v}_5$ to say that vector $\mathbf{v}$ has five components. Of course, for any n-dimensional vector $\mathbf{v}$, there is a one-to-one correspondence $\mathbf{v} \leftrightarrow \mathbf{v}^\top$.

A vector is therefore a single column of elements, while its transpose is given by the same elements disposed in a single row: in practice, the transposition of a vector is a counterclockwise rotation by 90 degrees of the original column vector. To avoid confusion, in some cases, it would be better to call the vector as column vectorand its transposed as row vector.

Any vector can be expressed in terms of unit (normalized) vectors $\mathbf{i}, \mathbf{j}, \mathbf{k}$ (in the case of vectors in $\mathbb{R}^3$), which are defined as follows:

$$
\mathbf{i} = \begin{pmatrix} 1 \\ 0 \\ 0 \end{pmatrix}; \quad \mathbf{j} = \begin{pmatrix} 0 \\ 1 \\ 0 \end{pmatrix}; \quad \mathbf{k} = \begin{pmatrix} 0 \\ 0 \\ 1 \end{pmatrix},
$$

M. Nichelatti, *Mathematical Tools for Telemedicine*, TELe-Health,
https://doi.org/10.1007/978-3-031-81709-0_20

representing three directions of axis x, y, and z, respectively, so that for a generic vector $\mathbf{v}$ we can write.

$$\mathbf{v} = \begin{pmatrix} v_1 \\ v_2 \\ v_3 \end{pmatrix} = v_1\mathbf{i} + v_2\mathbf{j} + v_3\mathbf{k}.$$

We can also obtain the unitary vector in the same direction of a given vector $\mathbf{a}$, since its unitary vector $\mathbf{u}$ will be

$$\mathbf{u_a} = \frac{\mathbf{a}}{\|\mathbf{a}\|},$$

$\|\mathbf{a}\|$ being the magnitude of the vector $\mathbf{a}$, e.g., its *norm*, $\|\mathbf{a}\| = \sqrt{a_1^2 + a_2^2 + a_3^2}$. For example, given $\mathbf{a} = 5\mathbf{i} + 4\mathbf{j} - 3\mathbf{k}$, its unitary vector is

$$\begin{aligned} \mathbf{u_a} &= \mathbf{a}\frac{1}{\sqrt{5^2 + 4^2 + (-3)^2}} \\ &= \mathbf{a}\frac{1}{5\sqrt{2}} \\ &= \frac{5}{5\sqrt{2}}\mathbf{i} + \frac{2}{5\sqrt{2}}\mathbf{j} - \frac{3}{5\sqrt{2}}\mathbf{k} \\ &= \frac{\sqrt{2}}{2}\mathbf{i} + \frac{\sqrt{2}}{5}\mathbf{j} - \frac{3\sqrt{2}}{10}\mathbf{k}, \end{aligned}$$

e.g., the vector having unitary length and lying on the same direction of $\mathbf{a}$.

The geometric meaning of vector can be explained considering a Cartesian system of coordinates in two dimensions: the vector $\mathbf{v}$ starts at the origin of axes and has its tip in the point $P(v_1, v_2)$; thus, the tip of the vector lies in the point having the first component of $\mathbf{v}$ as the x coordinate and the second component as the y coordinate. The sum of two vectors $\mathbf{v} + \mathbf{w}$ is a new vector starting at the origin, having its tip in the point $Q(v_1 + w_1, v_2 + w_2)$.

20.1 Basic Vector Operations

Two vectors $\mathbf{v}$ and $\mathbf{w}$ can be summed, provided that their dimension is the same; the vector sum is a new vector whose components are given by the elementwise sum of the components of $\mathbf{v}$ and $\mathbf{w}$. In the same way, we can obtain the difference between two vectors by elementwise subtraction of the elements, so as to have

$$\mathbf{v} \pm \mathbf{w} = \begin{pmatrix} v_1 \\ v_2 \\ \vdots \\ v_n \end{pmatrix} \pm \begin{pmatrix} w_1 \\ w_2 \\ \vdots \\ w_n \end{pmatrix} = \begin{pmatrix} v_1 \pm w_1 \\ v_2 \pm w_2 \\ \vdots \\ v_n \pm w_n \end{pmatrix}.$$

Notable vectors are the null vector $\mathbf{0}$ and the unitary vector $\mathbf{1}$, given as

$$\mathbf{0} = \begin{pmatrix} 0 \\ 0 \\ \vdots \\ 0 \end{pmatrix}, \qquad \mathbf{1} = \begin{pmatrix} 1 \\ 1 \\ \vdots \\ 1 \end{pmatrix};$$

in particular, the null vector $\mathbf{0}$ is the neutral element for the sum and difference, since for any n-dimensional vector $\mathbf{v}$, we have by the definition of vector sum and difference as

$$\mathbf{v} + \mathbf{0} = \mathbf{v}; \qquad \mathbf{v} - \mathbf{0} = \mathbf{v},$$

provided that the null vector has the same n dimensions.

The multiplication of a vector $\mathbf{v}$ by a scalar λ gives a new vector with components multiplied by λ, e.g.,

$$\lambda \mathbf{v} = \mathbf{v}\lambda = \lambda \begin{pmatrix} v_1 \\ \vdots \\ v_n \end{pmatrix} = \begin{pmatrix} \lambda v_1 \\ \vdots \\ \lambda v_n \end{pmatrix}.$$

20.2 Linear Forms

Two (column) vectors cannot by multiplied; however, it is possible to multiply a row vector $\mathbf{x}^\top$ by a column vector $\mathbf{y}$ and vice versa (e.g., $\mathbf{x}^\top \mathbf{y}$ and $\mathbf{y}^\top \mathbf{x}$), provided that $\mathbf{x}$ and $\mathbf{y}$ have the same dimensions: of course, a vector can be multiplied by its transposed vector; the result is a scalar anyway. This vector product is defined *dot product* (but also *scalar product* or *internal product* or even *minor product* in some textbooks) since it can be defined also with the equivalent formalism $\mathbf{x} \cdot \mathbf{y}$ (hence $\mathbf{x}^\top \mathbf{y} \equiv \mathbf{x} \cdot \mathbf{y}$). Indeed, another way to define the dot product, and the most useful for our purposes, is linear form.

Dealing with the three-component vectors $\mathbf{x}$ and $\mathbf{y}$, we may define the linear form

$$\mathbf{x}^\top \mathbf{y} = \begin{pmatrix} x_1 & x_2 & \cdots & x_n \end{pmatrix} \begin{pmatrix} y_1 \\ y_2 \\ \vdots \\ y_n \end{pmatrix}$$

$$= x_1 y_1 + x_2 y_2 + \cdots + x_n y_n$$

$$= \sum_{k=1}^{n} x_k y_k, \tag{20.2}$$

thus it is the sum of the products of the single vector components; it is evident that a linear form is defined if, and only if, the vectors have the same dimensions. Of course, given $\mathbf{x}$ we may also define the multiplication

$$\mathbf{x}^\top \mathbf{x} = \begin{pmatrix} x_1 & x_2 & \cdots & x_n \end{pmatrix} \begin{pmatrix} x_1 \\ x_2 \\ \vdots \\ x_n \end{pmatrix}$$

$$= x_1 x_1 + x_2 x_2 + \cdots + x_n x_n$$

$$= \sum_{k=1}^{n} x_k^2, \tag{20.3}$$

showing that $\mathbf{x}^\top \mathbf{x}$ is scalar equal to the sum of squares of the components of $\mathbf{x}$.

An example of calculus can be done by using the vectors

$$\mathbf{v} = \begin{pmatrix} 2 \\ 3 \\ -1 \end{pmatrix}, \qquad \mathbf{w} = \begin{pmatrix} 1 \\ -2 \\ 0 \end{pmatrix}$$

obtaining

$$\mathbf{v}^\top \mathbf{w} = \begin{pmatrix} 2 & 3 & -1 \end{pmatrix} \begin{pmatrix} 1 \\ -2 \\ 0 \end{pmatrix} = 2 \times 1 + 3 \times (-2) + (-1) \times 0 = -4$$

and

$$\mathbf{w}^\top \mathbf{v} = \begin{pmatrix} 1 & -2 & 0 \end{pmatrix} \begin{pmatrix} 2 \\ 3 \\ -1 \end{pmatrix} = 1 \times 2 + (-2) \times 3 + 0 \times (-1) = -4$$

where the commutative property $\mathbf{x}^\top \mathbf{y} = \mathbf{y}^\top \mathbf{x}$ of linear forms is verified.

We also have

$$\mathbf{v}^\top \mathbf{v} = \begin{pmatrix} 2 & 3 & -1 \end{pmatrix} \begin{pmatrix} 2 \\ 3 \\ -1 \end{pmatrix} = 2^2 + 3^2 + (-1)^2 = 14,$$

and

$$\mathbf{w}^\top \mathbf{w} = \begin{pmatrix} 1 & -2 & 0 \end{pmatrix} \begin{pmatrix} 1 \\ -2 \\ 0 \end{pmatrix} = 1^2 + (-2)^2 + 0^2 = 5.$$

e.g., the sum of squares of the components.

An interesting result is given by $\mathbf{1}_n^\top \mathbf{1}_n$, since it is

$$\mathbf{1}_n^\top \mathbf{1}_n = \sum_{i=1}^{n} 1_i^2 = n.$$

When $\mathbf{x}^\top \mathbf{y} = 0$ (excluding the trivial situations $\mathbf{x} = \mathbf{0}$ and $\mathbf{y} = \mathbf{0}$, giving always $x_k y_k = 0$), the vectors are said *orthogonal* ; for example, with

$$\mathbf{x} = \begin{pmatrix} 3 \\ 2 \\ 2 \end{pmatrix}; \quad \mathbf{y} = \begin{pmatrix} -2 \\ 1 \\ 2 \end{pmatrix},$$

we easily see that vectors are orthogonal since $\mathbf{x}^\top \mathbf{y} = 3 \times (-2) + 2 \times 1 + 2 \times 2 = -6 + 2 + 4 = 0$. When two vectors are orthogonal, their directions are perpendicular: for example, if

$$\mathbf{p} = \begin{pmatrix} a \\ b \end{pmatrix}, \quad \mathbf{q} = \begin{pmatrix} -b \\ a \end{pmatrix}, \quad \mathbf{r} = \begin{pmatrix} b \\ -a \end{pmatrix},$$

we can say that $\mathbf{p}$ is perpendicular to $\mathbf{q}$ and $\mathbf{s}$, since $\mathbf{p}^\top \mathbf{q} = \mathbf{q}^\top \mathbf{p} = 0$, and $\mathbf{p}^\top \mathbf{r} = \mathbf{r}^\top \mathbf{p} = 0$, while $\mathbf{q}$ and $\mathbf{r}$ ain't in general perpendicular, since $\mathbf{q}^\top \mathbf{r} = \mathbf{r}^\top \mathbf{q} = -b^2 - a^2$; indeed, $\mathbf{q}$ and $\mathbf{r}$ can be perpendicular (if their entries are complex numbers) in the particular case $a = ib$, or $a = -ib$, being $i = \sqrt{-1}$.

If for a set of orthogonal vectors $\mathbf{x}_{(1)}, \mathbf{x}_{(2)}, \ldots, \mathbf{x}_{(n)}$, in which $\mathbf{x}_{(j)}^\top \mathbf{x}_{(k)} = 0$ ($j \neq k$), and in which also we have $\mathbf{x}_{(k)}^\top \mathbf{x}_{(k)} = 1$, then these vectors are said *orthonormal*.

From the definition of linear form in Eq. (20.2), we immediately see that the Euclidean norm $\|\mathbf{v}\|$ of a given vector $\mathbf{v}$ may be written as

$$\|\mathbf{v}^\top - \mathbf{0}^\top\| = \sqrt{(\mathbf{v} - \mathbf{0})^\top (\mathbf{v} - \mathbf{0})},$$

or even in the more compact form

$$||\mathbf{v}|| = (\mathbf{v}^\top \mathbf{v})^{1/2},$$

which is equivalent to say that vector length is the square root of the sum of the squared components; thus, we infer that for an orthonormal vector, it must be $\mathbf{v}^\top \mathbf{v} = 1$ and also $||\mathbf{v}|| = (\mathbf{v}^\top \mathbf{v})^{1/2} = 1$.

If, for example,

$$\mathbf{v} = \begin{pmatrix} 3 \\ 4 \\ 5 \end{pmatrix},$$

then

$$||\mathbf{v}|| = (\mathbf{v}^\top \mathbf{v})^{1/2}$$

$$= \left((3\ 4\ 5) \begin{pmatrix} 3 \\ 4 \\ 5 \end{pmatrix} \right)^{1/2}$$

$$= \sqrt{9 + 16 + 25}$$

$$= 5\sqrt{2}.$$

20.3   Interesting Linear Forms

As previously observed, the definition of linear form allows to express any natural number $n \in \mathbb{N}$ using unit vectors, since

$$n = \mathbf{1}_n^\top \mathbf{1}_n;$$

for example,

$$(1\ 1\ 1) \begin{pmatrix} 1 \\ 1 \\ 1 \end{pmatrix} = 3,$$

and also the sum of first n natural numbers $m = 1 + 2 + \cdots + n - 1 + n$ in the form

$$\sum_{k=1}^{n} r_k = \mathbf{1}_n^\top \mathbf{r}_n = \mathbf{r}_n^\top \mathbf{1}_n,$$

being

$$\mathbf{r}_n = \begin{pmatrix} 1 \\ \vdots \\ n \end{pmatrix}$$

the vector having the first n natural numbers as components. For example,

$$(1\ 2\ 3) \begin{pmatrix} 1 \\ 1 \\ 1 \end{pmatrix} = (1\ 1\ 1) \begin{pmatrix} 1 \\ 2 \\ 3 \end{pmatrix} = 6,$$

since $1 + 2 + 3 = 6$. The equality $\mathbf{1}_n^{\top} \mathbf{r}_n = \mathbf{r}_n \mathbf{1}_n^{\top}$ is evident, since a linear form is a scalar.

Another important property of the linear forms is the capability to resume various statistical information of a set of measures. For example, if the components of a n-dimensional vector $\mathbf{h}$ are n measures h_i of height, taken on a sample of n subjects: the sum of all measured heights is $\mathbf{1}_n^{\top} \mathbf{h}_n$, and therefore its mean value is $\overline{h} = (h_1 + \cdots + h_n)/n$, which (omitting the subscripts) can be given also as:

$$\overline{h} = \frac{\mathbf{1}^{\top}\mathbf{h}}{n} = \frac{\mathbf{1}^{\top}\mathbf{h}}{\mathbf{1}^{\top}\mathbf{1}}. \tag{20.4}$$

Moreover, the sample variance of the n measures h_k is

$$s^2 = \frac{1}{n-1} \sum_{k=1}^{n} (h_k - \overline{h})^2$$

$$= \frac{1}{n-1} \sum_{k=1}^{n} (h_k - 2h_k\overline{h} + \overline{h})^2$$

$$= \frac{1}{n-1} \left(\sum_{k=1}^{n} h_k^2 - 2n\overline{h}^2 + n\overline{h}^2 \right)$$

$$= \frac{1}{n-1} \left(\sum_{k=1}^{n} h_k^2 - n\overline{h}^2 \right)$$

$$= \frac{1}{n-1} \left(\mathbf{h}^{\top}\mathbf{h} - n\left(\frac{\mathbf{1}^{\top}\mathbf{h}}{n}\right)^2 \right)$$

$$= \frac{1}{n-1} \left(\mathbf{h}^{\top}\mathbf{h} - \frac{1}{n}\left(\mathbf{1}^{\top}\mathbf{h}\right)^2 \right). \tag{20.5}$$

20.4   Linear Combination of Vectors

Assume we have the vector $\mathbf{w}$ given by the sum of n different vectors $\mathbf{v}_k$ belonging to a vector space $\mathbb{V}$, and all having the same dimensions, such that

$$\mathbf{w} = a_1\mathbf{v}_1 + a_2\mathbf{v}_2 + \cdots + a_n\mathbf{v}_n \tag{20.6}$$

in this case, we say that $\mathbf{w}$ is a *linear combination* of vectors $\mathbf{v}_1, \mathbf{v}_2, \mathbf{v}_3, \ldots, \mathbf{v}_n$ and that $\mathbf{v}_1, \mathbf{v}_2, \ldots, \mathbf{v}_n$ are *linearly independent* if

$$a_1\mathbf{v}_1 + a_2\mathbf{v}_2 + \cdots + a_n\mathbf{v}_n = \mathbf{0} \tag{20.7}$$

may be verified if, and only if, it is

$$a_1 = a_2 = a_3 = \cdots = a_n = 0. \tag{20.8}$$

Vectors $\mathbf{v}_j$ and $\mathbf{v}_k$ can't be linearly independent if they are proportional, e.g., if there is a scalar λ such that $\mathbf{v}_j = \lambda\mathbf{v}_k$; moreover, vectors can't be linearly independent if one of them is a linear combination of the others: in this case, vectors are *linearly dependent*; notably, any set of vectors including the null vector is always linearly dependent, since, in this case

$$a_1\mathbf{v}_1 + a_2\mathbf{v}_2 + \cdots + \lambda\mathbf{0} + \cdots + a_n\mathbf{v}_n = \mathbf{0}$$

is satisfied by letting $\lambda \neq 0$ while keeping all $a_k = 0$. Moreover, we can see that a set of n vectors that are m-dimensional can't be linearly independent if $m > n$, hence, for example, three vectors with two dimensions

$$\mathbf{p} = \begin{pmatrix} p_1 \\ p_2 \end{pmatrix}, \quad \mathbf{q} = \begin{pmatrix} q_1 \\ q_2 \end{pmatrix}, \quad \mathbf{r} = \begin{pmatrix} r_1 \\ r_2 \end{pmatrix},$$

are always linearly dependent, e.g.,

$$a_1 \begin{pmatrix} p_1 \\ p_2 \end{pmatrix} + a_2 \begin{pmatrix} q_1 \\ q_2 \end{pmatrix} = -a_3 \begin{pmatrix} r_1 \\ r_2 \end{pmatrix}$$

is always possible since (as we will see when discussing the reduced row echelon form of a matrix in the next chapter) above equation can be expressed as

$$\begin{pmatrix} a_1 \\ a_2 \end{pmatrix} = -a_3 \begin{pmatrix} -\frac{1}{p_1 q_2 - p_2 q_1}(q_1 r_2 - q_2 r_1) \\ \frac{1}{p_1 q_2 - p_2 q_1}(p_1 r_2 - p_2 r_1) \end{pmatrix}$$

meaning that vector $\mathbf{r}$ can be given as sum of vectors $\mathbf{p}$ and $\mathbf{q}$.

We note that for two vectors $\mathbf{x}$ and $\mathbf{y}$, the linear independence is satisfied if given a scalar λ, it is $\mathbf{x} \neq \lambda\mathbf{y}$, while if one can write $\mathbf{x} = \lambda\mathbf{y}$, then $\mathbf{x}$ and $\mathbf{y}$ are linearly dependent. In other words, if two vectors are multiple, they cannot be linearly independent.

20.5 Vector Product (Cross Product)

Assuming to have two vectors with the same number of components (e.g., three):

$$\mathbf{u} = \begin{pmatrix} u_x \\ u_y \\ u_z \end{pmatrix} ; \quad \mathbf{v} = \begin{pmatrix} v_x \\ v_y \\ v_z \end{pmatrix},$$

we define the vector product $\mathbf{w}$ between the two vectors as

$$\mathbf{w} = \mathbf{u} \times \mathbf{v}$$

$$= \begin{pmatrix} u_y v_z - u_z v_y \\ u_z v_x - u_x v_z \\ u_x v_y - u_y v_x \end{pmatrix},$$

hence $\mathbf{w}$ is itself a vector with the same dimensions of $\mathbf{u}$ and $\mathbf{w}$. The result can be obtained by calculating the *determinant*

$$\mathbf{w} = \det \begin{pmatrix} \mathbf{e}_x & \mathbf{e}_y & \mathbf{e}_z \\ u_x & u_y & u_z \\ v_x & v_y & v_z \end{pmatrix}$$

$$= \mathbf{e}_x \det \begin{pmatrix} u_y & u_z \\ v_y & v_z \end{pmatrix} - \mathbf{e}_y \det \begin{pmatrix} u_x & u_z \\ v_x & v_z \end{pmatrix} + \mathbf{e}_z \det \begin{pmatrix} u_x & u_y \\ v_x & v_y \end{pmatrix}$$

$$= \mathbf{e}_x(u_y v_z - u_z v_y) - \mathbf{e}_y(u_z v_x - u_x v_z) + \mathbf{e}_z(u_x v_y - u_y v_x)$$

where $\mathbf{e}_x, \mathbf{e}_y, \mathbf{e}_z$ are unit vectors in the x, y, z directions respectively. The concept and meaning of the determinant of a matrix will be discussed in the next chapter. Vector $\mathbf{w}$ is perpendicular to the plane where $\mathbf{u}$ and $\mathbf{v}$ are lying; $\mathbf{w}$ is directed upward with respect to that plane; the length of vector $\mathbf{w}$ is $\|\mathbf{u}\| \|\mathbf{v}\| \sin(\widehat{\mathbf{u}\mathbf{v}})$, while $\|\mathbf{u} \times \mathbf{v}\|$ is the area of the parallelogram defined by vectors $\mathbf{u}$ and $\mathbf{v}$.

From the definition, we understand that $\mathbf{u} \times \mathbf{v} = \mathbf{0}$ if $\mathbf{u}$ and $\mathbf{v}$ are parallel or when one or both vectors are null. Vector product does not commute unless changing the sign of $\mathbf{w}$, that is, $\mathbf{u} \times \mathbf{v} = -\mathbf{v} \times \mathbf{u}$ and behaves linearly, since given a scalar λ, we have $(\lambda\mathbf{u}) \times \mathbf{v} = \mathbf{u} \times (\lambda\mathbf{v}) = \lambda(\mathbf{u} \times \mathbf{v})$, and given a third vector $\mathbf{t}$, we have

$(\mathbf{t} + \mathbf{u}) \times \mathbf{v} = \mathbf{t} \times \mathbf{v} + \mathbf{t} \times \mathbf{v}$ and $(\mathbf{u} \times \mathbf{v}) \times \mathbf{t} = (\mathbf{uv})\mathbf{t} - (\mathbf{vt})\mathbf{u}$. Regarding the cross product of unit vectors, we infer

$$\|\mathbf{e}_x\| \, \|\mathbf{e}_y\| \sin(\widehat{\mathbf{e}_x \mathbf{e}_y}) = \|\mathbf{e}_y\| \, \|\mathbf{e}_z\| \sin(\widehat{\mathbf{e}_y \mathbf{e}_z}) = \|\mathbf{e}_z\| \, \|\mathbf{e}_x\| \sin(\widehat{\mathbf{e}_z \mathbf{e}_x})$$
$$= 1 \times 1 \times \sin\left(\frac{\pi}{2}\right) = 1,$$

as well as the following relations:

$$\mathbf{e}_x \times \mathbf{e}_x = \mathbf{e}_y \times \mathbf{e}_y = \mathbf{e}_z \times \mathbf{e}_z = \mathbf{0}$$
$$\mathbf{e}_x \times \mathbf{e}_y = \mathbf{e}_z; \quad \mathbf{e}_y \times \mathbf{e}_z = \mathbf{e}_x; \quad \mathbf{e}_z \times \mathbf{e}_x = \mathbf{e}_y$$
$$\mathbf{e}_y \times \mathbf{e}_x = -\mathbf{e}_z; \quad \mathbf{e}_z \times \mathbf{e}_y = -\mathbf{e}_x; \quad \mathbf{e}_x \times \mathbf{e}_z = -\mathbf{e}_y.$$

References

1. Banerjee S, Roy A. Linear algebra and matrix analysis for statistics. Boca Raton: CRC Press; 2014.
2. Brown WC. Matrices and vector spaces. New York: Marcel Dekker, Inc.; 1991.

Matrices

A generic matrix $\mathbf{A}_{m \times n}$ is an array of things (numbers, functions, objects) arranged in m rows and n columns: it can also be defined as an $m \times n$ matrix, or a matrix with dimensions $m \times n$. The notation $\mathbf{A}$ without subscripts can also be used when it is not necessary to specify the matrix dimensions. Each thing belonging to the matrix is called an *element* of the matrix $\mathbf{A}$ and is identified with a lowercase letter (in general it can be the same letter as the bold uppercase one used to define the matrix), and with a subscript with the numbers j and k, such that a_{jk} is the element of $\mathbf{A}_{m \times n}$ placed at the intersection of j-th row and k-th column. An $m \times n$ matrix is therefore written in the form:

$$\mathbf{A}_{m \times n} = \begin{pmatrix} a_{11} & a_{12} & \cdots & a_{1c} \\ a_{21} & a_{22} & \cdots & a_{2c} \\ \vdots & \vdots & \ddots & \vdots \\ a_{r1} & a_{r2} & \cdots & a_{mn} \end{pmatrix}. \tag{21.1}$$

or also, in the more general form $\mathbf{A} = \{a_{jk}\}$.

For example, if we take

$$\mathbf{B} = \begin{pmatrix} 2 & 3 & 1 & 5 \\ 3 & 7 & 4 & 3 \\ 6 & 2 & 0 & 3 \end{pmatrix} \tag{21.2}$$

we say that $\mathbf{B}$ is a 3×4 matrix, in which, from the definition, we may recognize the elements $a_{11} = 2$, $a_{32} = 4$, $a_{24} = 3$, and so on.

Each matrix $\mathbf{A}_{m \times n}$ corresponds to one, and only one, *transpose* $\mathbf{A}_{n \times m}^\top$ in which the rows and columns are exchanged, so that,

$$
\mathbf{A}_{n \times m}^\top =
\begin{pmatrix}
a_{11} & a_{12} & \cdots & a_{1n} \\
a_{21} & a_{22} & \cdots & a_{2n} \\
\vdots & \vdots & \ddots & \vdots \\
a_{m1} & a_{m2} & \cdots & a_{mn}
\end{pmatrix}^\top
=
\begin{pmatrix}
a_{11} & a_{21} & \cdots & a_{n1} \\
a_{12} & a_{22} & \cdots & a_{n2} \\
\vdots & \vdots & \ddots & \vdots \\
a_{1n} & a_{2m} & \cdots & a_{nm}
\end{pmatrix}
$$

where, if $\mathbf{A}$ is $m \times n$, then $\mathbf{A}^\top$ is $n \times m$; thus, the transpose of matrix (21.2) is

$$
\mathbf{B}^\top =
\begin{pmatrix}
2 & 3 & 6 \\
3 & 7 & 2 \\
1 & 4 & 0 \\
5 & 3 & 3
\end{pmatrix} ;
$$

hence, $\mathbf{B}$ is a 3×4 matrix, while $\mathbf{B}^\top$ is a 4×3 matrix, and the element b_{jk} of $\mathbf{B}$ is the element b_{kj} of $\mathbf{B}^\top$. Obviously, the transposition of the transpose of a matrix returns the matrix itself, that is, $(\mathbf{A}^\top)^\top = \mathbf{A}$.

A *square matrix* is a matrix with the number of rows equal to the number of columns, so that it can be given as $\mathbf{A}_{nn}$ (in some textbooks simply as $\mathbf{A}_n$); otherwise, we are dealing with a *rectangular matrix*. In a square matrix, all elements a_{jk} with $j = k$ are defined *diagonal elements*, while elements with $j \neq k$ are *nondiagonal*. If in a square matrix we find $a_{jk} = 0$ for $j \neq k$, then the matrix is diagonal if we have at least a diagonal element $a_{jj} \neq 0$. Moreover, if in a square matrix we have $a_{jk} = a_{kj}$, then the matrix is *symmetric*, while if $a_{jk} = -a_{kj}$, then the matrix is *skew-symmetric*.

Three examples of square matrices are given below: we recognize a diagonal matrix $\mathbf{D}$, a symmetric matrix $\mathbf{S}$, and a skew-symmetric: matrix $\mathbf{Z}$

$$
\mathbf{D} =
\begin{pmatrix}
0 & 0 & 0 \\
0 & -2 & 0 \\
0 & 0 & 7
\end{pmatrix} ; \quad
\mathbf{S} =
\begin{pmatrix}
2 & 4 & 1 \\
4 & 1 & 3 \\
1 & 3 & 5
\end{pmatrix} ; \quad
\mathbf{Z} =
\begin{pmatrix}
0 & 3 & 7 \\
-3 & 0 & 4 \\
-7 & -4 & 0
\end{pmatrix} ,
$$

and we see that $d_{jk} = 0$ if $j \neq k$, $s_{jk} = s_{kj}$ and that $z_{jk} = -z_{kj}$. As expected, we also see that $\mathbf{D} = \mathbf{D}^\top$, $\mathbf{S} = \mathbf{S}^\top$ (thus diagonal matrices are also symmetric) and $\mathbf{Z} = -\mathbf{Z}^\top$.

Notably, we observe that the diagonal elements of $\mathbf{Z}$ are all zero: this is because the only possibility to have $z_{jj} = -z_{jj}$ in a square matrix is $z_{jj} = 0$. Indeed, things aren't so simple: we must also assume that $\mathbf{T}$ belongs to a *field* with characteristic different from 2; in algebra, the characteristic is the minimum number of multiplicative identities to be summed to obtain the additive identity (however, here we are far beyond the scope of this book). For evident reasons, rectangular matrices cannot be diagonal, nor symmetric or skew-symmetric.

A generalization of the transpose is the *Hermitian matrix* $\mathbf{A}^H$, which is defined when some entries are complex numbers. In a Hermitian matrix, the diagonal elements are real, while the off-diagonal elements are defined as $a_{jk} = \alpha + i\beta$ and $a_{kj} = \alpha - i\beta$; thus, a_{jk} is the complex conjugate of a_{kj}. An example of Hermitian matrix is

$$\begin{pmatrix} 2 & \alpha - i\beta & \zeta + i\eta \\ \alpha + i\beta & 1 & \kappa + i\lambda \\ \zeta - i\eta & \kappa - i\lambda & 3 \end{pmatrix} = \begin{pmatrix} 2 & \alpha & \zeta \\ \alpha & 1 & \kappa \\ \zeta & \kappa & 3 \end{pmatrix} + i \begin{pmatrix} 0 & -\beta & \eta \\ \beta & 0 & \lambda \\ -\eta & -\lambda & 0 \end{pmatrix}$$

so that, in general we may write a Hermitian matrix as the sum of a symmetric matrix $\mathbf{P}$ plus a skew-symmetric matrix $\mathbf{Q}$ as follows:

$$\mathbf{A}^H = \mathbf{P} + i\mathbf{Q},$$

where $i = \sqrt{-1}$.

The diagonal elements of a Hermitian matrix must be real since a complex number is equal to its complex conjugate if its imaginary part is zero, e.g., if the number is real. Of course, if all entries of a Hermitian matrix are real, then the Hermitian matrix is symmetric.

Other matrices to be considered are the *triangular matrices*, which can be *upper trigular* or *lower triangular*. These are square matrices in which all elements, respectively below or above the diagonal, are zero. Examples of an upper triangular matrix $\mathbf{A}$ and of a lower triangular matrix $\mathbf{B}$ respectively are

$$\mathbf{A} = \begin{pmatrix} a_{11} & a_{21} & a_{31} & a_{41} \\ 0 & a_{22} & a_{23} & a_{24} \\ 0 & 0 & a_{33} & a_{34} \\ 0 & 0 & 0 & a_{44} \end{pmatrix}; \quad \mathbf{B} = \begin{pmatrix} b_{11} & 0 & 0 & 0 \\ b_{21} & b_{22} & 0 & 0 \\ b_{31} & b_{32} & b_{33} & 0 \\ b_{41} & b_{42} & b_{43} & b_{44} \end{pmatrix}.$$

In most cases, working with matrices, it is not necessary to use the subscript reporting the number of row and columns, but in some other cases, the subscript must be used to better specify the properties of a given matrix and its *conformability*. As we will see soon, not all matrices are always suitable for an operation; thus, we define a matrix *conformable* if it is suitable for that given operation, and conformability strictly depends on the matrix dimensions.

Important matrices are the *identity matrix* $\mathbf{I}_n$, a diagonal matrix (hence, it is also a square matrix) with $d_{jk} = 1$ if $j = k$ and $d_{jk} = 0$ if $j \neq k$; thus,

$$\mathbf{I}_n = \begin{pmatrix} 1 & 0 & \cdots & 0 \\ 0 & 1 & \cdots & 0 \\ \vdots & \vdots & \ddots & \vdots \\ 0 & 0 & \cdots & 1 \end{pmatrix},$$

the *null matrix* $\mathbf{O}_{m \times n}$ (may or may not be a square matrix) with all entries $d_{jk} = 0$, and the *unit matrix* $\mathbf{U}_{m \times n}$ (also may or may not be a square matrix) with all entries $d_{jk} = 1$; if $\mathbf{U}$ is a non-square unit matrix, the notation $\mathbf{1}_{m \times n}$ can also be found in some textbooks: in this case, one must be aware of the risk of confusing it with the unit vector.

21.1   Matrices as Data Tables

A matrix is a table of numbers, and we can think it is an extension of the concept of vector. Assume we are collecting some data from a sample of five people, and assume these data are given in the following table.

Gender (1=M, 2=F)	Height (cm)	Weight (kg)	Age (y)
1	179	82	34
2	166	54	41
2	172	56	37
1	182	79	46
1	176	75	35

This table is a matrix $\mathbf{M}$, with five rows (the number of subjects) and four columns (the number of variables): in other words, we can write the above table as follows.

$$\mathbf{M} = \begin{pmatrix} 1 & 179 & 82 & 34 \\ 2 & 166 & 54 & 41 \\ 2 & 172 & 56 & 37 \\ 1 & 182 & 79 & 46 \\ 1 & 176 & 75 & 35 \end{pmatrix}$$

which is a 5×4 matrix. Thus, any row represents a subject, and any column represents a variable; moreover, any column is a vector of measures.

21.2   Matrix Sum

Given two matrices $\mathbf{A}_{mn}$ and $\mathbf{B}_{mn}$, their sum $\mathbf{C}_{mn}$ is the matrix $c_{jk} = a_{jk} + b_{jk}$; hence, if

$$\mathbf{A} = \begin{pmatrix} a_{11} & a_{12} & \cdots & a_{1n} \\ a_{21} & a_{22} & \cdots & a_{2n} \\ \vdots & \vdots & \ddots & \vdots \\ a_{m1} & a_{m2} & \cdots & a_{mn} \end{pmatrix}, \quad \mathbf{B} = \begin{pmatrix} b_{11} & b_{12} & \cdots & b_{1n} \\ b_{21} & b_{22} & \cdots & b_{2n} \\ \vdots & \vdots & \ddots & \vdots \\ b_{m1} & b_{m2} & \cdots & b_{mn} \end{pmatrix},$$

then

$$\mathbf{A} \pm \mathbf{B} = \mathbf{C}$$

$$= \begin{pmatrix} a_{11} \pm b_{11} & a_{12} \pm b_{12} & \cdots & a_{1n} \pm b_{1n} \\ a_{21} \pm b_{21} & a_{22} \pm b_{22} & \cdots & a_{2n} \pm b_{2n} \\ \vdots & & \vdots & \ddots & \vdots \\ a_{m1} \pm b_{m1} & a_{m2} \pm b_{m2} & \cdots & a_{mn} \pm b_{mn} \end{pmatrix}. \tag{21.3}$$

From (21.3), one immediately realizes that the sum of matrices is defined if, and only if, the matrices have the same number of rows and columns, or, in other words if they are conformable for sum. Indeed, matrices $\mathbf{A}_{rc}$ and $\mathbf{B}_{mn}$ are conformable for sum only if $r = m$ and $c = n$. From (21.3) we also see that the matrix sum commutes, so that $\mathbf{A}_{mn} + \mathbf{B}_{mn} = \mathbf{B}_{mn} + \mathbf{A}_{mn}$, since also the elementwise sums commute, e.g., $c_{jk} = a_{jk} + b_{jk} = b_{jk} + a_{jk}$. Moreover, from definition, we also infer that the sum of matrices must be associative; thus,

$$(\mathbf{A}_{mn} + \mathbf{B}_{mn}) + \mathbf{C}_{mn} = \mathbf{A}_{mn} + (\mathbf{B}_{mn} + \mathbf{C}_{mn}).$$

The difference $\mathbf{A}_{mn} - \mathbf{B}_{mn} = \mathbf{Z}_{mn}$ is a matrix whose elements are $z_{jk} = a_{jk} - b_{jk}$; thus, it is equivalent to the sum of matrices in which the second one has the negative sign. One must recall that the difference of matrices does not commute, that is, in general $\mathbf{A}_{mn} - \mathbf{B}_{mn} \neq \mathbf{B}_{mn} - \mathbf{A}_{mn}$ (unless $\mathbf{A}_{mn} = \mathbf{B}_{mn}$), while $\mathbf{A}_{mn} - \mathbf{B}_{mn} = -(\mathbf{B}_{mn} - \mathbf{A}_{mn})$ is always true; this seems evident, since $a_{jk} - b_{jk} \neq b_{jk} - a_{jk}$ (again, unless $a_{jk} - b_{jk}$) and $(a_{jk} - b_{jk}) = -(b_{jk} - a_{jk})$.

The null matrix $\mathbf{O}$ is the *neutral element for matrix sum* and difference, since it is always $o_{jk} = 0$; hence $\mathbf{A}_{mn} + \mathbf{O}_{mn} = \mathbf{A}_{mn} - \mathbf{O}_{mn} = \mathbf{A}_{mn}$. In other words, since

$$\mathbf{O}_{m \times n} = \begin{pmatrix} 0 & \cdots & 0 \\ \vdots & \ddots & \vdots \\ 0 & \cdots & 0 \end{pmatrix}.$$

then $\mathbf{A} \pm \mathbf{O} = \mathbf{A}$, always bearing in mind that $\mathbf{A}_{m \times n} + \mathbf{O}_{m \times n} = \mathbf{A}_{m \times n} - \mathbf{O}_{m \times n} = -(\mathbf{O}_{m \times n} - \mathbf{A}_{m \times n})$.

21.3 Multiplication of a Matrix by a Scalar

As we already saw for vectors, given the matrix $\mathbf{A}_{m \times n}$ and the scalar λ, we have $\lambda \mathbf{A} = \mathbf{A} \lambda$, in which any element a_{jk} is multiplied times λ; hence,

$$\lambda \mathbf{A} = \mathbf{A}\lambda = \lambda \begin{pmatrix} a_{11} & a_{12} & \cdots & a_{1n} \\ a_{21} & a_{22} & \cdots & a_{2n} \\ \vdots & \vdots & \ddots & \vdots \\ a_{m1} & a_{m2} & \cdots & a_{mn} \end{pmatrix} = \begin{pmatrix} \lambda a_{11} & \lambda a_{12} & \cdots & \lambda a_{1n} \\ \lambda a_{21} & \lambda a_{22} & \cdots & \lambda a_{2n} \\ \vdots & \vdots & \ddots & \vdots \\ \lambda a_{m1} & \lambda a_{m2} & \cdots & \lambda a_{mn} \end{pmatrix}.$$

21.4 Matrix Product

The product of two arbitrary matrices $\mathbf{X}$ and $\mathbf{Y}$ is not always defined: more precisely, if $\mathbf{X}$ is $m \times n$ and $\mathbf{Y}$ is $p \times q$, then the product $\mathbf{XY} = \mathbf{Z}$ is defined if, and only if, $n = p$, and the resulting matrix $\mathbf{Z}$ will be $m \times q$. In practice, the matrix product $\mathbf{XY}$ is defined if the number of columns of $\mathbf{X}$ (the premultiplying matrix) is equal to the number of rows of $\mathbf{Y}$ (the postmultiplying matrix): in this case, we say that $\mathbf{X}$ and $\mathbf{Y}$ are conformable for multiplication. In the case $n \neq p$, the product $\mathbf{Z} = \mathbf{XY}$ does not exist.

The product of conformable matrices is associative, e.g.,

$$(\mathbf{X}_{m \times n} \mathbf{Y}_{n \times p}) \mathbf{W}_{p \times q} = \mathbf{X}_{m \times n} (\mathbf{Y}_{n \times p} \mathbf{W}_{p \times q}) = \mathbf{Z}_{m \times q}$$

and is also distributive, so that

$$(\mathbf{X}_{m \times n} + \mathbf{Y}_{m \times n}) \mathbf{W}_{n \times p} = (\mathbf{XW})_{m \times p} + (\mathbf{YW})_{m \times p} = \mathbf{Z}_{m \times p};$$

$$\mathbf{X}_{m \times n} (\mathbf{Y}_{n \times p} + \mathbf{W}_{n \times p}) = (\mathbf{XY})_{m \times p} + (\mathbf{XW})_{m \times p} = \mathbf{Z}_{m \times p},$$

but the matrix product does not commute.

This last statement is very important: when dealing with scalars α and β, we are facing a product which is commutative, so that $\alpha\beta = \beta\alpha$, but when dealing with matrices, the product is not commutative, and therefore, in general, assuming that matrices are conformable, $\mathbf{XY} \neq \mathbf{YX}$ even if $\mathbf{XY}$ and $\mathbf{YX}$ are both defined. For example, let $\mathbf{X}$ be 5×3, and let $\mathbf{Y}$ be 2×5; in this case, only $\mathbf{YX}$ would be defined, while $\mathbf{XY}$ would not. Or also, let $\mathbf{X}$ be 7×4 and let $\mathbf{Y}$ be 4×7; both $\mathbf{XY}$ and $\mathbf{YX}$ would be defined, but $\mathbf{XY}$ would be a 7×7 matrix, while $\mathbf{YX}$ would be a 4×4 one, such that, in any case we would have $\mathbf{XY} \neq \mathbf{YX}$. The situation is different if $\mathbf{X}$ and $\mathbf{Y}$ are square matrices: in this case both products $\mathbf{XY}$ and $\mathbf{YX}$ will be defined, but again in general, we will find $\mathbf{XY} \neq \mathbf{YX}$, unless some particular cases, like when $\mathbf{X} = \mathbf{Y}$, from which we would have a commutative product. Thus, in any case, one must pay attention at the order of factors before evaluating a matrix product.

If we have to multiply three matrices (but this situation may be generalized in the case of a product with a higher number of matrices), we must consider the problem of conformability since, for example, the product $\mathbf{Z} = \mathbf{A}_{4 \times 6} \mathbf{B}_{6 \times 2} \mathbf{C}_{2 \times 3}$ is defined, and $\mathbf{Z}$ is 4×3, whereas we cannot obtain the product $\mathbf{A}_{4 \times 6} \mathbf{C}_{2 \times 3} \mathbf{B}_{6 \times 2}$ since it is undefined.

The matrix product generalizes the dot product we have seen for vectors: each element w_{ij} of the product matrix $\mathbf{W} = \mathbf{XY}$ is the dot product obtained by multiplicating the i-th row vector of the premultiplying matrix times the j-th column vector of the postmultiplying matrix, and this product is the element placed at the intersection between the i-th row and the j-th column of the product matrix $\mathbf{W}$. Thus, the element w_{ij} of matrix $\mathbf{W}$ is

$$w_{ij} = \sum_{k=1}^{n} x_{ik} y_{kj},$$

where x_{ik} is the (i, k)-th element of $\mathbf{X}$ and y_{kj} is the (k, j)-th element of $\mathbf{Y}$.

For example, let

$$\mathbf{X} = \begin{pmatrix} 1 & 2 & 4 \\ 3 & 1 & 3 \\ 2 & 1 & 4 \\ 0 & 2 & 1 \end{pmatrix}, \quad \mathbf{Y} = \begin{pmatrix} 1 & 2 \\ 3 & 0 \\ 2 & 1 \end{pmatrix};$$

since $\mathbf{X}$ is 4×3 and $\mathbf{Y}$ is 3×2; then, the number of columns of $\mathbf{X}$ is equal to the number of rows of $\mathbf{Y}$; thus, the matrices are conformable, and the product $\mathbf{XY}$ is defined (and the product $\mathbf{YX}$ is not), and will have the same number of row as $\mathbf{X}$ and the same number of columns as $\mathbf{Y}$; hence, $\mathbf{XY} = \mathbf{W}$ will be 4×2. The multiplication will give

$$\mathbf{X}_{4 \times 3} \mathbf{Y}_{3 \times 2} = \begin{pmatrix} 1 & 2 & 4 \\ 3 & 1 & 3 \\ 2 & 1 & 4 \\ 0 & 2 & 1 \end{pmatrix} \begin{pmatrix} 1 & 2 \\ 3 & 0 \\ 2 & 1 \end{pmatrix}$$

$$= \begin{pmatrix} 1 \times 1 + 2 \times 3 + 4 \times 2 & 1 \times 2 + 2 \times 0 + 4 \times 1 \\ 3 \times 1 + 1 \times 3 + 3 \times 2 & 3 \times 2 + 1 \times 0 + 3 \times 1 \\ 2 \times 1 + 1 \times 3 + 4 \times 2 & 2 \times 2 + 1 \times 0 + 4 \times 1 \\ 0 \times 1 + 2 \times 3 + 1 \times 2 & 0 \times 2 + 2 \times 0 + 1 \times 1 \end{pmatrix}$$

$$= \begin{pmatrix} 15 & 6 \\ 12 & 9 \\ 13 & 8 \\ 8 & 1 \end{pmatrix}$$

$$= \mathbf{W}_{4 \times 2}.$$

In other words, if we take two conformable matrices $\mathbf{X}_{m \times n}$ and $\mathbf{Y}_{n \times p}$, and writing them in terms respectively of row and column vectors such that

$$X = \begin{pmatrix} \mathbf{r}_1 \\ \mathbf{r}_2 \\ \vdots \\ \mathbf{r}_m \end{pmatrix}; \quad Y = \begin{pmatrix} \mathbf{c}_1 \ \mathbf{c}_2 \ \cdots \ \mathbf{c}_p \end{pmatrix},$$

then the product $\mathbf{XY}$ is the matrix $m \times p$:

$$\mathbf{XY} = \begin{pmatrix} \mathbf{r}_1\mathbf{c}_1 & \mathbf{r}_1\mathbf{c}_2 & \cdots & \mathbf{r}_1\mathbf{c}_p \\ \mathbf{r}_2\mathbf{c}_1 & \mathbf{r}_2\mathbf{c}_2 & \cdots & \mathbf{r}_2\mathbf{c}_p \\ \vdots & \vdots & \ddots & \vdots \\ \mathbf{r}_m\mathbf{c}_1 & \mathbf{r}_m\mathbf{c}_2 & \cdots & \mathbf{r}_m\mathbf{c}_p \end{pmatrix},$$

where each element $\mathbf{r}_j\mathbf{c}_k$ is a scalar, e.g., the linear form given by the j-th n-dimensional row vector $\mathbf{r}j$ of $\mathbf{X}$, times the k-th n-dimensional column vector $\mathbf{c}_k$ of $\mathbf{Y}$: note that we omit the transposition sign as superscript of the symbols of vectors $\mathbf{r}j$ since $\mathbf{r}j$ vectors are row vectors by definition.

By the way, we observe that if $\mathbf{r}_j$ a $\mathbf{c}_k$ are orthogonal vectors, one has $\mathbf{r}_j\mathbf{c}_k = 0$ and that if this true for all $\mathbf{r}_j\mathbf{c}_k$ linear forms, then we argue that the product of two matrices may be equal to the null matrix $\mathbf{O}$, even if $\mathbf{X} \neq \mathbf{O}$ and $\mathbf{Y} \neq \mathbf{O}$.

The identity matrix $\mathbf{I}$ is the neutral element of the matrix product, that is, assuming the conformability, $\mathbf{AI} = \mathbf{A}$ and $\mathbf{IA} = \mathbf{A}$. One must always consider matrix dimensions, since

$$\mathbf{A}_{m\times n}\mathbf{I}_n = \mathbf{A}_{m\times n},$$

whereas

$$\mathbf{I}_m\mathbf{A}_{m\times n} = \mathbf{A}_{m\times n},$$

so that we must use the identity matrix $\mathbf{I}_m$ to premultiplicate $\mathbf{A}_{m\times n}$ and the identity matrix $\mathbf{I}_n$ to postmultiplicate $\mathbf{A}_{m\times n}$ (we assume $m \neq n$); thus, the hypothesis $\mathbf{AI} = \mathbf{IA} = \mathbf{A}$ is verified only if $\mathbf{A}$ is a square matrix.

As a practical example, we can observe that

$$\mathbf{A}_{3\times 2}\mathbf{I}_2 = \begin{pmatrix} a_{11} & a_{12} \\ a_{21} & a_{22} \\ a_{31} & a_{32} \end{pmatrix} \begin{pmatrix} 1 & 0 \\ 0 & 1 \end{pmatrix}$$

$$= \begin{pmatrix} 1a_{11} + 0a_{12} & 0a_{11} + 1a_{12} \\ 1a_{21} + 0a_{22} & 0a_{21} + 1a_{22} \\ 1a_{31} + 0a_{32} & 0a_{31} + 0a_{32} \end{pmatrix} = \begin{pmatrix} a_{11} & a_{12} \\ a_{21} & a_{22} \\ a_{31} & a_{32} \end{pmatrix}$$

$$= \mathbf{A}_{3\times 2};$$

and that

$$\mathbf{I}_3\mathbf{A}_{3\times2} = \begin{pmatrix} 1 & 0 & 0 \\ 0 & 1 & 0 \\ 0 & 0 & 1 \end{pmatrix} \begin{pmatrix} a_{11} & a_{12} \\ a_{21} & a_{22} \\ a_{31} & a_{32} \end{pmatrix}$$

$$= \begin{pmatrix} 1a_{11} + 0a_{21} + 0a_{31} & 1a_{12} + 0a_{22} + 0a_{32} \\ 0a_{11} + 1a_{21} + 0a_{31} & 0a_{12} + 1a_{22} + 0a_{32} \\ 0a_{11} + 0a_{21} + 1a_{31} & 0a_{12} + 0a_{22} + 1a_{32} \end{pmatrix} = \begin{pmatrix} a_{11} & a_{12} \\ a_{21} & a_{22} \\ a_{31} & a_{32} \end{pmatrix}$$

$$= \mathbf{A}_{3\times2},$$

where we note that the matrix products give the same result, but matrix $\mathbf{A}_{3\times2}$ had to be postmultiplied by $\mathbf{I}_2$ and premultiplied by $\mathbf{I}_3$ to get that result.

The identity matrix is also the neutral element for the transformation of any vector $\mathbf{v}_n$, since we may easily verify that $\mathbf{I}_n\mathbf{v}_n = \mathbf{v}_{n\times1}$, for example, taking a three-dimensional vector, as follows:

$$\begin{pmatrix} 1 & 0 & 0 \\ 0 & 1 & 0 \\ 0 & 0 & 1 \end{pmatrix} \begin{pmatrix} a \\ b \\ c \end{pmatrix} = \begin{pmatrix} 1a + 0b + 0c \\ 0a + 1b + 0c \\ 0a + 0b + 1c \end{pmatrix}$$

$$= \begin{pmatrix} a \\ b \\ c \end{pmatrix},$$

while obviously the product $\mathbf{v}_{n\times1}\mathbf{I}_n$ is not defined.

In practice, the matrix $\mathbf{I}$ and the matrix $\mathbf{O}$ are equivalent to the scalar 1 and to the scalar 0, respectively, corresponding, in arithmetic, to the neutral elements for multiplication and addition.

If a square matrix $\mathbf{A}$ possess an inverse $\mathbf{A}^{-1}$ (we will discuss this topic in a next section), then $\mathbf{A}$ is said an *invertible matrix* or a *nonsingular matrix* (sometimes a *regular matrix*) and $\mathbf{A}\mathbf{A}^{-1} = \mathbf{I}$.

A square matrix $\mathbf{M}_{nn}$ may be obtained as the product of the multiplication of two n-dimensional vectors $\mathbf{x}_{n\times1}$ and $\mathbf{y}_{n\times1}$ since $\mathbf{M}_{n\times n} = \mathbf{x}_{n\times1}\mathbf{y}_{1\times n}^\top$, e.g.,

$$\mathbf{x}\mathbf{y}^\top = \begin{pmatrix} x_1 \\ x_2 \\ \vdots \\ x_n \end{pmatrix} \begin{pmatrix} y_1 & y_2 & \cdots & y_n \end{pmatrix}$$

$$= \begin{pmatrix} x_1y_1 & x_1y_2 & \cdots & x_1y_n \\ x_2y_1 & x_2y_2 & \cdots & x_2y_n \\ \vdots & \vdots & \ddots & \vdots \\ x_ny_1 & x_ny_2 & \cdots & x_ny_n \end{pmatrix} = \mathbf{M}.$$

21.5 Where the Matrix Product Comes From

When approaching the matrix product for first time, one may feel that something apparently unnatural is going to happen: indeed, if one has to multiply a 2×3 matrix $\mathbf{A}$ by a 3×2 matrix $\mathbf{P}$, the result will be the 2×2 matrix $\mathbf{AB}$, such that, if

$$\mathbf{A} = \begin{pmatrix} a & b & c \\ d & e & f \end{pmatrix}; \quad \mathbf{P} = \begin{pmatrix} p & q \\ r & s \\ t & u \end{pmatrix} \tag{21.4}$$

then

$$\mathbf{AP} = \begin{pmatrix} a & b & c \\ d & e & f \end{pmatrix} \begin{pmatrix} p & q \\ r & s \\ t & u \end{pmatrix} \tag{21.5}$$

$$= \begin{pmatrix} ap + br + ct & aq + bs + cu \\ re + dp + ft & se + dq + fu \end{pmatrix} \tag{21.6}$$

and one would ask on which basis, for example, the element in the first row and second column of the matrix $\mathbf{AP}$ must be $aq + bs + cu$.

To understand where the result of a matrix multiplication is coming from, we could hypothesized an experiment. Pretend you are a biologist feeding two groups of rats (let's call them 1 and 2, respectively), with three different experimental foods (let us call them y_1, y_2, and y_3), such that the daily intake z_1 of a rat in the group 1 is given by a units of y_1, b units of y_2, and c units of y_3, while the daily intake z_2 of a rat belonging to group 2 is d units of y_1, e units of y_2, and f units of y_3; in other words:

$$\begin{cases} z_1 = ay_1 + by_2 + cy_3 \\ z_2 = dy_1 + ey_2 + fy_3 \end{cases} \tag{21.7}$$

Now, assume that any of the foods y_1, y_2, and y_3 contains different amounts, say, x_1 and x_2, of two given proteins, such that the food daily protein amount is

$$\begin{cases} y_1 = px_1 + qx_2 \\ y_2 = rx_1 + sx_2 \\ y_3 = tx_1 + ux_2 \end{cases} \tag{21.8}$$

Now, question is: "which amount of the two proteins is assumed daily by the two groups of rats?" The most intuitive and simple way is to insert the values y_1, y_2, y_3 given in the system (21.8) into system (21.7), such that one gets

$$\begin{cases} z_1 = a(px_1 + qx_2) + b(rx_1 + sx_2) + c(tx_1 + ux_2) \\ z_2 = d(px_1 + qx_2) + e(rx_1 + sx_2) + f(tx_1 + ux_2) \end{cases} \tag{21.9}$$

hence

$$\begin{cases} z_1 = apx_1 + aqx_2 + brx_1 + bsx_2 + ctx_1 + cux_2 \\ z_2 = dpx_1 + dqx_2 + erx_1 + esx_2 + ftx_1 + fux_2 \end{cases} \quad (21.10)$$

thus

$$\begin{cases} z_1 = (ap + br + ct)x_1 + (aq + bs + cu)x_2 \\ z_2 = (dp + er + ft)x_1 + (dq + es + fu)x_2 \end{cases} \cdot \quad (21.11)$$

In practice, we have found that

$$\mathbf{z} = \mathbf{APx} \quad (21.12)$$

which reads

$$\begin{pmatrix} z_1 \\ z_2 \end{pmatrix} = \begin{pmatrix} ap + br + ct & aq + bs + cu \\ re + dp + ft & se + dq + fu \end{pmatrix} \begin{pmatrix} x_1 \\ x_2 \end{pmatrix} \quad (21.13)$$

$$= \begin{pmatrix} a & b & c \\ d & e & f \end{pmatrix} \begin{pmatrix} p & q \\ r & s \\ t & u \end{pmatrix} \begin{pmatrix} x_1 \\ x_2 \end{pmatrix} \quad (21.14)$$

where we find the definition of matrix multiplication, since the matrix in Eq. (21.13) is exactly equal to the product of the two matrices in Eq. (21.14), e.g.,

$$\begin{pmatrix} a & b & c \\ d & e & f \end{pmatrix} \begin{pmatrix} p & q \\ r & s \\ t & u \end{pmatrix} = \begin{pmatrix} ap + br + ct & aq + bs + cu \\ re + dp + ft & se + dq + fu \end{pmatrix} \cdot$$

21.6 Mutually Orthogonal Matrices

Matrix multiplication may give some apparently disappointing results, even if absolutely coherent with its definition. As we already mentioned previously, we may have $\mathbf{AW} = \mathbf{O}$, even if $\mathbf{A} \neq \mathbf{O}$ and $\mathbf{W} \neq \mathbf{O}$. In this case, $\mathbf{A}$ and $\mathbf{W}$ are said *mutually orthogonal matrices*. Indeed, let us take two arbitrary 2×2 matrices:

$$\mathbf{A} = \begin{pmatrix} a & b \\ c & d \end{pmatrix}; \quad \mathbf{W} = \begin{pmatrix} w & x \\ y & z \end{pmatrix},$$

the product is

$$\mathbf{AW} = \begin{pmatrix} aw + by & ax + bz \\ cw + dy & cx + dz \end{pmatrix};$$

thus, to get $\mathbf{AW} = \mathbf{O}$ it must be

$$\begin{cases} aw = -by \\ ax = -bz \\ cw = -dy \\ cx = -dz \end{cases},$$

thus, excluding the trivial cases $\mathbf{A} = \mathbf{O}$ or $\mathbf{W} = \mathbf{O}$, the above conditions for a null matrix product are verified—for example—if (but not only if), we have $ad - bc = 0$ and $a \neq 0$, with $w = -\frac{by}{a}, x = -\frac{bz}{a}$, for arbitrary values y and z.

As an example using the cited necessary conditions, we may take the matrices:

$$\mathbf{A} = \begin{pmatrix} 3 & 1 \\ 2 & \frac{2}{3} \end{pmatrix}; \quad \mathbf{W} = \begin{pmatrix} -\frac{4}{3} & -\frac{7}{3} \\ 4 & 7 \end{pmatrix}, \tag{21.15}$$

from which we obtain

$$\mathbf{AW} = \begin{pmatrix} 3 & 1 \\ 2 & \frac{2}{3} \end{pmatrix} \begin{pmatrix} -\frac{4}{3} & -\frac{7}{3} \\ 4 & 7 \end{pmatrix}$$

$$= \begin{pmatrix} 3 \times \left(-\frac{4}{3}\right) + 1 \times 4 & 3 \times \left(-\frac{7}{3}\right) + 1 \times 7 \\ 2 \times \left(-\frac{4}{3}\right) + \frac{2}{3} \times 4 & 2 \times \left(-\frac{7}{3}\right) + \frac{2}{3} \times 7 \end{pmatrix}$$

$$= \begin{pmatrix} 0 & 0 \\ 0 & 0 \end{pmatrix}$$

$$= \mathbf{O}.$$

Much attention must be paid to noncommutativity of matrix product even for square matrices of the same order: indeed, if the matrix product of the matrices defined in (21.15) gives $\mathbf{AW} = \mathbf{O}$, we also see that $\mathbf{WA} \neq \mathbf{O}$, since

$$\mathbf{WA} = \begin{pmatrix} -\frac{4}{3} & -\frac{7}{3} \\ 4 & 7 \end{pmatrix} \begin{pmatrix} 3 & 1 \\ 2 & \frac{2}{3} \end{pmatrix}$$

$$= \begin{pmatrix} \left(-\frac{4}{3}\right) \times 3 + \left(-\frac{7}{3}\right) \times 2 & \left(-\frac{4}{3}\right) \times 1 + \left(-\frac{7}{3}\right) \times \frac{2}{3} \\ 4 \times 3 + 7 \times 2 & 4 \times 1 + 7 \times \frac{2}{3} \end{pmatrix}$$

$$= \begin{pmatrix} -\frac{26}{3} & -\frac{26}{9} \\ 26 & \frac{26}{3} \end{pmatrix}.$$

21.7   A Note About Associativity of Matrix Product

It is interesting to briefly discuss some topics related to associativity of matrix multiplication; associativity of matrix product implies $\mathbf{ABC} = (\mathbf{AB})\mathbf{C} = \mathbf{A}(\mathbf{BC})$, assuming all matrices are conformable. The choice of the product to be calculated for first was crucial in terms of time needed for the operations to be carried out when modern computers were not available and all single multiplications had to be done with paper and pencil. However, when the involved matrices are large, computation time may be also very important. In practice, any matrix multiplication involves a specific number of scalar multiplication, e.g., if $\mathbf{A}$ is $m \times n$ and $\mathbf{B}$ is $n \times p$, to obtain $\mathbf{AB}$, which will be a matrix $m \times p$, one must calculate $m \times n \times p$ scalar products, that is, if both $\mathbf{A}$ and $\mathbf{B}$ are 2×2, then to obtain $\mathbf{AB}$ will require $2 \times 2 \times 2 = 8$ scalar multiplications.

For example, if $\mathbf{Z}_{4 \times 3} = \mathbf{A}_{4 \times 6}\mathbf{B}_{6 \times 2}\mathbf{C}_{2 \times 3}$, we see that $\mathbf{AB}$ is a 4×2 matrix obtained by calculating $4 \times 6 \times 2 = 48$ scalar products, while $\mathbf{BC}$ is 6×3 and is obtained by calculating $6 \times 2 \times 3 = 36$ scalar products. Thus, if we want $\mathbf{Z}$ as $\mathbf{Z} = (\mathbf{AB})\mathbf{C}$, we must calculate $48 + 4 \times 2 \times 3 = 72$ scalar products, whereas, if we want $\mathbf{Z}$ as $\mathbf{Z} = \mathbf{A}(\mathbf{BC})$, the scalar products to be calculated are $36 + 4 \times 6 \times 3 = 108$. In practice, we would need exactly a 50% more scalar multiplications (since $72 = 108 - 36$) to get $\mathbf{Z}$ as $\mathbf{A}(\mathbf{BC})$ than $\mathbf{Z}$ as $(\mathbf{AB})\mathbf{C}$. These differences become more and more important as the order of matrices increases and also as the number of matrice increases.

As a general rule, the more time-sparing approach is to avoid to multiplicate first the matrices for which the number of scalar products $m \times n \times p$ is smaller; hence, the more profitable approach is to first multiplicate the consecutive with the highest row-column number: in our case, where $\mathbf{Z}_{4 \times 3} = \mathbf{A}_{4 \times 6}\mathbf{B}_{6 \times 2}\mathbf{C}_{2 \times 3}$ is therefore preferable to first obtain $\mathbf{A}_{4 \times 6}\mathbf{B}_{6 \times 2}$, which is characterized by a higher common row-column value, equal to 6, since $\mathbf{A}$ has 6 columns and $\mathbf{B}$ has 6 rows.

21.8   Transpose of a Product

Take two conformable matrices, $\mathbf{A}_{3 \times 2}$ and $\mathbf{Z}_{2 \times 2}$, such that $\mathbf{AZ}$ is defined, but $\mathbf{ZA}$ is not, and take also the respective transpose matrices $\mathbf{A}_{2 \times 3}^{\top}$ and $\mathbf{Z}_{2 \times 2}^{\top}$, such that $\mathbf{Z}^{\top}\mathbf{A}^{\top}$ is defined, but $\mathbf{A}^{\top}\mathbf{Z}^{\top}$ is not:

$$\mathbf{A} = \begin{pmatrix} a & b \\ c & d \\ e & f \end{pmatrix}; \quad \mathbf{Z} = \begin{pmatrix} w & x \\ y & z \end{pmatrix};$$

$$\mathbf{A}^{\top} = \begin{pmatrix} a & c & e \\ b & d & f \end{pmatrix}; \quad \mathbf{Z}^{\top} = \begin{pmatrix} w & y \\ x & z \end{pmatrix}.$$

We may obtain the products:

$$\mathbf{AZ} = \begin{pmatrix} a & b \\ c & d \\ e & f \end{pmatrix} \begin{pmatrix} w & x \\ y & z \end{pmatrix}$$

$$= \begin{pmatrix} aw + by & ax + bz \\ cw + dy & cx + dz \\ ew + fy & ex + fz \end{pmatrix},$$

and

$$\mathbf{Z}^\top \mathbf{A}^\top = \begin{pmatrix} w & y \\ x & z \end{pmatrix} \begin{pmatrix} a & c & e \\ b & d & f \end{pmatrix}$$

$$= \begin{pmatrix} aw + by & cw + dy & ew + fy \\ ax + bz & cx + dz & ex + fz \end{pmatrix}. \tag{21.16}$$

Now, if we take the transpose of $\mathbf{AZ}$, we get:

$$(\mathbf{AZ})^\top = \begin{pmatrix} aw + by & cw + dy & ew + fy \\ ax + bz & cx + dz & ex + fz \end{pmatrix}; \tag{21.17}$$

hence, comparing Eqs. (21.16) and (21.17), we note that $(\mathbf{AZ})^\top = \mathbf{Z}^\top \mathbf{A}^\top$. This property holds in general for any couple of conformable matrices, and so we can tell that given the conformable matrices $\mathbf{A}_{m \times n}$ and $\mathbf{Z}_{n \times p}$, the transpose of the product is equal to the product of the transposed in the inverse order, such that $(\mathbf{AZ})^\top = \mathbf{Z}^\top \mathbf{A}^\top$. The proof of this statement may be obtained by considering that the element of the product $\mathbf{V}_{m \times p} = \mathbf{A}_{m \times n} \mathbf{Z}_{n \times p}$ found at the intersection of the i-th row with the j-th column is $v_{ij} = \sum_{k=1}^{n} a_{ik} z_{kj}$; hence, the element of matrix $\mathbf{W}_{p \times m} = \mathbf{V}^\top = (\mathbf{AZ})^\top$ will be $w_{ij} = v_{ji} = \sum_{k=1}^{n} a_{jk} z_{ki} = \sum_{k=1}^{n} z_{ki} a_{jk}$, and therefore $(\mathbf{AZ})^\top = \mathbf{Z}^\top \mathbf{A}^\top$.

Thus, generalizing this equality, we may also verify that

$$(\mathbf{A}_{(1)} \mathbf{A}_{(2)} \cdots \mathbf{A}_{(n-1)} \mathbf{A}_{(n)})^\top = \mathbf{A}_{(n)}^\top \mathbf{A}_{(n-1)}^\top \cdots \mathbf{A}_{(2)}^\top \mathbf{A}_{(1)}^\top.$$

21.9   Tensor Product for Vectors and Matrices

For two vectors $\mathbf{a}$ in $\mathbb{R}^m$ and $\mathbf{b}$ in $\mathbb{R}^n$, we define the tensor product $\mathbf{a} \otimes \mathbf{b}$ in $\mathbb{R}^m \otimes \mathbb{R}^n$ as the new vector whose entries are the pairwise products of their components; thus,

$$\mathbf{a} \otimes \mathbf{b} = \begin{pmatrix} a_1 b_1 \\ a_1 b_2 \\ \vdots \\ a_m b_{n-1} \\ a_m b_n \end{pmatrix};$$

for example, given

$$\mathbf{a} = \begin{pmatrix} 4 \\ 5 \end{pmatrix}; \quad \mathbf{b} = \begin{pmatrix} 3 \\ 1 \\ 2 \end{pmatrix},$$

then

$$\mathbf{a} \otimes \mathbf{b} = \begin{pmatrix} 4 \times 3 \\ 4 \times 1 \\ 4 \times 2 \\ 5 \times 3 \\ 5 \times 1 \\ 5 \times 2 \end{pmatrix} = \begin{pmatrix} 12 \\ 4 \\ 8 \\ 15 \\ 5 \\ 10 \end{pmatrix};$$

note that

$$\mathbf{a} \otimes \mathbf{b} = \begin{pmatrix} 4 \times 3 \\ 4 \times 1 \\ 4 \times 2 \\ 5 \times 3 \\ 5 \times 1 \\ 5 \times 2 \end{pmatrix} \neq \begin{pmatrix} 3 \times 4 \\ 3 \times 5 \\ 1 \times 4 \\ 1 \times 5 \\ 2 \times 4 \\ 2 \times 5 \end{pmatrix} = \mathbf{b} \otimes \mathbf{a};$$

thus, in general the tensor product is not commutative. In our example $(\mathbf{a}_2 \otimes \mathbf{b}_3) \in \mathbb{R}^6$, and in general $(\mathbf{a}_m \otimes \mathbf{b}_n) \in \mathbb{R}^{m \times n}$. Note also that

$$\begin{pmatrix} \alpha \\ \beta \end{pmatrix} \otimes \begin{pmatrix} \gamma \\ \delta \end{pmatrix} \otimes \begin{pmatrix} \varepsilon \\ \zeta \end{pmatrix} = \begin{pmatrix} \alpha \begin{pmatrix} \gamma \begin{pmatrix} \varepsilon \\ \zeta \end{pmatrix} \\ \delta \begin{pmatrix} \varepsilon \\ \zeta \end{pmatrix} \end{pmatrix} \\ \beta \begin{pmatrix} \gamma \begin{pmatrix} \varepsilon \\ \zeta \end{pmatrix} \\ \delta \begin{pmatrix} \varepsilon \\ \zeta \end{pmatrix} \end{pmatrix} \end{pmatrix} = \begin{pmatrix} \alpha\gamma\varepsilon \\ \alpha\gamma\zeta \\ \alpha\delta\varepsilon \\ \alpha\delta\zeta \\ \beta\gamma\varepsilon \\ \beta\gamma\zeta \\ \beta\delta\varepsilon \\ \beta\delta\zeta \end{pmatrix}.$$

It must be pointed out that the tensor product of a vector $\mathbf{v}$ with a transpose vector $\mathbf{w}^\top$ is a matrix, since we have

$$
\mathbf{v} \otimes \mathbf{w}^\top = \begin{pmatrix} v_1 \\ v_2 \\ \vdots \\ v_m \end{pmatrix} \otimes \begin{pmatrix} w_1 & w_2 & \cdots & w_n \end{pmatrix}
$$

$$
= \begin{pmatrix} v_1 w_1 & v_1 w_2 & \cdots & v_1 w_n \\ v_2 w_1 & v_2 w_2 & \cdots & v_2 w_n \\ \vdots & \vdots & \ddots & \vdots \\ v_m w_1 & v_m v_2 & \cdots & v_m w_n \end{pmatrix},
$$

so that, if we are dealing with the very particular case $\mathbf{v} \otimes \mathbf{v}^\top$, then we easily verify that

$$
\mathbf{v} \otimes \mathbf{v}^\top = \mathbf{v}\mathbf{v}^\top.
$$

Given two matrices $\mathbf{A}_{m \times n}$ and $\mathbf{B}_{p \times q}$, the *tensor product* (a.k.a. the *Kronecker product*) $\mathbf{A} \otimes \mathbf{B}$ is defined as

$$
\mathbf{A} \otimes \mathbf{B} = \begin{pmatrix} a_{11}\mathbf{B} & a_{12}\mathbf{B} & \cdots & a_{1n}\mathbf{B} \\ a_{21}\mathbf{B} & a_{22}\mathbf{B} & \cdots & a_{2n}\mathbf{B} \\ \vdots & \vdots & \ddots & \vdots \\ a_{m1}\mathbf{B} & a_{m2}\mathbf{B} & \cdots & a_{mn}\mathbf{B} \end{pmatrix}
$$

thus

$$
\mathbf{A} \otimes \mathbf{B} = \begin{pmatrix} a_{11}\begin{pmatrix} b_{11} & \cdots & b_{1q} \\ \vdots & \ddots & \vdots \\ b_{p1} & \cdots & b_{pq} \end{pmatrix} & \cdots & a_{1n}\begin{pmatrix} b_{11} & \cdots & b_{1q} \\ \vdots & \ddots & \vdots \\ b_{p1} & \cdots & b_{pq} \end{pmatrix} \\ \vdots & \ddots & \vdots \\ a_{m1}\begin{pmatrix} b_{11} & \cdots & b_{1q} \\ \vdots & \ddots & \vdots \\ b_{p1} & \cdots & b_{pq} \end{pmatrix} & \cdots & a_{mn}\begin{pmatrix} b_{11} & \cdots & b_{1q} \\ \vdots & \ddots & \vdots \\ b_{p1} & \cdots & b_{pq} \end{pmatrix} \end{pmatrix}
$$

and therefore the Kronecker product is the $mp \times nq$ block matrix:

$$\mathbf{A} \otimes \mathbf{B} = \begin{pmatrix} \begin{pmatrix} a_{11}b_{11} & \cdots & a_{11}b_{1q} \\ \vdots & \ddots & \vdots \\ a_{11}b_{p1} & \cdots & a_{11}b_{pq} \end{pmatrix} & \cdots & \begin{pmatrix} a_{1n}b_{11} & \cdots & a_{1n}b_{1q} \\ \vdots & \ddots & \vdots \\ a_{1n}b_{p1} & \cdots & a_{1n}b_{pq} \end{pmatrix} \\ \vdots & \ddots & \vdots \\ \begin{pmatrix} a_{m1}b_{11} & \cdots & a_{m1}b_{1q} \\ \vdots & \ddots & \vdots \\ a_{m1}b_{p1} & \cdots & a_{m1}b_{pq} \end{pmatrix} & \cdots & \begin{pmatrix} a_{mn}b_{11} & \cdots & a_{mn}b_{1q} \\ \vdots & \ddots & \vdots \\ a_{mn}b_{p1} & \cdots & a_{mn}b_{pq} \end{pmatrix} \end{pmatrix}.$$

Obviously, the tensor product is not commutative: even if $\mathbf{B} \otimes \mathbf{A}$ is also $mp \times nq$, the elements differ, since

$$\mathbf{B} \otimes \mathbf{A} = \begin{pmatrix} \begin{pmatrix} b_{11}a_{11} & \cdots & b_{11}a_{1n} \\ \vdots & \ddots & \vdots \\ b_{11}a_{m1} & \cdots & b_{11}a_{mn} \end{pmatrix} & \cdots & \begin{pmatrix} b_{1q}a_{11} & \cdots & b_{1q}a_{1n} \\ \vdots & \ddots & \vdots \\ b_{1q}a_{m1} & \cdots & b_{1q}a_{mn} \end{pmatrix} \\ \vdots & \ddots & \vdots \\ \begin{pmatrix} b_{p1}a_{11} & \cdots & b_{p1}a_{1n} \\ \vdots & \ddots & \vdots \\ b_{p1}a_{m1} & \cdots & b_{p1}a_{mn} \end{pmatrix} & \cdots & \begin{pmatrix} b_{pq}a_{11} & \cdots & b_{pq}a_{1n} \\ \vdots & \ddots & \vdots \\ b_{pq}a_{m1} & \cdots & b_{pq}a_{mn} \end{pmatrix} \end{pmatrix}.$$

The tensor product is linear and associative, since we can easily demonstrate that

$$\lambda(\mathbf{A} \otimes \mathbf{B}) = \lambda\mathbf{A} \otimes \mathbf{B} = \mathbf{A} \otimes \lambda\mathbf{B}$$

and

$$\mathbf{A} \otimes (\mathbf{B} \otimes \mathbf{C}) = (\mathbf{A} \otimes \mathbf{B}) \otimes \mathbf{C}$$
$$\mathbf{A} \otimes (\mathbf{B} + \mathbf{C}) = \mathbf{A} \otimes \mathbf{B} + \mathbf{A} \otimes \mathbf{C}$$

provided $\mathbf{B}$ and $\mathbf{C}$ conformable for matrix sum.

Moreover, we may also demonstrate that the inverse of the tensor product is the tensor product of the inverses, e.g.,

$$(\mathbf{A} \otimes \mathbf{A})^{-1} = \mathbf{A}^{-1} \otimes \mathbf{B}^{-1}$$

provided both $\mathbf{A}$ and $\mathbf{B}$ invertible, and that the matrix multiplication of two tensor products (*mixed product*) is given as

$$(\mathbf{A} \otimes \mathbf{B})(\mathbf{C} \otimes \mathbf{D}) = \mathbf{AC} \otimes \mathbf{BD}$$

provided **A,C** and **B,D** respectively conformable for the matrix products.

Notably, there is not a neutral element for the tensor product, e.g., there is not a matrix **X** such that $\mathbf{X} \otimes \mathbf{A} = \mathbf{A}$, unless taking $\mathbf{X} = \lambda$ as a 1×1 matrix.

21.10 Linear Transformations

As a general rule, we must recall that a matrix **T** which premultiplies an n-dimensional vector **x** returns an m-dimensional vector **y**, provided that the number of rows of **x** is equal to the number of columns of **T**; thus, **T** must be $m \times n$; otherwise, the product is not defined. Indeed, **T** is not only a matrix, since it can be considered a *linear transformation*, since, when applied at n-dimensional vector **x**, transforms **x** in the new m-dimensional vector **y**, thus

$$\mathbf{T}_{m \times n} \mathbf{x}_{n \times 1} = \mathbf{y}_{m \times 1},$$

in which the j-th element of **y** is

$$y_j = \sum_{k=1}^{n} t_{jk} x_k.$$

An example of a generic linear transformation can be given by taking

$$\mathbf{T} = \begin{pmatrix} -1 & 4 & -3 \\ 7 & 2 & 1 \end{pmatrix}; \quad \mathbf{x} = \begin{pmatrix} 2 \\ 1 \\ -1 \end{pmatrix}$$

thus

$$\mathbf{y} = \mathbf{T}\mathbf{x}$$

$$= \begin{pmatrix} -1 & 4 & -3 \\ 7 & 2 & 1 \end{pmatrix} \begin{pmatrix} 2 \\ 1 \\ -1 \end{pmatrix} = \begin{pmatrix} -2+4+3 \\ 14+2-1 \end{pmatrix}$$

$$= \begin{pmatrix} 5 \\ 15 \end{pmatrix}$$

where the three-dimensional vector **x** is transformed into the two-dimensional vector **y**. In other words, we have had the transformation $\mathbf{T} : \mathbb{R}^3 \rightarrow \mathbb{R}^2$.

If **T** is a square matrix, the transformation does not change the dimensions of the vector to be transformed; thus, $\mathbf{T} : \mathbb{R}^n \rightarrow \mathbb{R}^n$, but it does change its length and direction. An example of a linear transformation with a square matrix can be given by taking

$$\mathbf{V} = \begin{pmatrix} 1 & -2 & 2 \\ 7 & 1 & 4 \\ 3 & 0 & 3 \end{pmatrix}; \quad \mathbf{x} = \begin{pmatrix} 2 \\ 1 \\ -1 \end{pmatrix} \quad (21.18)$$

thus

$$\mathbf{z} = \mathbf{V}\mathbf{x}$$

$$= \begin{pmatrix} 1 & -2 & 2 \\ 7 & 1 & 4 \\ 3 & 0 & 3 \end{pmatrix} \begin{pmatrix} 2 \\ 1 \\ -1 \end{pmatrix} = \begin{pmatrix} 2-2-2 \\ 14+1-4 \\ 6+0-3 \end{pmatrix}$$

$$= \begin{pmatrix} -2 \\ 11 \\ 3 \end{pmatrix}$$

where the three-dimensional vector $\mathbf{x}$ is transformed into another three-dimensional vector $\mathbf{z}$, so as to have a transformation $\mathbf{T} : \mathbb{R}^3 \rightarrow \mathbb{R}^3$. Going back to definitions (21.18), we see that the inverse of $\mathbf{V}$ is

$$\mathbf{V}^{-1} = \begin{pmatrix} \frac{1}{5} & \frac{2}{5} & -\frac{2}{3} \\ -\frac{3}{5} & -\frac{1}{5} & \frac{2}{3} \\ -\frac{1}{5} & -\frac{2}{5} & 1 \end{pmatrix}$$

and that applying the $\mathbf{V}^{-1}$ transformation to the transformed vector $\mathbf{z}$, we have

$$\begin{pmatrix} \frac{1}{5} & \frac{2}{5} & -\frac{2}{3} \\ -\frac{3}{5} & -\frac{1}{5} & \frac{2}{3} \\ -\frac{1}{5} & -\frac{2}{5} & 1 \end{pmatrix} \begin{pmatrix} -2 \\ 11 \\ 3 \end{pmatrix} = \begin{pmatrix} 2 \\ 1 \\ -1 \end{pmatrix};$$

hence, the inverse of the transformation (provided the transformation is invertible) applied to the transformed vector $\mathbf{z}$ returns the original vector $\mathbf{x}$ before the transformation. We will soon return to present the inverse matrices in a next section.

Among the most important linear transformation, we may recall the rotation and the projection.

The counterclockwise rotation of a two-dimensional vector by an angle θ is governed by the *rotation matrix*:

$$\mathbf{R} = \begin{pmatrix} \cos\theta & \sin\theta \\ -\sin\theta & \cos\theta \end{pmatrix},$$

such that a vector $\mathbf{x}$ is transformed into

$$\mathbf{y} = \mathbf{Rx}$$

$$= \begin{pmatrix} \cos\theta & \sin\theta \\ -\sin\theta & \cos\theta \end{pmatrix} \begin{pmatrix} x_1 \\ x_2 \end{pmatrix}$$

$$= \begin{pmatrix} x_1\cos\theta + x_2\sin\theta \\ x_2\cos\theta - x_1\sin\theta \end{pmatrix};$$

for example, taking the vector $\mathbf{x}$ and the counterclockwise rotation

$$\mathbf{x} = \begin{pmatrix} 1 \\ 1 \end{pmatrix}; \quad \mathbf{R} = \begin{pmatrix} \cos\left(\frac{\pi}{2}\right) & \sin\left(\frac{\pi}{2}\right) \\ -\sin\left(\frac{\pi}{2}\right) & \cos\left(\frac{\pi}{2}\right) \end{pmatrix}$$

we see that the $\frac{\pi}{2}$ (i.e., $90°$) counterclockwise rotation of $\mathbf{x}$ produces

$$\mathbf{y} = \begin{pmatrix} \cos\left(\frac{\pi}{2}\right) & \sin\left(\frac{\pi}{2}\right) \\ -\sin\left(\frac{\pi}{2}\right) & \cos\left(\frac{\pi}{2}\right) \end{pmatrix} \begin{pmatrix} 1 \\ 1 \end{pmatrix}$$

$$= \begin{pmatrix} 1 \\ -1 \end{pmatrix};$$

or, considering a π (i.e., $180°$) counterclockwise rotation:

$$\mathbf{y} = \begin{pmatrix} \cos(\pi) & \sin(\pi) \\ -\sin(\pi) & \cos(\pi) \end{pmatrix} \begin{pmatrix} 1 \\ 1 \end{pmatrix}$$

$$= \begin{pmatrix} -1 \\ -1 \end{pmatrix},$$

as expected.

Examples of *projection matrices* are

$$\mathbf{P} = \begin{pmatrix} 1 & 0 \\ 0 & 0 \end{pmatrix}; \quad \mathbf{Q} = \begin{pmatrix} 0 & 0 \\ 0 & 1 \end{pmatrix}$$

which take a two-dimensional vector $\mathbf{v}$ and map it onto the x and y Cartesian axis, respectively, so as, if

$$\mathbf{v} = \begin{pmatrix} 2 \\ -3 \end{pmatrix}$$

we see that

$$\mathbf{Pv} = \begin{pmatrix} 1 & 0 \\ 0 & 0 \end{pmatrix} \begin{pmatrix} 2 \\ -3 \end{pmatrix} = \begin{pmatrix} 2 \\ 0 \end{pmatrix};$$

$$\mathbf{Qv} = \begin{pmatrix} 0 & 0 \\ 0 & 1 \end{pmatrix} \begin{pmatrix} 2 \\ -3 \end{pmatrix} = \begin{pmatrix} 0 \\ -3 \end{pmatrix}.$$

In the case of a three-dimensional vector, say,

$$\mathbf{w} = \begin{pmatrix} 2 \\ -3 \\ 4 \end{pmatrix}$$

we can take some of the possible projection matrices in $\mathbb{R}^3$, like

$$\mathbf{A} = \begin{pmatrix} 1 & 0 & 0 \\ 0 & 0 & 0 \\ 0 & 0 & 0 \end{pmatrix}; \ \mathbf{B} = \begin{pmatrix} 1 & 0 & 0 \\ 0 & 1 & 0 \\ 0 & 0 & 0 \end{pmatrix}; \ \mathbf{C} = \begin{pmatrix} 0 & 0 & 0 \\ 0 & 0 & 0 \\ 0 & 0 & 1 \end{pmatrix}; \ \mathbf{D} = \begin{pmatrix} 1 & 0 & 0 \\ 0 & 0 & 0 \\ 0 & 0 & 1 \end{pmatrix}$$

to see how they take the vector $\mathbf{w}$ and map it respectively: (1) on the x-axis; (2) on the xy-plane; (3) on the z-axis; (4) on the xz-plane, as follows:

$$\mathbf{Aw} = \begin{pmatrix} 1 & 0 & 0 \\ 0 & 0 & 0 \\ 0 & 0 & 0 \end{pmatrix} \begin{pmatrix} 2 \\ -3 \\ 4 \end{pmatrix} = \begin{pmatrix} 2 \\ 0 \\ 0 \end{pmatrix};$$

$$\mathbf{Bw} = \begin{pmatrix} 1 & 0 & 0 \\ 0 & 1 & 0 \\ 0 & 0 & 0 \end{pmatrix} \begin{pmatrix} 2 \\ -3 \\ 4 \end{pmatrix} = \begin{pmatrix} 2 \\ -3 \\ 0 \end{pmatrix};$$

$$\mathbf{Cw} = \begin{pmatrix} 0 & 0 & 0 \\ 0 & 0 & 0 \\ 0 & 0 & 1 \end{pmatrix} \begin{pmatrix} 2 \\ -3 \\ 4 \end{pmatrix} = \begin{pmatrix} 0 \\ 0 \\ 4 \end{pmatrix};$$

$$\mathbf{Dw} = \begin{pmatrix} 1 & 0 & 0 \\ 0 & 0 & 0 \\ 0 & 0 & 1 \end{pmatrix} \begin{pmatrix} 2 \\ -3 \\ 4 \end{pmatrix} = \begin{pmatrix} 2 \\ 0 \\ 4 \end{pmatrix}.$$

As one would expect, the projection is an *idempotent operation*, that is, applying two times the same projection to a vector, the result will be the same obtained after the first projection. For example,

$$\mathbf{DDw} = \mathbf{D}^2\mathbf{w} = \begin{pmatrix} 1 & 0 & 0 \\ 0 & 0 & 0 \\ 0 & 0 & 1 \end{pmatrix} \begin{pmatrix} 1 & 0 & 0 \\ 0 & 0 & 0 \\ 0 & 0 & 1 \end{pmatrix} \begin{pmatrix} 2 \\ -3 \\ 4 \end{pmatrix}$$

$$= \begin{pmatrix} 2 \\ 0 \\ 4 \end{pmatrix}$$

which implies

$$\mathbf{D}^2 = \begin{pmatrix} 1 & 0 & 0 \\ 0 & 0 & 0 \\ 0 & 0 & 1 \end{pmatrix} \begin{pmatrix} 1 & 0 & 0 \\ 0 & 0 & 0 \\ 0 & 0 & 1 \end{pmatrix} = \begin{pmatrix} 1 & 0 & 0 \\ 0 & 0 & 0 \\ 0 & 0 & 1 \end{pmatrix} = \mathbf{D};$$

we also observe that

$$\mathbf{D}^\top = \begin{pmatrix} 1 & 0 & 0 \\ 0 & 0 & 0 \\ 0 & 0 & 1 \end{pmatrix} = \mathbf{D}$$

and when, like in this case, the transpose of a projection matrix is equal to the projection matrix itself, we are dealing with an *orthogonal projection matrix*. We will analyze the properties of the projection matrices—with particular emphasis on their idempotence—in a next section.

21.11 Bilinear and Quadratic Forms

Given a matrix $\mathbf{A}_{m \times n}$ and two vectors $\mathbf{x}_m$ and $\mathbf{y}_n$, we define *bilinear form* the product $\mathbf{x}^\top \mathbf{A}\mathbf{y}$. Since $\mathbf{x}^\top$ is $1 \times m$ and $\mathbf{A}$ is $m \times n$, the product $\mathbf{x}^\top \mathbf{A}$ is $1 \times n$; moreover since $\mathbf{y}$ is $n \times 1$, the final product $\mathbf{x}^\top \mathbf{A}\mathbf{y}$ is 1×1, so a bilinear form is a scalar.

As an example, let us take the vectors $\mathbf{x}$ and $\mathbf{y}$, and the matrix $\mathbf{A}$ as follows:

$$\mathbf{x} = \begin{pmatrix} x_1 \\ x_2 \\ x_3 \end{pmatrix}; \quad \mathbf{A} = \begin{pmatrix} a_{11} & a_{12} & a_{13} & a_{14} \\ a_{21} & a_{22} & a_{23} & a_{24} \\ a_{31} & a_{32} & a_{33} & a_{34} \end{pmatrix}; \quad \mathbf{y} = \begin{pmatrix} y_1 \\ y_2 \\ y_3 \\ y_4 \end{pmatrix},$$

so as to have

$$\mathbf{x}^\top \mathbf{A} \mathbf{y} = \begin{pmatrix} x_1 & x_2 & x_3 \end{pmatrix} \begin{pmatrix} a_{11} & a_{12} & a_{13} & a_{14} \\ a_{21} & a_{22} & a_{23} & a_{24} \\ a_{31} & a_{32} & a_{33} & a_{34} \end{pmatrix} \begin{pmatrix} y_1 \\ y_2 \\ y_3 \\ y_4 \end{pmatrix}$$

$$= \sum_{k=1}^{n} \left(\sum_{j=1}^{m} a_{jk} x_j \right) y_k$$

$$= y_1 \left(a_{11} x_1 + a_{21} x_2 + a_{31} x_3 \right) + y_2 \left(a_{12} x_1 + a_{22} x_2 + a_{32} x_3 \right)$$

$$+ y_3 \left(a_{13} x_1 + a_{23} x_2 + a_{33} x_3 \right) + y_4 \left(a_{14} x_1 + a_{24} x_2 + a_{34} x_3 \right)$$

$$= a_{11} x_1 y_1 + a_{12} x_1 y_2 + a_{13} x_1 y_3 + a_{14} x_1 y_4 + a_{21} x_2 y_1 + a_{22} x_2 y_2$$

$$+ a_{23} x_2 y_3 + a_{24} x_2 y_4 + a_{31} x_3 y_1 + a_{32} x_3 y_2 + a_{33} x_3 y_3 + a_{34} x_3 y_4;$$

hence, we may verify that assuming $\mathbf{x}$ and $\mathbf{y}$ having variable components and that the elements of $\mathbf{A}$ are coefficients, we may consider a bilinear form as a second-degree function in x_k and y_k. In some textbooks, a bilinear form is defined only if $\mathbf{A}$ is a square matrix, and therefore if vectors $\mathbf{x}$ and $\mathbf{y}$, although different, have the same dimensions: however, we use the more general definition, for which $\mathbf{A}$ must not be necessarily a square matrix.

The algebraic meaning of a bilinear form can be understood if we look at some very simple situations, for example, letting $\mathbf{A}_{2\times 3} = \mathbf{U}_{2\times 3}$, so that

$$\begin{pmatrix} a & b \end{pmatrix} \begin{pmatrix} 1 & 1 & 1 \\ 1 & 1 & 1 \end{pmatrix} \begin{pmatrix} x \\ y \\ z \end{pmatrix} = \begin{pmatrix} a+b & a+b & a+b \end{pmatrix} \begin{pmatrix} x \\ y \\ z \end{pmatrix}$$

$$= (a+b)(x+y+z)$$

and with $\mathbf{A}_{2\times 3} = n\mathbf{U}_{2\times 3}$

$$\begin{pmatrix} a & b \end{pmatrix} \begin{pmatrix} n & n & n \\ n & n & n \end{pmatrix} \begin{pmatrix} x \\ y \\ z \end{pmatrix} = \begin{pmatrix} na+nb & na+nb & na+nb \end{pmatrix} \begin{pmatrix} x \\ y \\ z \end{pmatrix}$$

$$= n(a+b)(x+y+z)$$

and in the case

$$\mathbf{A}_{2\times 3} = \begin{pmatrix} 1 & 2 & 3 \\ 4 & 5 & 6 \end{pmatrix}$$

then

$$\begin{pmatrix} a & b \end{pmatrix} \begin{pmatrix} 1 & 2 & 3 \\ 4 & 5 & 6 \end{pmatrix} \begin{pmatrix} x \\ y \\ z \end{pmatrix} = \begin{pmatrix} a + 4b & 2a + 5b & 3a + 6b \end{pmatrix} \begin{pmatrix} x \\ y \\ z \end{pmatrix}$$

$$= (a + 4b)\, x + (2a + 5b)\, y + (3a + 6b)\, z;$$

thus, for example, we may write a function:

$$f(x, y, z) = (M\alpha)x + (P\alpha + Q\beta)\, y + (S\beta)z$$

as the bilinear form

$$(M\alpha)x + (P\alpha + Q\beta)\, y + (S\beta)z = (M\alpha + 0\beta)\, x + (P\alpha + Q\beta)\, y + (0\alpha + S\beta)\, z$$

$$= \begin{pmatrix} \alpha & \beta \end{pmatrix} \begin{pmatrix} M & P & 0 \\ 0 & Q & S \end{pmatrix} \begin{pmatrix} x \\ y \\ z \end{pmatrix}.$$

A particular case of bilinear form arises when $\mathbf{y} = \mathbf{x}$. Here the bilinear form $\mathbf{x}^{\top}\mathbf{A}\mathbf{x}$ is called a *quadratic form*, which, from the previous example, must be calculated as

$$\mathbf{x}^{\top}\mathbf{A}\mathbf{x} = \begin{pmatrix} x_1 & x_2 & x_3 \end{pmatrix} \begin{pmatrix} a_{11} & a_{12} & a_{13} \\ a_{21} & a_{22} & a_{23} \\ a_{31} & a_{32} & a_{33} \end{pmatrix} \begin{pmatrix} x_1 \\ x_2 \\ x_3 \end{pmatrix}$$

$$= \sum_{k=1}^{n} \left(\sum_{j=1}^{n} a_{jk} x_j \right) x_k$$

$$= (a_{11}x_1 + a_{21}x_2 + a_{31}x_3)\, x_1 + (a_{12}x_1 + a_{22}x_2 + a_{32}x_3)\, x_2$$

$$+ (a_{13}x_1 + a_{23}x_2 + a_{33}x_3)\, x_3$$

$$= a_{11}x_1^2 + a_{21}x_1 x_2 + a_{31}x_1 x_3 + a_{12}x_1 x_2 + a_{22}x_2^2 + a_{32}x_2 x_3$$

$$+ a_{13}x_1 x_3 + a_{23}x_2 x_3 + a_{33}x_3^2,$$

where we see that also a quadratic form is a scalar given as

$$\mathbf{x}^{\top}\mathbf{A}\mathbf{x} = \sum_{j=1}^{n}\sum_{k=1}^{n} a_{jk} x_j x_k = \sum_{j,k=1}^{n} a_{jk} x_j x_k.$$

As a simple example of calculus of a quadratic form, we can take the vector:

$$\mathbf{v} = \begin{pmatrix} x \\ y \end{pmatrix}$$

and the matrices

$$\mathbf{I} = \begin{pmatrix} 1 & 0 \\ 0 & 1 \end{pmatrix}; \mathbf{Z} = \begin{pmatrix} 0 & 1 \\ 1 & 0 \end{pmatrix}; \mathbf{U} = \begin{pmatrix} 1 & 1 \\ 1 & 1 \end{pmatrix}; \qquad (21.19)$$

$$\mathbf{G} = \begin{pmatrix} 1 & 0 \\ 0 & -1 \end{pmatrix}; \mathbf{W} = \begin{pmatrix} 1 & -1 \\ -1 & 1 \end{pmatrix}, \qquad (21.20)$$

we see that

$$\mathbf{v}^\top \mathbf{I} \mathbf{v} = \begin{pmatrix} x & y \end{pmatrix} \begin{pmatrix} 1 & 0 \\ 0 & 1 \end{pmatrix} \begin{pmatrix} x \\ y \end{pmatrix}$$
$$= x^2 + y^2$$
$$= \mathbf{v}^\top \mathbf{v},$$

which is not unexpected, since $\mathbf{I}$ is the neutral element in the vector and matrix multiplication. We also obtain:

$$\mathbf{v}^\top \mathbf{Z} \mathbf{v} = \begin{pmatrix} x & y \end{pmatrix} \begin{pmatrix} 0 & 1 \\ 1 & 0 \end{pmatrix} \begin{pmatrix} x \\ y \end{pmatrix}$$
$$= 2xy;$$

$$\mathbf{v}^\top \mathbf{U} \mathbf{v} = \begin{pmatrix} x & y \end{pmatrix} \begin{pmatrix} 1 & 1 \\ 1 & 1 \end{pmatrix} \begin{pmatrix} x \\ y \end{pmatrix}$$
$$= x^2 + 2xy + y^2$$
$$= (x + y)^2;$$

$$\mathbf{v}^\top \mathbf{G} \mathbf{v} = \begin{pmatrix} x & y \end{pmatrix} \begin{pmatrix} 1 & 0 \\ 0 & -1 \end{pmatrix} \begin{pmatrix} x \\ y \end{pmatrix}$$
$$= x^2 - y^2$$
$$= (x + y)(x - y);$$

$$\mathbf{v}^\top \mathbf{W} \mathbf{v} = (x \; y) \begin{pmatrix} 1 & -1 \\ -1 & 1 \end{pmatrix} \begin{pmatrix} x \\ y \end{pmatrix}$$

$$= x^2 - 2xy + y^2$$

$$= (x - y)^2.$$

Thus, it is immediate to realize also that from definitions (21.19) and (21.20), we get:

$$\mathbf{v}^\top \mathbf{I} \mathbf{v} + \mathbf{v}^\top \mathbf{Z} \mathbf{v} = \mathbf{v}^\top (\mathbf{I} + \mathbf{Z}) \mathbf{v} = \mathbf{v}^\top \mathbf{U} \mathbf{v},$$

so that

$$\mathbf{v}^\top \begin{pmatrix} 1 & 0 \\ 0 & 1 \end{pmatrix} \mathbf{v} + \mathbf{v}^\top \begin{pmatrix} 0 & 1 \\ 1 & 0 \end{pmatrix} \mathbf{v} = \mathbf{v}^\top \left[\begin{pmatrix} 1 & 0 \\ 0 & 1 \end{pmatrix} + \begin{pmatrix} 0 & 1 \\ 1 & 0 \end{pmatrix} \right] \mathbf{v}$$

$$= \mathbf{v}^\top \begin{pmatrix} 1 & 1 \\ 1 & 1 \end{pmatrix} \mathbf{v}$$

and

$$\mathbf{v}^\top \mathbf{I} \mathbf{v} - \mathbf{v}^\top \mathbf{Z} \mathbf{v} = \mathbf{v}^\top (\mathbf{I} - \mathbf{Z}) \mathbf{v} = \mathbf{v}^\top \mathbf{W} \mathbf{v},$$

so that

$$\mathbf{v}^\top \begin{pmatrix} 1 & 0 \\ 0 & 1 \end{pmatrix} \mathbf{v} - \mathbf{v}^\top \begin{pmatrix} 0 & 1 \\ 1 & 0 \end{pmatrix} \mathbf{v} = \mathbf{v}^\top \left[\begin{pmatrix} 1 & 0 \\ 0 & 1 \end{pmatrix} - \begin{pmatrix} 0 & 1 \\ 1 & 0 \end{pmatrix} \right] \mathbf{v}$$

$$= \mathbf{v}^\top \begin{pmatrix} 1 & -1 \\ -1 & 1 \end{pmatrix} \mathbf{v};$$

therefore, the algebraic sum of two quadratic forms characterized by the same vector $\mathbf{v}$ is a new quadratic form with the same vector $\mathbf{v}$, in which the matrix is the algebraic sum of the matrices of the quadratic forms.

21.12 Applications of Quadratic Forms to Statistics

We already saw in Eq. (20.4) that the mean μ of n measures x_k in a population can be written as

$$\mu = \frac{\mathbf{1}^\top \mathbf{x}}{n}$$

and, in Eq. (20.5), that the variance may be written as

$$\sigma^2 = \frac{\mathbf{x}^\top \mathbf{x}}{n} - \left(\frac{\mathbf{1}^\top \mathbf{x}}{n}\right)^2; \tag{21.21}$$

this value can also approximate the sample variance s^2 in the case n is big enough to write $n + 1 \approx n$.

Incidentally, we note that the sample variance of the j-th variable is

$$s_{jj} = \frac{1}{n-1} \sum_{i=1}^{n} (x_{ij} - \bar{x}_i)^2$$

whereas the covariance between the j-th and the k-th variables is

$$s_{jk} = \frac{1}{n-1} \sum_{i=1}^{n} (x_{ij} - \bar{x}_i)(x_{ik} - \bar{x}_k);$$

thus, the variance-covariance matrix $\mathbf{S}$ can be always be represented as

$$\mathbf{S} = \frac{1}{n-1} \sum_{i=1}^{n} (\mathbf{x}_i - \bar{\mathbf{x}})(\mathbf{x}_i - \bar{\mathbf{x}})^\top.$$

Now we can use the quadratic forms to redefine the variance in Eq. (21.21) as follows:

$$\begin{aligned}
\sigma^2 &= \frac{\mathbf{x}^\top \mathbf{x}}{n} - \left(\frac{\mathbf{1}^\top \mathbf{x}}{n}\right)^2 \\
&= \frac{\mathbf{x}^\top \mathbf{x}}{n} - \frac{\mathbf{1}^\top \mathbf{x}}{n}\frac{\mathbf{1}^\top \mathbf{x}}{n} \\
&= \frac{\mathbf{x}^\top \mathbf{I} \mathbf{x}}{n} - \frac{\mathbf{x}^\top \mathbf{1}\mathbf{1}^\top \mathbf{x}}{n^2} \\
&= \frac{1}{n}\left(\mathbf{x}^\top \mathbf{I} \mathbf{x} - \mathbf{x}^\top \frac{\mathbf{1}\mathbf{1}^\top}{n}\mathbf{x}\right) \\
&= \frac{1}{n}\left(\mathbf{x}^\top \mathbf{I} \mathbf{x} - \mathbf{x}^\top \frac{\mathbf{U}}{n}\mathbf{x}\right) \\
&= \frac{1}{n}\mathbf{x}^\top \left(\mathbf{I} \mathbf{x} - \frac{\mathbf{U}}{n}\mathbf{x}\right) \\
&= \frac{1}{n}\mathbf{x}^\top \left(\mathbf{I} - \frac{\mathbf{U}}{n}\right)\mathbf{x}, \tag{21.22}
\end{aligned}$$

where we used the equality $\mathbf{1}_{n \times 1} \mathbf{1}_{1 \times n}^{\top} = \mathbf{U}_{n \times n}$, being $\mathbf{U}$ the square unity matrix, already defined as

$$\mathbf{U} = \begin{pmatrix} 1 \cdots 1 \\ \vdots \ddots \vdots \\ 1 \cdots 1 \end{pmatrix},$$

and characterized by the property

$$\mathbf{U}_n^m = \begin{pmatrix} n^{m-1} & n^{m-1} & \cdots & n^{m-1} \\ n^{m-1} & n^{m-1} & \cdots & n^{m-1} \\ \vdots & \vdots & \ddots & \vdots \\ n^{m-1} & n^{m-1} & \cdots & n^{m-1} \end{pmatrix} = n^{m-1} \mathbf{U}_n,$$

from which we get the particular case

$$\mathbf{U}_n^2 = n \mathbf{U}_n.$$

Hence,

$$\mathbf{I} - \frac{\mathbf{U}}{n} = \begin{pmatrix} 1 & 0 & \cdots & 0 \\ 0 & 1 & \cdots & 0 \\ \vdots & \vdots & \ddots & \vdots \\ 0 & 0 & \cdots & 1 \end{pmatrix} - \begin{pmatrix} \frac{1}{n} & \frac{1}{n} & \cdots & \frac{1}{n} \\ \frac{1}{n} & \frac{1}{n} & \cdots & \frac{1}{n} \\ \vdots & \vdots & \ddots & \vdots \\ \frac{1}{n} & \frac{1}{n} & \cdots & \frac{1}{n} \end{pmatrix}$$

$$= \begin{pmatrix} 1-\frac{1}{n} & -\frac{1}{n} & \cdots & -\frac{1}{n} \\ -\frac{1}{n} & 1-\frac{1}{n} & \cdots & -\frac{1}{n} \\ \vdots & \vdots & \ddots & \vdots \\ -\frac{1}{n} & -\frac{1}{n} & \cdots & 1-\frac{1}{n} \end{pmatrix}, \tag{21.23}$$

Equation (21.22) may be rewritten as

$$\sigma^2 = \frac{1}{n} \mathbf{x}^{\top} \left(\mathbf{I} - \frac{\mathbf{U}}{n} \right) \mathbf{x}$$

$$= \frac{1}{n} \begin{pmatrix} x_1 & x_2 & \cdots & x_n \end{pmatrix} \begin{pmatrix} 1-\frac{1}{n} & -\frac{1}{n} & \cdots & -\frac{1}{n} \\ -\frac{1}{n} & 1-\frac{1}{n} & \cdots & -\frac{1}{n} \\ \vdots & \vdots & \ddots & \vdots \\ -\frac{1}{n} & -\frac{1}{n} & \cdots & 1-\frac{1}{n} \end{pmatrix} \begin{pmatrix} x_1 \\ x_2 \\ \vdots \\ x_n \end{pmatrix},$$

which depends on the deviation from the mean of the observations.

We may verify this proposition by first taking into account the matrix $\mathbf{I} - \mathbf{U}/n$, to observe a peculiar property, that is its *idempotence*: to say that a square matrix $\mathbf{A}_n$ is idempotent means to say $\mathbf{A}_n^2 = \mathbf{A}_n$. In the set of real numbers, we know only two idempotents, 0 and 1 (in fact $0^2 = 0$ e $1^2 = 1$), whereas in the set of square matrices of order n, the number of idempotent ones is virtually infinite (we will extensively come back to idempotent matrices in a later chapter).

To verify the idempotence of $\mathbf{I} - \mathbf{U}/n$ defined in Eq. (21.23), we may calculate:

$$\left(\mathbf{I} - \frac{\mathbf{U}}{n}\right)^2 = \mathbf{I}^2 - 2\frac{\mathbf{IU}}{n} + \frac{\mathbf{U}^2}{n^2} = \mathbf{I} - 2\frac{\mathbf{U}}{n} + \frac{\mathbf{U}}{n}$$

$$= \mathbf{I} - \frac{\mathbf{U}}{n};$$

thus, the variance could be rewritten as

$$\sigma^2 = \frac{1}{n}\mathbf{x}^\top \left(\mathbf{I} - \frac{\mathbf{U}}{n}\right)\mathbf{x}$$

$$= \frac{1}{n}\mathbf{x}^\top \left(\mathbf{I} - \frac{\mathbf{U}}{n}\right)\left(\mathbf{I} - \frac{\mathbf{U}}{n}\right)\mathbf{x};$$

hence, we have:

$$\mathbf{x}^\top \left(\mathbf{I} - \frac{\mathbf{U}}{n}\right) = (x_1 \; x_2 \; \cdots \; x_n) \begin{pmatrix} 1 - \frac{1}{n} & -\frac{1}{n} & \cdots & -\frac{1}{n} \\ -\frac{1}{n} & 1 - \frac{1}{n} & \cdots & -\frac{1}{n} \\ \vdots & \vdots & \ddots & \vdots \\ -\frac{1}{n} & -\frac{1}{n} & \cdots & 1 - \frac{1}{n} \end{pmatrix}$$

$$= \left(x_1 - \frac{x_1}{n} - \frac{x_2}{n} - \cdots - \frac{x_n}{n} \quad \cdots \quad -\frac{x_1}{n} - \frac{x_2}{n} - \cdots + x_n - \frac{x_n}{n}\right)$$

$$= \left(x_1 - \sum_{k=1}^{n} \frac{x_k}{n} \quad \cdots \quad x_n - \sum_{k=1}^{n} \frac{x_k}{n}\right);$$

and

$$\left(\mathbf{I} - \frac{\mathbf{U}}{n}\right)\mathbf{x} = \begin{pmatrix} 1 - \frac{1}{n} & -\frac{1}{n} & \cdots & -\frac{1}{n} \\ -\frac{1}{n} & 1 - \frac{1}{n} & \cdots & -\frac{1}{n} \\ \vdots & \vdots & \ddots & \vdots \\ -\frac{1}{n} & -\frac{1}{n} & \cdots & 1 - \frac{1}{n} \end{pmatrix} \begin{pmatrix} x_1 \\ x_2 \\ \vdots \\ x_n \end{pmatrix}$$

$$= \begin{pmatrix} x_1(1 - \frac{1}{n}) - \frac{x_2}{n} - \cdots - \frac{x_n}{n} \\ \vdots \\ -\frac{x_1}{n} - \frac{x_2}{n} - \cdots + x_n(1 - \frac{1}{n}) \end{pmatrix}$$

$$= \begin{pmatrix} x_1 - \sum_{k=1}^{n} \frac{x_k}{n} \\ \vdots \\ x_n - \sum_{k=1}^{n} \frac{x_k}{n} \end{pmatrix};$$

therefore

$$\sigma^2 = \frac{1}{n} \mathbf{x}^{\top} \left(\mathbf{I} - \frac{\mathbf{U}}{n} \right) \left(\mathbf{I} - \frac{\mathbf{U}}{n} \right) \mathbf{x}$$

$$= \frac{1}{n} \left(x_1 - \sum_{k=1}^{n} \frac{x_k}{n} \cdots x_n - \sum_{k=1}^{n} \frac{x_k}{n} \right) \begin{pmatrix} x_1 - \sum_{k=1}^{n} \frac{x_k}{n} \\ \vdots \\ x_n - \sum_{k=1}^{n} \frac{x_k}{n} \end{pmatrix}$$

$$= \frac{1}{n} \left(\left(x_1 - \sum_{k=1}^{n} \frac{x_k}{n} \right)^2 + \cdots + \left(x_n - \sum_{k=1}^{n} \frac{x_k}{n} \right)^2 \right)$$

$$= \frac{1}{n} \sum_{i=1}^{n} \left(x_i - \sum_{k=1}^{n} \frac{x_k}{n} \right)^2.$$

In practice, defining the vector of the deviation from average $\mathbf{d}$, having a generic element

$$\delta_i = x_i - \sum_{k=1}^{n} \frac{x_k}{n},$$

the variance may be written in the simple form:

$$\sigma^2 = \frac{\mathbf{d}^{\top} \mathbf{d}}{n},$$

i.e., in terms of the internal product $\mathbf{d}^{\top} \mathbf{d}$.

21.13 The Product $\mathbf{A}^{\top}\mathbf{A}$

The product $\mathbf{A}^{\top}\mathbf{A}$ of a matrix $\mathbf{A}_{m \times n}$ premultiplied by its transpose $\mathbf{A}_{n \times m}^{\top}$ is of great interest in statistics, in particular when dealing with linear regression. Given $\mathbf{A}_{m \times n}$, the product $\mathbf{A}^{\top}\mathbf{A}$ is always a symmetric $n \times n$ square matrix, since $\mathbf{A}$ is $m \times n$, and $\mathbf{A}^{\top}$ is $n \times m$.

Taking

$$\mathbf{A} = \begin{pmatrix} a_{11} & a_{12} & \cdots & a_{1n} \\ a_{21} & a_{22} & \cdots & a_{2n} \\ \vdots & \vdots & \ddots & \vdots \\ a_{m1} & a_{m2} & \cdots & a_{mn} \end{pmatrix},$$

then

$$\mathbf{A}^\top \mathbf{A} = \begin{pmatrix} a_{11} & a_{21} & \cdots & a_{m1} \\ a_{12} & a_{22} & \cdots & a_{m2} \\ \vdots & \vdots & \ddots & \vdots \\ a_{1n} & a_{2n} & \cdots & a_{nm} \end{pmatrix} \begin{pmatrix} a_{11} & a_{12} & \cdots & a_{1n} \\ a_{21} & a_{22} & \cdots & a_{2n} \\ \vdots & \vdots & \ddots & \vdots \\ a_{m1} & a_{m2} & \cdots & a_{mn} \end{pmatrix}$$

$$= \begin{pmatrix} A_{11} & A_{12} & \cdots & A_{1c} \\ A_{21} & A_{22} & \cdots & A_{2c} \\ \vdots & \vdots & \ddots & \vdots \\ A_{r1} & A_{r2} & \cdots & A_{rc} \end{pmatrix}. \tag{21.24}$$

where

$$A_{11} = a_{11}^2 + \ldots + a_{m1}^2$$
$$A_{12} = a_{11}a_{12} + \cdots + a_{m1}a_{m2}$$
$$A_{1c} = a_{11}a_{1n} + \cdots + a_{m1}a_{mn}$$
$$A_{21} = a_{11}a_{12} + \cdots + a_{m1}a_{m2}$$
$$A_{22} = a_{12}^2 + \cdots + a_{m2}^2$$
$$A_{2c} = a_{12}a_{1n} + \cdots + a_{m2}a_{mn}$$
$$A_{r1} = a_{11}a_{1n} + \cdots + a_{m1}a_{mn}$$
$$A_{r2} = a_{12}a_{1n} + \cdots + a_{m2}a_{mn}$$
$$A_{rc} = a_{1n}^2 + \cdots + a_{mn}^2,$$

hence

$$\mathbf{A}^\top \mathbf{A} = \begin{pmatrix} \sum_{k=1}^m a_{k1}^2 & \sum_{k=1}^m a_{k1}a_{k2} & \cdots & \sum_{k=1}^m a_{k1}a_{kn} \\ \sum_{k=1}^m a_{k1}a_{k2} & \sum_{k=1}^m a_{k2}^2 & \cdots & \sum_{k=1}^m a_{k2}a_{kn} \\ \vdots & \vdots & \ddots & \vdots \\ \sum_{k=1}^m a_{k1}a_{kn} & \sum_{k=1}^m a_{k2}a_{kn} & \cdots & \sum_{k=1}^m a_{kn}^2 \end{pmatrix}.$$

Note that $\mathbf{A}^\top\mathbf{A}$ is symmetric and that its k-th diagonal element is given by the sum of the squared elements of the k-th column of $\mathbf{A}_{m\times n}$ (or also of the k-th row of $\mathbf{A}^\top$). This may be verified by writing the matrices $\mathbf{A}^\top$ and $\mathbf{A}$ in terms of their column vectors; hence as

$$\mathbf{A}^\top = \begin{pmatrix} \mathbf{c}_1^\top \\ \mathbf{c}_2^\top \\ \vdots \\ \mathbf{c}_n^\top \end{pmatrix}; \quad \mathbf{A} = \begin{pmatrix} \mathbf{c}_1 & \mathbf{c}_2 & \cdots & \mathbf{c}_n \end{pmatrix},$$

so that $\mathbf{A}^\top\mathbf{A}$ is the $n \times n$ matrix

$$\mathbf{A}^\top\mathbf{A} = \begin{pmatrix} \mathbf{c}_1^\top\mathbf{c}_1 & \mathbf{c}_1^\top\mathbf{c}_2 & \cdots & \mathbf{c}_1^\top\mathbf{c}_n \\ \mathbf{c}_2^\top\mathbf{c}_1 & \mathbf{c}_2^\top\mathbf{c}_2 & \cdots & \mathbf{c}_2^\top\mathbf{c}_n \\ \vdots & \vdots & \ddots & \vdots \\ \mathbf{c}_n^\top\mathbf{c}_1 & \mathbf{c}_n^\top\mathbf{c}_2 & \cdots & \mathbf{c}_n^\top\mathbf{c}_n \end{pmatrix}$$

$$= \begin{pmatrix} \mathbf{c}_1^\top\mathbf{c}_1 & \mathbf{c}_1^\top\mathbf{c}_2 & \cdots & \mathbf{c}_1^\top\mathbf{c}_n \\ \mathbf{c}_1^\top\mathbf{c}_2 & \mathbf{c}_2^\top\mathbf{c}_2 & \cdots & \mathbf{c}_2^\top\mathbf{c}_n \\ \vdots & \vdots & \ddots & \vdots \\ \mathbf{c}_1^\top\mathbf{c}_n & \mathbf{c}_2^\top\mathbf{c}_n & \cdots & \mathbf{c}_n^\top\mathbf{c}_n \end{pmatrix},$$

where all elements are scalars; hence, the matrix is symmetric.

As we can observe, the diagonal elements are sums of squares: any k-the diagonal element is the sum of the squares of elements belonging to the k-th column of $\mathbf{A}$, or the k-th row of $\mathbf{A}^\top$, while the *subdiagonal and superdiagonal elements* (i.e., the elements respectively lying immediately below and above the diagonal elements) are sums of products. Indeed, any subdiagonal element $s_{i,i-1}$ placed in the k-th row and in the $(k-1)$-th column of $\mathbf{A}^\top\mathbf{A}$ is the sum of the products of the elements in the $(k-1)$-th column multiplied by the corresponding element of the k-th column of $\mathbf{A}$, and any element $s_{i-1,i}$ placed in the k-th column and in the $(k-1)$-th row of $\mathbf{A}^\top\mathbf{A}$ is the sum of the products of any element in the $(k-1)$-th row multiplied by the corresponding element in the k-th row of $\mathbf{A}^\top$; obviously, since $\mathbf{A}^\top\mathbf{A}$ is symmetric, we will have $s_{i,i-1} = s_{i-1,i}$. What seen above is valid also for the sub-subdiagonal and the super-superdiagonal elements, and so on.

Clearly, the product $\mathbf{A}^\top\mathbf{A}$ does not commute if $\mathbf{A}$ is $m \times n$ with $m \neq n$: in this case, indeed, $\mathbf{A}^\top\mathbf{A}$ is $n \times n$, while $\mathbf{A}\mathbf{A}^\top$ is $m \times m$. However, even in the case of a square matrix $n \times n$ (thus, even $\mathbf{A}^\top\mathbf{A}$ and $\mathbf{A}\mathbf{A}^\top$ would be $n \times n$ square matrices), the product will not necessarily commute, so that, in general, $\mathbf{A}^\top\mathbf{A} \neq \mathbf{A}\mathbf{A}^\top$.

21.14 The Determinant

To any square matrix $\mathbf{A}_n$ it associates a number, called the *determinant of* $\mathbf{A}$, written as det($\mathbf{A}$), or also as $|\mathbf{A}|$; thus, we can write:

$$\det \begin{pmatrix} a_{11} & a_{12} & a_{13} \\ a_{21} & a_{22} & a_{23} \\ a_{31} & a_{32} & a_{33} \end{pmatrix} = \begin{vmatrix} a_{11} & a_{12} & a_{13} \\ a_{21} & a_{22} & a_{23} \\ a_{31} & a_{32} & a_{33} \end{vmatrix}$$

since the two notations are perfectly equivalent.

The determinant is a scalar function with matrix argument: in other words if we are dealing with real numbers, then, $\det(\cdot) : \mathbb{R}^{n,n} \to \mathbb{R}$.

The determinant is a number with a specific geometric significance, but it is also an indispensable mathematical tool to obtain the inverse of a matrix (see in the next sections) and also for more advanced calculations. To obtain the determinant of a square matrix, there may be several methods; for our purposes, we will start from its mathematical definition.

The determinant det($\mathbf{A}$) of a square matrix $\mathbf{A}_n$ is defined as

$$\det(\mathbf{A}) = \sum_{j=1}^{n} a_{jk}c_{jk} = \sum_{k=1}^{n} a_{jk}c_{jk} \qquad (21.25)$$

where a_{jk} is the element of $\mathbf{A}$ found in the j-th row and in the k-th column, while c_{jk} is the *algebraic complement* of a_{jk}, e.g., the determinant of the *adjoint matrix* of $\mathbf{A}$; this last (also called the *adjugate matrix,* or also the *minor* of $\mathbf{A}$) is the matrix resulting after eliminating the row and the column of the element a_{jk} of $\mathbf{A}$, multiplied by $(-1)^{j+k}$. It is not important which row and column is chosen to calculate the determinant of a matrix: the result will be always the same, as we will see.

We also will see in a next section that there are some very simple shortcuts to calculate the determinant of a 2×2 and of a 3×3 matrix.

All possible algebraic complements c_{jk} of square matrix $\mathbf{A}_{n \times n}$ are the elements of a matrix $\mathbf{C_A}$, which is the *matrix of the cofactors* of $\mathbf{A}$, e.g., a $n \times n$ square matrix defined as

$$\mathbf{C_A} = \begin{pmatrix} (-1)^{1+1} \det(A_{[11]}) & (-1)^{1+2} \det(A_{[12]}) & \cdots & (-1)^{1+n} \det(A_{[1n]}) \\ (-1)^{2+1} \det(A_{[21]}) & (-1)^{2+2} \det(A_{[22]}) & \cdots & (-1)^{2+n} \det(A_{[2n]}) \\ \vdots & \vdots & \ddots & \vdots \\ (-1)^{n+1} \det(A_{[n1]}) & (-1)^{n+2} \det(A_{[n2]}) & \cdots & (-1)^{n+n} \det(A_{[nn]}) \end{pmatrix},$$

$$(21.26)$$

where, as already mentioned,

$$\det(\mathbf{A}_{[jk]}) = \begin{vmatrix} a_{11} & \cdots & a_{1,k-1} & a_{1,k+1} & \cdots & a_{1n} \\ \vdots & \ddots & \vdots & \vdots & & \vdots \\ a_{j-1,1} & \cdots & a_{j-1,k-1} & a_{j-1,k+1} & \cdots & a_{j-1,n} \\ a_{j+1,1} & \cdots & a_{j+1,k-1} & a_{j+1,k+1} & \cdots & a_{j+1,n} \\ \vdots & & \vdots & \vdots & \ddots & \vdots \\ a_{n1} & \cdots & a_{n,k-1} & a_{n,k+1} & \cdots & a_{nn} \end{vmatrix} \qquad (21.27)$$

is the determinant of the adjoint matrix $\mathbf{A}_{[jk]}$, which is the matrix $\mathbf{A}$ deprived of the j-th row and of the k-th column. Obviously, being $\mathbf{A}$ a $n \times n$ matrix, then $\mathbf{A}_{[jk]}$ is $(n-1) \times (n-1)$.

By definition, if a matrix is 1×1, its determinant is equal to the unique element of the matrix; thus, if $\mathbf{A} = (a_{11})$, we have $\det(\mathbf{A}) = a_{11}$.

Given the definition, we easily understand that its calculus may be obtained recursively; thus, for example, extracting the elements of the first column of $\mathbf{A}$ as

$$\det(\mathbf{A}) = a_{11}\det(\mathbf{A}_{[11]}) - a_{21}\det(\mathbf{A}_{[21]}) + \cdots + (-1)^{n+1}a_{n1}\det(\mathbf{A}_{[n1]})$$

and then one may obtain the single determinants $\det(\mathbf{A}_{[k1]})$ exactly in the same way.

Taking an arbitrary 4×4 matrix, we could write:

$$\det(\mathbf{A}) = \begin{vmatrix} a_{11} & a_{12} & a_{13} & a_{14} \\ a_{21} & a_{22} & a_{23} & a_{24} \\ a_{31} & a_{32} & a_{33} & a_{34} \\ a_{41} & a_{42} & a_{43} & a_{44} \end{vmatrix}$$

$$= a_{11}\begin{vmatrix} a_{22} & a_{23} & a_{24} \\ a_{32} & a_{33} & a_{34} \\ a_{42} & a_{43} & a_{44} \end{vmatrix} - a_{21}\begin{vmatrix} a_{12} & a_{13} & a_{14} \\ a_{32} & a_{33} & a_{34} \\ a_{42} & a_{43} & a_{44} \end{vmatrix}$$

$$+ a_{31}\begin{vmatrix} a_{12} & a_{13} & a_{14} \\ a_{22} & a_{23} & a_{24} \\ a_{42} & a_{43} & a_{44} \end{vmatrix} - a_{41}\begin{vmatrix} a_{12} & a_{13} & a_{14} \\ a_{22} & a_{23} & a_{24} \\ a_{32} & a_{33} & a_{34} \end{vmatrix}$$

$$= a_{11}\left(a_{22}\begin{vmatrix} a_{33} & a_{34} \\ a_{43} & a_{44} \end{vmatrix} - a_{32}\begin{vmatrix} a_{23} & a_{24} \\ a_{43} & a_{44} \end{vmatrix} + a_{42}\begin{vmatrix} a_{23} & a_{24} \\ a_{33} & a_{34} \end{vmatrix}\right)$$

$$- a_{21}\left(a_{12}\begin{vmatrix} a_{33} & a_{34} \\ a_{43} & a_{44} \end{vmatrix} - a_{32}\begin{vmatrix} a_{13} & a_{14} \\ a_{43} & a_{44} \end{vmatrix} + a_{42}\begin{vmatrix} a_{13} & a_{14} \\ a_{33} & a_{34} \end{vmatrix}\right)$$

$$+ a_{31}\left(a_{12}\begin{vmatrix} a_{23} & a_{24} \\ a_{43} & a_{44} \end{vmatrix} - a_{22}\begin{vmatrix} a_{13} & a_{14} \\ a_{43} & a_{44} \end{vmatrix} + a_{42}\begin{vmatrix} a_{13} & a_{14} \\ a_{23} & a_{24} \end{vmatrix}\right)$$

$$- a_{41}\left(a_{12}\begin{vmatrix} a_{23} & a_{24} \\ a_{33} & a_{34} \end{vmatrix} - a_{22}\begin{vmatrix} a_{13} & a_{14} \\ a_{33} & a_{34} \end{vmatrix} + a_{32}\begin{vmatrix} a_{13} & a_{14} \\ a_{23} & a_{24} \end{vmatrix}\right)$$

$$= a_{11}\left(a_{22}(a_{33}a_{44} - a_{43}a_{34}) - a_{32}(a_{23}a_{44} - a_{43}a_{24})\right.$$

$$+ a_{42}(a_{23}a_{34} - a_{33}a_{24})) - a_{21}\left(a_{12}(a_{33}a_{44} - a_{43}a_{34})\right.$$

$$- a_{32}(a_{13}a_{44} - a_{43}a_{14}) + a_{42}(a_{13}a_{34} - a_{33}a_{14}))$$

$$+ a_{31}\left(a_{12}(a_{23}a_{44} - a_{43}a_{24}) - a_{22}(a_{13}a_{44} - a_{43}a_{14})\right.$$

$$+ a_{42}(a_{13}a_{24} - a_{23}a_{14})) - a_{41}\left(a_{12}(a_{23}a_{34} - a_{33}a_{24})\right.$$

$$- a_{22}(a_{13}a_{34} - a_{33}a_{14}) + a_{32}(a_{13}a_{24} - a_{23}a_{14})),$$

where we see that the calculus has been always done using the adjoint matrices, which have been obtained by eliminating the first column of any matrix and then the rows crossing the same first column.

Indeed, as we saw before, the calculus of the determinant may be carried out by eliminating any column or row: in particular, there may be situations suggesting the more suitable rows and columns to be excluded.

As a practical example, let us take the matrix:

$$\mathbf{X} = \begin{pmatrix} 1 & 2 & 1 & 3 \\ 3 & 2 & 1 & 1 \\ 1 & 0 & 2 & 1 \\ 1 & 2 & 1 & 1 \end{pmatrix}, \tag{21.28}$$

where we have

$$\det \begin{pmatrix} 1 & 2 & 1 & 3 \\ 3 & 2 & 1 & 1 \\ 1 & 0 & 2 & 1 \\ 1 & 2 & 1 & 1 \end{pmatrix} = 1 \begin{vmatrix} 2 & 1 & 1 \\ 0 & 2 & 1 \\ 2 & 1 & 1 \end{vmatrix} - 3 \begin{vmatrix} 2 & 1 & 3 \\ 0 & 2 & 1 \\ 2 & 1 & 1 \end{vmatrix}$$

$$+ 1 \begin{vmatrix} 2 & 1 & 3 \\ 2 & 1 & 1 \\ 2 & 1 & 1 \end{vmatrix} - 1 \begin{vmatrix} 2 & 1 & 3 \\ 2 & 1 & 1 \\ 0 & 2 & 1 \end{vmatrix}$$

$$= 1 \left(2 \begin{vmatrix} 2 & 1 \\ 1 & 1 \end{vmatrix} - 0 \begin{vmatrix} 1 & 1 \\ 1 & 1 \end{vmatrix} + 2 \begin{vmatrix} 1 & 1 \\ 2 & 1 \end{vmatrix} \right)$$

$$- 3 \left(2 \begin{vmatrix} 2 & 1 \\ 1 & 1 \end{vmatrix} - 0 \begin{vmatrix} 1 & 3 \\ 1 & 1 \end{vmatrix} + 2 \begin{vmatrix} 1 & 3 \\ 2 & 1 \end{vmatrix} \right)$$

$$+ 1 \left(2 \begin{vmatrix} 1 & 1 \\ 1 & 1 \end{vmatrix} - 2 \begin{vmatrix} 1 & 3 \\ 1 & 1 \end{vmatrix} + 2 \begin{vmatrix} 1 & 3 \\ 1 & 1 \end{vmatrix} \right)$$

$$- 1 \left(2 \begin{vmatrix} 1 & 1 \\ 2 & 1 \end{vmatrix} - 2 \begin{vmatrix} 1 & 3 \\ 2 & 1 \end{vmatrix} + 0 \begin{vmatrix} 1 & 3 \\ 1 & 1 \end{vmatrix} \right)$$

$$= 1 \times (2 \times (2 \times 1 - 1 \times 1) - 0 \times (1 \times 1 - 1 \times 1)$$
$$+ 2 \times (2 \times 1 - 2 \times 1)) - 3 \times (2 \times (2 \times 1 - 1 \times 1)$$
$$- 0 \times (1 \times 1 - 1 \times 3) + 2 \times (1 \times 1 - 2 \times 3))$$
$$+ 1 \times (2 \times (1 \times 1 - 1 \times 1) - 2 \times (1 \times 1 - 1 \times 3) + 2$$
$$\times (1 \times 1 - 1 \times 3)) - 1 \times (2 \times (1 \times 1 - 2 \times 1)$$
$$- 2 \times (1 \times 1 - 2 \times 3) + 0 \times (1 \times 1 - 1 \times 3))$$
$$= 2 + 24 + 0 - 8$$
$$= 16.$$

21.15 Determinant of a 2 × 2 Matrix

A simple case of determinant calculus may be seen in the 2×2 matrices, where the determinant is given by $a_{11}a_{22} - a_{21}a_{12}$; thus, by the product of the diagonal elements a_{11}, a_{22}, minus the product of the elements a_{21}, a_{12}, lying off-diagonal. For example, given the matrices

$$\mathbf{X} = \begin{pmatrix} 1 & 2 \\ 3 & 4 \end{pmatrix}, \quad \mathbf{Y} = \begin{pmatrix} 3 & 5 \\ -2 & 3 \end{pmatrix}, \quad \mathbf{Z} = \begin{pmatrix} 5 & 4 \\ \frac{5}{2} & 2 \end{pmatrix},$$

their respective determinants are

$$\det(\mathbf{X}) = (1 \times 4) - (3 \times 2) = 4 - 6 = -2;$$
$$\det(\mathbf{Y}) = (3 \times 3) - ((-2) \times 5) = 9 - (-10) = 19;$$
$$\det(\mathbf{Z}) = (5 \times 2) - (\tfrac{5}{2} \times 4) = 10 - 10 = 0.$$

It is just a particular case of the calculus obtained from the general formula (21.25): in fact, given a matrix

$$\mathbf{A} = \begin{pmatrix} a_{11} & a_{12} \\ a_{21} & a_{22} \end{pmatrix},$$

we see that its adjoint matrices are

$$\mathbf{A}_{[11]} = a_{22}; \quad \mathbf{A}_{[12]} = a_{21}; \quad \mathbf{A}_{[21]} = a_{12}; \quad \mathbf{A}_{[22]} = a_{11},$$

e.g., all adjoints are 1×1 matrices; hence, the respective algebraic complements are

$$c_{11} = (-1)^{1+1} \det(\mathbf{A}_{[11]}) = \det(a_{22}) = a_{22},$$

$$c_{12} = (-1)^{1+2} \det(\mathbf{A}_{[12]}) = -\det(a_{21}) = -a_{21},$$

$$c_{21} = (-1)^{2+1} \det(\mathbf{A}_{[21]}) = -\det(a_{12}) = -a_{12},$$

$$c_{22} = (-1)^{2+2} \det(\mathbf{A}_{[22]}) = \det(a_{11}) = a_{11};$$

therefore, using Eq. (21.25), we have:

$$\det(\mathbf{A}) = a_{11}c_{11} + a_{21}c_{21}$$
$$= a_{11} \times a_{22} + a_{21} \times (-a_{12})$$
$$= a_{11}a_{22} - a_{21}a_{12},$$

where we extracted the elements of the first column. In fact, if we had extracted the elements in the first row, the result would have been the same, since

$$\det(\mathbf{A}) = a_{11}c_{11} + a_{12}c_{12}$$
$$= a_{11} \times a_{22} + a_{12} \times (-a_{21})$$
$$= a_{11}a_{22} - a_{21}a_{12}.$$

The result does not change even with the extraction of the elements of the second row:

$$\det(\mathbf{A}) = a_{21}c_{21} + a_{22}c_{22}$$
$$= a_{21} \times (-a_{12}) + a_{22} \times a_{11}$$
$$= a_{11}a_{22} - a_{21}a_{12},$$

or those of the second column

$$\det(\mathbf{A}) = a_{12}c_{12} + a_{22}c_{22}$$
$$= a_{12} \times (-a_{21}) + a_{22} \times a_{11}$$
$$= a_{11}a_{22} - a_{21}a_{12}.$$

The geometrical significance of the determinant is very simple in a 2×2 matrix: its absolute value is the surface area of a parallelogram having the vertices in the points $(0, 0)$, (a, c), (b, d) and $(a + b, c + d)$ of a system of Cartesian axes.

21.16 Determinant of a 3 × 3 Matrix

The determinant of a generic 3×3 matrix is

$$\det \begin{pmatrix} l & m & n \\ p & q & r \\ s & u & v \end{pmatrix} = lqv + mrs + npu - sqn - url - vpm,$$

which is equivalent to the addition and subtraction of the "virtual diagonals" starting from the principal one, so as to add the diagonals "top to bottom," and to subtract the "bottom to top" ones, always moving from left to right

$$\begin{array}{ccccc} l & m & n & l & m \\ & q & r & p & \\ s & u & v & s & u \end{array} \implies \begin{cases} \text{top to bottom diagonals } lqv, mrs, npu \\ \text{bottom to top diagonals } sqn, url, vpm \end{cases}.$$

This shortcut to obtain the determinant is called the *rule of Sarrus*; it works only with the 3×3 matrices. For the matrices of higher order, one must use the standard method involving the adjoint and the cofactor matrices in the calculus.

In a 3×3 matrix, the geometrical significance of the determinant is the volume of a polyhedron having the vertices in the eight points of coordinates respectively $(0, 0, 0)$, (a_{11}, a_{21}, a_{31}), (a_{12}, a_{22}, a_{23}), (a_{13}, a_{23}, a_{33}), $(a_{11} + a_{12}, a_{21} + a_{22}, a_{31} + a_{32})$, $(a_{11} + a_{13}, a_{21} + a_{23}, a_{31} + a_{33})$, $(a_{12} + a_{13}, a_{22} + a_{23}, a_{32} + a_{33})$, and $(a_{11} + a_{12} + a_{13}, a_{21} + a_{22} + a_{23}, a_{31} + a_{32} + a_{33})$, or—still better—considering the matrix as column vectors:

$$\mathbf{A} = \begin{pmatrix} a_{11} & a_{12} & a_{13} \\ a_{21} & a_{22} & a_{23} \\ a_{31} & a_{32} & a_{33} \end{pmatrix} = \begin{pmatrix} \mathbf{a_1} & \mathbf{a_2} & \mathbf{a_3} \end{pmatrix}$$

so that

$$\mathbf{a_1} = \begin{pmatrix} a_{11} \\ a_{21} \\ a_{31} \end{pmatrix} ; \quad \mathbf{a_2} = \begin{pmatrix} a_{12} \\ a_{22} \\ a_{32} \end{pmatrix} ; \quad \mathbf{a_3} = \begin{pmatrix} a_{13} \\ a_{23} \\ a_{33} \end{pmatrix} ;$$

then, starting from the origin $(0, 0, 0)$ of a three-dimensional system of Cartesian axes, the polyhedron will have the vertices at the end of vectors $\mathbf{a_1}, \mathbf{a_2}, \mathbf{a_3}, \mathbf{a_1} + \mathbf{a_2}$, $\mathbf{a_1} + \mathbf{a_3}, \mathbf{a_2} + \mathbf{a_3}$, and $\mathbf{a_1} + \mathbf{a_2} + \mathbf{a_3}$.

The geometrical significance of the determinant will remain the same also for square matrices of order higher than 3: in this case we will more appropriately speak about a hypervolume.

21.17 Gauss Elimination

The Gauss elimination is used to transform a square matrix into another one of the same dimensions but much more applicable for some given purposes, like the solution of linear systems. It works by means of some *Gauss moves*, as we will see here.

To understand how the Gauss elimination works, let us take as example an arbitrary 3×3 square matrix; we will perform some row operations, like switch, multiplication, addition, ad so on, and we will use the notation r_n to indicate the n-th row of the matrix, so that we will write $r_m \leftrightarrow r_n$ to say that we have exchanged the position of the m-th and the n-th rows, as well as we will use a notation like $r_j = \alpha r_m + \beta r_n$ to say that we are swapping the j-th row with the m-th row multiplied by α plus the n-th row multiplied by β, and so on.

Thus, consider the matrix

$$\mathbf{M} = \begin{pmatrix} 0 & 2 & 3 \\ 2 & 5 & 2 \\ 3 & 3 & 1 \end{pmatrix},$$

and let us try the task to transform it into a step matrix. The operations we use are as follows: first we swap row 1 and row 3:

$$\begin{pmatrix} 0 & 2 & 3 \\ 2 & 5 & 2 \\ 3 & 3 & 1 \end{pmatrix} \xrightarrow{r_1 \leftrightarrow r_3} \begin{pmatrix} 3 & 3 & 1 \\ 2 & 5 & 2 \\ 0 & 2 & 3 \end{pmatrix}$$

then we subtract $\frac{2}{3}r_1$ from r_2:

$$\begin{pmatrix} 3 & 3 & 1 \\ 2 & 5 & 2 \\ 0 & 2 & 3 \end{pmatrix} \xrightarrow{r_2 - \frac{2}{3}r_1} \begin{pmatrix} 3 & 3 & 1 \\ 0 & 3 & \frac{4}{3} \\ 0 & 2 & 3 \end{pmatrix}$$

and then we subtract $\frac{2}{3}r_2$ from r_3:

$$\begin{pmatrix} 3 & 3 & 1 \\ 0 & 3 & \frac{4}{3} \\ 0 & 2 & 3 \end{pmatrix} \xrightarrow{r_3 - \frac{2}{3}r_1} \begin{pmatrix} 3 & 3 & 1 \\ 0 & 3 & \frac{4}{3} \\ 0 & 0 & \frac{19}{9} \end{pmatrix}.$$

We can go ahead multiplying r_3 by $\frac{9}{19}$

$$\begin{pmatrix} 3 & 3 & 1 \\ 0 & 3 & \frac{4}{3} \\ 0 & 0 & \frac{19}{9} \end{pmatrix} \xrightarrow{r_3 = \frac{9}{19}r_3} \begin{pmatrix} 3 & 3 & 1 \\ 0 & 3 & \frac{4}{3} \\ 0 & 0 & 1 \end{pmatrix},$$

and subtracting $\frac{4}{3}r_3$ from r_2

$$\begin{pmatrix} 3 & 3 & 1 \\ 0 & 3 & \frac{4}{3} \\ 0 & 0 & 1 \end{pmatrix} \xrightarrow{r_2 - \frac{4}{3}r_3} \begin{pmatrix} 3 & 3 & 1 \\ 0 & 3 & 0 \\ 0 & 0 & 1 \end{pmatrix},$$

then r_3 from r_1

$$\begin{pmatrix} 3 & 3 & 1 \\ 0 & 3 & 0 \\ 0 & 0 & 1 \end{pmatrix} \xrightarrow{r_1 - r_3} \begin{pmatrix} 3 & 3 & 0 \\ 0 & 3 & 0 \\ 0 & 0 & 1 \end{pmatrix},$$

so that we can first divide r_2 by 3

$$\begin{pmatrix} 3 & 3 & 0 \\ 0 & 3 & 0 \\ 0 & 0 & 1 \end{pmatrix} \xrightarrow{r_2 = \frac{1}{3}r_2} \begin{pmatrix} 3 & 3 & 0 \\ 0 & 1 & 0 \\ 0 & 0 & 1 \end{pmatrix},$$

and then subtract $3r_2$ from r_1

$$\begin{pmatrix} 3 & 3 & 0 \\ 0 & 1 & 0 \\ 0 & 0 & 1 \end{pmatrix} \xrightarrow{r_1 - 3r_2} \begin{pmatrix} 3 & 0 & 0 \\ 0 & 1 & 0 \\ 0 & 0 & 1 \end{pmatrix},$$

so that, dividing r_1 by 3, we obtain the identity matrix

$$\begin{pmatrix} 3 & 0 & 0 \\ 0 & 1 & 0 \\ 0 & 0 & 1 \end{pmatrix} \xrightarrow{r_1 = \frac{1}{3}r_1} \begin{pmatrix} 1 & 0 & 0 \\ 0 & 1 & 0 \\ 0 & 0 & 1 \end{pmatrix},$$

which is the matrix in its *reduced echelon form*. To be more precise, and defining the *pivot* any first nonzero element in a matrix row, a matrix in its reduced echelon form, is a matrix having the *pivots* equal to 1 and with any of the pivots is on the right of the pivot above it.

We first have seen a square matrix; let us now see what can happen with a non-square matrix like

$$\mathbf{N} = \begin{pmatrix} 3 & 7 & 3 & 1 \\ 7 & 5 & 2 & 3 \\ 2 & 5 & 3 & 1 \end{pmatrix};$$

in this case we can do as follows:

$$\begin{pmatrix} 3 & 7 & 3 & 1 \\ 7 & 5 & 2 & 3 \\ 2 & 5 & 3 & 1 \end{pmatrix} \quad \xrightarrow{r_1 \leftrightarrow r_2} \quad \begin{pmatrix} 7 & 5 & 2 & 3 \\ 3 & 7 & 3 & 1 \\ 2 & 5 & 3 & 1 \end{pmatrix},$$

then

$$\begin{pmatrix} 7 & 5 & 2 & 3 \\ 3 & 7 & 3 & 1 \\ 2 & 5 & 3 & 1 \end{pmatrix} \quad \xrightarrow{r_2 - \frac{3}{7}r_1} \quad \begin{pmatrix} 7 & 5 & 2 & 3 \\ 0 & \frac{34}{7} & \frac{15}{7} & -\frac{2}{7} \\ 2 & 5 & 3 & 1 \end{pmatrix},$$

and

$$\begin{pmatrix} 7 & 5 & 2 & 3 \\ 0 & \frac{34}{7} & \frac{15}{7} & -\frac{2}{7} \\ 2 & 5 & 3 & 1 \end{pmatrix} \quad \xrightarrow{r_3 - \frac{2}{7}r_1} \quad \begin{pmatrix} 7 & 5 & 2 & 3 \\ 0 & \frac{34}{7} & \frac{15}{7} & -\frac{2}{7} \\ 0 & \frac{25}{7} & \frac{17}{7} & \frac{1}{7} \end{pmatrix},$$

and again

$$\begin{pmatrix} 7 & 5 & 2 & 3 \\ 0 & \frac{34}{7} & \frac{15}{7} & -\frac{2}{7} \\ 0 & \frac{25}{7} & \frac{17}{7} & \frac{1}{7} \end{pmatrix} \quad \xrightarrow{r_3 - \frac{25}{34}r_2} \quad \begin{pmatrix} 7 & 5 & 2 & 3 \\ 0 & \frac{34}{7} & \frac{15}{7} & -\frac{2}{7} \\ 0 & 0 & \frac{29}{34} & \frac{6}{17} \end{pmatrix},$$

so that

$$\begin{pmatrix} 7 & 5 & 2 & 3 \\ 0 & \frac{34}{7} & \frac{15}{7} & -\frac{2}{7} \\ 0 & 0 & \frac{29}{34} & \frac{6}{17} \end{pmatrix} \quad \xrightarrow{r_3 = \frac{34}{29}r_3} \quad \begin{pmatrix} 7 & 5 & 2 & 3 \\ 0 & \frac{34}{7} & \frac{15}{7} & -\frac{2}{7} \\ 0 & 0 & 1 & \frac{12}{29} \end{pmatrix},$$

and

$$\begin{pmatrix} 7 & 5 & 2 & 3 \\ 0 & \frac{34}{7} & \frac{15}{7} & -\frac{2}{7} \\ 0 & 0 & 1 & \frac{12}{29} \end{pmatrix} \quad \xrightarrow{r_2 - \frac{15}{7}r_3} \quad \begin{pmatrix} 7 & 5 & 2 & 3 \\ 0 & \frac{34}{7} & 0 & -\frac{34}{29} \\ 0 & 0 & 1 & \frac{12}{29} \end{pmatrix},$$

thus

$$\begin{pmatrix} 7 & 5 & 2 & 3 \\ 0 & \frac{34}{7} & 0 & -\frac{34}{29} \\ 0 & 0 & 1 & \frac{12}{29} \end{pmatrix} \quad \xrightarrow{r_1 - 2r_3} \quad \begin{pmatrix} 7 & 5 & 0 & \frac{63}{29} \\ 0 & \frac{34}{7} & 0 & -\frac{34}{29} \\ 0 & 0 & 1 & \frac{12}{29} \end{pmatrix},$$

and

$$
\begin{pmatrix} 7 & 5 & 0 & \frac{63}{29} \\ 0 & \frac{34}{7} & 0 & -\frac{34}{29} \\ 0 & 0 & 1 & \frac{12}{29} \end{pmatrix} \quad \xrightarrow{r_2 = \frac{7}{24}r_2} \quad \begin{pmatrix} 7 & 5 & 0 & \frac{63}{29} \\ 0 & 1 & 0 & -\frac{7}{29} \\ 0 & 0 & 1 & \frac{12}{29} \end{pmatrix},
$$

therefore

$$
\begin{pmatrix} 7 & 5 & 0 & \frac{63}{29} \\ 0 & 1 & 0 & -\frac{7}{29} \\ 0 & 0 & 1 & \frac{12}{29} \end{pmatrix} \quad \xrightarrow{r_1 - 5r_2} \quad \begin{pmatrix} 7 & 0 & 0 & \frac{98}{29} \\ 0 & 1 & 0 & -\frac{7}{29} \\ 0 & 0 & 1 & \frac{12}{29} \end{pmatrix},
$$

and finally

$$
\begin{pmatrix} 7 & 0 & 0 & \frac{98}{29} \\ 0 & 1 & 0 & -\frac{7}{29} \\ 0 & 0 & 1 & \frac{12}{29} \end{pmatrix} \quad \xrightarrow{r_1 = \frac{1}{7}r_1} \quad \begin{pmatrix} 1 & 0 & 0 & \frac{14}{29} \\ 0 & 1 & 0 & -\frac{7}{29} \\ 0 & 0 & 1 & \frac{12}{29} \end{pmatrix};
$$

hence, we have a reduced matrix in which, again, all pivots are 1 and all pivots are at the right of the pivots above them.

Now, we may try to see how Gauss elimination is useful to solve the linear systems: let us take

$$
\begin{cases} 3x + 2y - 4z = 2 \\ x + 2z \quad\;\; = 1 \\ x - 3y + z \;\; = 4 \end{cases} \tag{21.29}
$$

where the coefficient matrix and the *augmented matrix* respectively are

$$
\begin{pmatrix} 3 & 2 & -4 \\ 1 & 0 & 2 \\ 1 & -3 & 1 \end{pmatrix}; \quad \begin{pmatrix} 3 & 2 & -4 & 2 \\ 1 & 0 & 2 & 1 \\ 1 & -3 & 1 & 4 \end{pmatrix}.
$$

Let us work on the augmented matrix, to obtain its row echelon form:

$$
\begin{pmatrix} 3 & 2 & -4 & 2 \\ 1 & 0 & 2 & 1 \\ 1 & -3 & 1 & 4 \end{pmatrix} \quad \xrightarrow{r_1 \leftrightarrow r_2} \quad \begin{pmatrix} 1 & 0 & 2 & 1 \\ 3 & 2 & -4 & 2 \\ 1 & -3 & 1 & 4 \end{pmatrix};
$$

$$
\begin{pmatrix} 1 & 0 & 2 & 1 \\ 3 & 2 & -4 & 2 \\ 1 & -3 & 1 & 4 \end{pmatrix} \quad \xrightarrow{r_2 - 3r_1} \quad \begin{pmatrix} 1 & 0 & 2 & 1 \\ 0 & 2 & -10 & -1 \\ 1 & -3 & 1 & 4 \end{pmatrix};
$$

$$
\begin{pmatrix} 1 & 0 & 2 & 1 \\ 0 & 2 & -10 & -1 \\ 1 & -3 & 1 & 4 \end{pmatrix} \xrightarrow{\ r_3 - r_1\ } \begin{pmatrix} 1 & 0 & 2 & 1 \\ 0 & 2 & -10 & -1 \\ 0 & -3 & -1 & 3 \end{pmatrix} ;
$$

$$
\begin{pmatrix} 1 & 0 & 2 & 1 \\ 0 & 2 & -10 & -1 \\ 0 & -3 & -1 & 3 \end{pmatrix} \xrightarrow{\ r_2 \leftrightarrow r_3\ } \begin{pmatrix} 1 & 0 & 2 & 1 \\ 0 & -3 & -1 & 3 \\ 0 & 2 & -10 & -1 \end{pmatrix} ;
$$

$$
\begin{pmatrix} 1 & 0 & 2 & 1 \\ 0 & -3 & -1 & 3 \\ 0 & 2 & -10 & -1 \end{pmatrix} \xrightarrow{\ r_3 + \frac{2}{3} r_2\ } \begin{pmatrix} 1 & 0 & 2 & 1 \\ 0 & -3 & -1 & 3 \\ 0 & 0 & -\frac{32}{3} & 1 \end{pmatrix} ;
$$

$$
\begin{pmatrix} 1 & 0 & 2 & 1 \\ 0 & -3 & -1 & 3 \\ 0 & 0 & -\frac{32}{3} & 1 \end{pmatrix} \xrightarrow{\ r_3 = -\frac{3}{32} r_3\ } \begin{pmatrix} 1 & 0 & 2 & 1 \\ 0 & -3 & -1 & 3 \\ 0 & 0 & 1 & -\frac{3}{32} \end{pmatrix} ;
$$

$$
\begin{pmatrix} 1 & 0 & 2 & 1 \\ 0 & -3 & -1 & 3 \\ 0 & 0 & 1 & -\frac{3}{32} \end{pmatrix} \xrightarrow{\ r_2 + r_3\ } \begin{pmatrix} 1 & 0 & 2 & 1 \\ 0 & -3 & 0 & \frac{93}{32} \\ 0 & 0 & 1 & -\frac{3}{32} \end{pmatrix} ;
$$

$$
\begin{pmatrix} 1 & 0 & 2 & 1 \\ 0 & -3 & 0 & \frac{93}{32} \\ 0 & 0 & 1 & -\frac{3}{32} \end{pmatrix} \xrightarrow{\ r_1 - 2r_3\ } \begin{pmatrix} 1 & 0 & 0 & \frac{19}{16} \\ 0 & -3 & 0 & \frac{93}{32} \\ 0 & 0 & 1 & -\frac{3}{32} \end{pmatrix} ;
$$

and

$$
\begin{pmatrix} 1 & 0 & 0 & \frac{19}{16} \\ 0 & -3 & 0 & \frac{93}{32} \\ 0 & 0 & 1 & -\frac{3}{32} \end{pmatrix} \xrightarrow{\ r_2 = -\frac{1}{3} r_3\ } \begin{pmatrix} 1 & 0 & 0 & \frac{19}{16} \\ 0 & 1 & 0 & -\frac{31}{32} \\ 0 & 0 & 1 & -\frac{3}{32} \end{pmatrix} .
$$

Now, let us rewrite the system (21.29) according to its row echelon form we found above: we have

$$
\begin{cases} 3x + 2y - 4z = 2 \\ x + 2z = 1 \\ x - 3y + z = 4 \end{cases} \implies \begin{cases} x = \frac{19}{16} \\ y = -\frac{31}{32} \\ z = -\frac{3}{32} \end{cases}
$$

so that the reduced row echelon form allows us to get the solution of the system only by means of some linear changes in the rows of the augmented matrix of the system.

21.18 Properties of the Determinant

To go ahead, we first must bear in mind that if we use the Gauss elimination to get a matrix $\mathbf{B}$ from $\mathbf{A}$, then, since the Gauss elimination preserves the determinant, it must also be $\det(\mathbf{A}) = \det(\mathbf{B})$. Indeed, the determinant of $\mathbf{A}$ is the same determinant of $\mathbf{B}$, obtained after the Gauss elimination, since this last is a triangular matrix with a determinant given by the product of the pivots. For example, by Gaussian elimination (here we avoid the intermediate steps), we have:

$$\mathbf{A} = \begin{pmatrix} 3 & 2 & 4 \\ 1 & 2 & 3 \\ 6 & 1 & 3 \end{pmatrix} \longrightarrow \begin{pmatrix} 1 & 2 & 3 \\ 0 & -11 & -15 \\ 0 & 0 & \frac{5}{11} \end{pmatrix} = \mathbf{B}$$

such that

$$\det(\mathbf{A}) = -5 = 1 \times (-11) \times \frac{5}{11} = \det(\mathbf{B}).$$

An important property of the determinant is that selecting any k rows from a square matrix $\mathbf{A}_n$, then calculate all the minors multiplied by the respective cofactors, and then sum all the results; then, we get $\det(\mathbf{A})$, as we already saw. Now, we may verify that for two square matrices $\mathbf{A}$ and $\mathbf{B}$, $\det(\mathbf{AB}) = \det(\mathbf{A})\det(\mathbf{B})$ (this is the *Binet theorem*), since taking

$$\mathbf{A} = \begin{pmatrix} a_{11} & a_{12} \\ a_{21} & a_{22} \end{pmatrix}; \quad \mathbf{B} = \begin{pmatrix} b_{11} & b_{12} \\ b_{21} & b_{22} \end{pmatrix}$$

we have

$$\det(\mathbf{A}) = a_{11}a_{22} - a_{12}a_{21}$$
$$\det(\mathbf{B}) = b_{11}b_{22} - b_{12}b_{21}$$

while

$$\mathbf{AB} = \begin{pmatrix} a_{11} & a_{12} \\ a_{21} & a_{22} \end{pmatrix} \begin{pmatrix} b_{11} & b_{12} \\ b_{21} & b_{22} \end{pmatrix}$$
$$= \begin{pmatrix} a_{11}b_{11} + a_{12}b_{21} & a_{11}b_{12} + a_{12}b_{22} \\ a_{21}b_{11} + a_{22}b_{21} & a_{21}b_{12} + a_{22}b_{22} \end{pmatrix}$$

and

$$\det(\mathbf{AB}) = \det \begin{pmatrix} a_{11}b_{11} + a_{12}b_{21} & a_{11}b_{12} + a_{12}b_{22} \\ a_{21}b_{11} + a_{22}b_{21} & a_{21}b_{12} + a_{22}b_{22} \end{pmatrix}$$

$$= a_{11}a_{22}b_{11}b_{22} + a_{12}a_{21}b_{12}b_{21}$$
$$- (a_{11}a_{22}b_{12}b_{21} + a_{12}a_{21}b_{11}b_{22}) \qquad (21.30)$$

so we can see that

$$\det(\mathbf{A})\det(\mathbf{B}) = (a_{11}a_{22} - a_{12}a_{21})(b_{11}b_{22} - b_{12}b_{21})$$
$$= a_{11}a_{22}b_{11}b_{22} + a_{12}a_{21}b_{12}b_{21}$$
$$- (a_{11}a_{22}b_{12}b_{21} + a_{12}a_{21}b_{11}b_{22}); \qquad (21.31)$$

thus, the results of (21.30) and (21.31) are identical.

However, it can be convenient to test Binet's theorem in a more general way: let us take a matrix:

$$\mathbf{M} = \begin{pmatrix} j & k & l & m \\ n & o & p & q \\ s & t & u & v \\ w & x & y & z \end{pmatrix} :$$

excluding the third and fourth rows, we have six possible minors, e.g.,

$$\begin{pmatrix} j & k \\ n & o \end{pmatrix} ; \begin{pmatrix} j & l \\ n & p \end{pmatrix} ; \begin{pmatrix} j & m \\ n & q \end{pmatrix} ;$$

$$\begin{pmatrix} k & l \\ o & p \end{pmatrix} ; \begin{pmatrix} k & m \\ o & q \end{pmatrix} ; \begin{pmatrix} l & m \\ p & q \end{pmatrix} ;$$

with

$$\det \begin{pmatrix} j & k \\ n & o \end{pmatrix} = jo - kn; \quad \det \begin{pmatrix} j & l \\ n & p \end{pmatrix} = jp - lm;$$

$$\det \begin{pmatrix} j & m \\ n & q \end{pmatrix} = jq - mn; \quad \det \begin{pmatrix} k & l \\ o & p \end{pmatrix} = kp - lo;$$

$$\det \begin{pmatrix} k & m \\ o & q \end{pmatrix} = kq - mo; \quad \det \begin{pmatrix} l & m \\ p & q \end{pmatrix} = lq - mp.$$

Thus, by means of the Laplace theorem, we can write:

$$\det \mathbf{M} = \det \begin{pmatrix} j & k \\ n & o \end{pmatrix} (-1)^{1+2+1+2} \det \begin{pmatrix} u & v \\ y & z \end{pmatrix}$$

$$+ \det \begin{pmatrix} j & l \\ n & p \end{pmatrix} (-1)^{1+2+1+3} \det \begin{pmatrix} t & u \\ x & z \end{pmatrix}$$

$$+ \det \begin{pmatrix} j & m \\ n & q \end{pmatrix} (-1)^{1+2+1+4} \det \begin{pmatrix} t & u \\ x & y \end{pmatrix}$$

$$+ \det \begin{pmatrix} k & l \\ o & p \end{pmatrix} (-1)^{1+2+2+3} \det \begin{pmatrix} s & v \\ w & z \end{pmatrix}$$

$$+ \det \begin{pmatrix} k & m \\ o & q \end{pmatrix} (-1)^{1+2+2+4} \det \begin{pmatrix} s & u \\ w & y \end{pmatrix}$$

$$+ \det \begin{pmatrix} l & m \\ p & q \end{pmatrix} (-1)^{1+2+3+4} \det \begin{pmatrix} s & t \\ w & x \end{pmatrix}.$$

Now, if we take any $2n \times 2n$ square matrix with the form

$$\mathbf{P} = \begin{pmatrix} \mathbf{A}_n & \mathbf{O}_n \\ -\mathbf{I}_n & \mathbf{B}_n \end{pmatrix}$$

$$= \begin{pmatrix} a_{11} & \cdots & a_{n1} & 0 & \cdots & 0 \\ \vdots & \ddots & \vdots & \vdots & \ddots & \vdots \\ a_{1n} & \cdots & a_{nn} & 0 & \cdots & 0 \\ -1 & \cdots & 0 & b_{11} & \cdots & b_{1n} \\ \vdots & \ddots & \vdots & \vdots & \ddots & \vdots \\ 0 & \cdots & -1 & b_{n1} & \cdots & b_{nn} \end{pmatrix},$$

we see that $\det(\mathbf{P}) = \det(\mathbf{A}) \det(\mathbf{B})$; moreover, after a little algebra, one obtains:

$$\mathbf{Q} = \begin{pmatrix} \mathbf{A}_n & \mathbf{AB} \\ -\mathbf{I}_n & \mathbf{O}_n \end{pmatrix}$$

with $\det(\mathbf{Q}) = \det(\mathbf{P}) = \det(\mathbf{A}) \det(\mathbf{B})$. But if we calculate the determinant using the Laplace theorem, we have:

$$\det(\mathbf{A}) \det(\mathbf{B}) = \det(\mathbf{Q})$$

$$= \det(-\mathbf{I}_n)(-1)^{n(1+2n)} \det(\mathbf{AB})$$

$$= (-1)^n (-1)^{2n^2+n} \det(\mathbf{AB})$$

$$= (-1)^{2n^2+2n} \det(\mathbf{AB})$$

$$= \det(\mathbf{AB}),$$

since $2n^2 + 2n$ is always even for all values of n.

21.19 Rank of a Matrix

The rank $\rho(\mathbf{A})$ of a matrix $\mathbf{A}_{m \times n}$ is the number of the column vectors of $\mathbf{A}$ which are linearly independent, or, even, the number of row vectors of $\mathbf{A}$ which are linearly independent. For any matrix $\mathbf{A}_{m \times n}$, it is always verified $\rho(\mathbf{A}) \leq \min(m, n)$; thus, for $\mathbf{X}_{5 \times 4}$, we always will find that $\min(5, 4) = 4 \geq \rho(\mathbf{X}_{5 \times 4})$, and, in particular, for a $n \times n$ square matrix $\mathbf{A}_n$ we will have

$$\min(n, n) = n \geq \rho(\mathbf{A}_n)$$

When a matrix has the highest possible rank (e.g., when a square matrix $\mathbf{Y}_n$ has $\rho(\mathbf{Y}_n) = n$), then that matrix is said a *full rank matrix*.

For any matrix $\mathbf{A}_{m \times n}$, the rank $\rho_{\text{col}}(\mathbf{A})$ obtained from the column vectors and the rank $\rho_{\text{row}}(\mathbf{A})$ obtained from the row vectors are always equal, so that

$$\rho_{\text{col}}(\mathbf{A}) = \rho_{\text{row}}(\mathbf{A}) = \rho(\mathbf{A}),$$

and therefore also $\rho(\mathbf{A}) = \rho(\mathbf{A}^\top)$.

In fact, given $\mathbf{A}_{m \times n}$, taking any possible basis of $\mathbf{A}$, we can write $\mathbf{A} = \mathbf{X}\mathbf{Y}$, where $\mathbf{X}$ is a $m \times r$ matrix such that the column vectors of $\mathbf{A}$ are a linear combination of the column vectors of $\mathbf{X}$, while $\mathbf{Y}$ is a $r \times n$ matrix such that the row vectors of $\mathbf{A}$ are a linear combination of the row vectors of $\mathbf{Y}$. Therefore, $\rho_{\text{row}}(\mathbf{A}) \leq \rho_{\text{row}}(\mathbf{Y})$, and since $\mathbf{Y}$ is $r \times n$, then also $\rho_{\text{row}}(\mathbf{Y}) \leq r = \rho_{\text{col}}(\mathbf{A})$, thus

$$\rho_{\text{row}}(\mathbf{A}) \leq \rho_{\text{col}}(\mathbf{A}),$$

but taking the transpose $\mathbf{A}_{n \times m}^\top$ we must also have:

$$\rho_{\text{row}}(\mathbf{A}^\top) = \rho_{\text{col}}(\mathbf{A}) \leq \rho_{\text{col}}(\mathbf{A}^\top) = \rho_{\text{row}}(\mathbf{A});$$

hence, the only case simultaneously allowing the conditions

$$\begin{cases} \rho_{\text{row}}(\mathbf{A}) \leq \rho_{\text{col}}(\mathbf{A}) \\ \rho_{\text{col}}(\mathbf{A}) \leq \rho_{\text{row}}(\mathbf{A}) \end{cases}$$

is the equality

$$\rho_{\text{row}}(\mathbf{A}) = \rho_{\text{col}}(\mathbf{A}).$$

21.20 Inverse Matrix

For a given square matrix $\mathbf{A}_n$, we define, if it exists, the *inverse matrix* $\mathbf{A}_n^{-1}$, such that

$$\mathbf{A}_n \mathbf{A}_n^{-1} = \mathbf{A}_n^{-1} \mathbf{A}_n = \mathbf{I}_n.$$

If a square matrix $\mathbf{A}$ has the inverse, then $\mathbf{A}$ is said invertible. An inverse matrix, if exists, is unique, and is also always invertible. Inverting an inverse matrix produces the original matrix: in other words, $(\mathbf{A}^{-1})^{-1} = \mathbf{A}$. The condition for $\mathbf{A}$ to be invertible is $\det(\mathbf{A}) \neq 0$; hence, $\mathbf{A}$ must be nonsingular. In the following pages, we will see that this condition is equivalent to say that $\mathbf{A}$ must have all rows (or all columns) linearly independent.

To find the inverse of a 2×2 matrix is not a particularly difficult task. In practice, given

$$\mathbf{A} = \begin{pmatrix} a & b \\ c & d \end{pmatrix}$$

(here a, b, c, and d are known), we must search for the generic matrix:

$$\mathbf{A}^{-1} = \begin{pmatrix} w & x \\ y & z \end{pmatrix}$$

such that $\mathbf{A}\mathbf{A}^{-1} = \mathbf{I}$.

Therefore, we must have

$$\mathbf{I} = \begin{pmatrix} a & b \\ c & d \end{pmatrix} \begin{pmatrix} w & x \\ y & z \end{pmatrix}$$

$$= \begin{pmatrix} aw + by & ax + bz \\ cw + dy & cx + dz; \end{pmatrix}$$

thus, we must impose the condition:

$$\begin{cases} aw + by = 1 \\ ax + bz = 0 \\ cw + dy = 0 \\ cx + dz = 1 \end{cases},$$

from which we calculate the unknown values w, x, y, and z as

$$\begin{cases} w = \dfrac{d}{ad-bc} \\ x = -\dfrac{b}{ad-bc} \\ y = -\dfrac{c}{ad-bc} \\ z = \dfrac{a}{ad-bc} \end{cases}, \tag{21.32}$$

hence

$$\mathbf{A}^{-1} = \begin{pmatrix} \dfrac{d}{ad-bc} & -\dfrac{b}{ad-bc} \\ -\dfrac{c}{ad-bc} & \dfrac{a}{ad-bc} \end{pmatrix},$$

and since all elements of $\mathbf{A}^{-1}$ show the same denominator $ad - bc$, then

$$\mathbf{A}^{-1} = \frac{1}{ad - bc} \begin{pmatrix} d & -b \\ -c & a \end{pmatrix}$$

but we immediately realize that $ad - bc$ is the determinant of $\mathbf{A}$; therefore

$$\mathbf{A}^{-1} = \frac{1}{\det(\mathbf{A})} \begin{pmatrix} d & -b \\ -c & a \end{pmatrix}.$$

Here is the reason why the matrix $\mathbf{A}$ must have a nonzero determinant to be invertible. In the case $\det(\mathbf{A}) = 0$, all elements of $\mathbf{A}^{-1}$ would be fractions with zero denominator, and thus not evaluable.

We therefore have also found a simple practical rule to obtain the inverse of a 2×2 matrix. We must: (1) to exchange the diagonal elements of the matrix; (2) to change the sign of the nondiagonal elements; (3) to divide the value of the elements thus obtained by the determinant of the matrix to be inverted, provided the determinant is nonzero.

21.21 Inverse of a Generic Square Matrix

The calculation of the inverse of a square matrix of order greater than 2 is in general more complicated: in fact, one must first calculate the determinant of the matrix, verifying that it is nonzero, and then one must calculate the *cofactor matrix*, and from this the *adjoint matrix*, which is also defined *the minor (matrix)*. We shall see that the computation of the inverse of a 2×2 matrix is only a special case of this general case.

Given a matrix $\mathbf{A}_{n\times n}$, we already seen that its cofactor matrix $\mathbf{C}_{n\times n}$ is a matrix whose elements c_{jk} are the determinants of the submatrices obtained by eliminating the rows and the columns in which the elements a_{jk} of $\mathbf{A}$ are placed, multiplied times $(-1)^{j+k}$. In other words,

$$\mathbf{C} = \begin{pmatrix} (-1)^{1+1} \det(\mathbf{A}_{[11]}) & (-1)^{1+2} \det(\mathbf{A}_{[12]}) & \cdots & (-1)^{1+n} \det(\mathbf{A}_{[1n]}) \\ (-1)^{2+1} \det(\mathbf{A}_{[21]}) & (-1)^{2+2} \det(\mathbf{A}_{[22]}) & \cdots & (-1)^{2+n} \det(\mathbf{A}_{[2n]}) \\ \vdots & \vdots & \ddots & \vdots \\ (-1)^{n+1} \det(\mathbf{A}_{[n1]}) & (-1)^{n+2} \det(\mathbf{A}_{[n2]}) & \cdots & (-1)^{n+n} \det(\mathbf{A}_{[nn]}) \end{pmatrix},$$

where

$$\det(\mathbf{A}_{[jk]}) = \det \begin{pmatrix} a_{11} & \cdots & a_{1,k-1} & a_{1,k+1} & \cdots & a_{1n} \\ \vdots & \ddots & \vdots & \vdots & & \vdots \\ a_{j-1,1} & \cdots & a_{j-1,k-1} & a_{j-1,k+1} & \cdots & a_{j-1,n} \\ a_{j+1,1} & \cdots & a_{j+1,k-1} & a_{j+1,k+1} & \cdots & a_{j+1,n} \\ \vdots & & \vdots & \vdots & \ddots & \vdots \\ a_{n1} & \cdots & a_{n,k-1} & a_{n,k+1} & \cdots & a_{nn} \end{pmatrix}.$$

At this point, we will obtain the inverse of $\mathbf{A}$ by multiplying the reciprocal of its determinant $\det(\mathbf{A})$ times the transpose $\mathbf{C}_{\mathbf{A}}^{\top}$ of its cofactor matrix.

For example, if

$$\mathbf{X} = \begin{pmatrix} 1 & 2 & 1 \\ 3 & 2 & 1 \\ 1 & 0 & 2 \end{pmatrix}$$

then $\mathbf{C}_{\mathbf{X}}$, also taking into account the various factors $(-1)^{j+k}$ is

$$\mathbf{C}_{\mathbf{X}} = \begin{pmatrix} \det(\mathbf{X}_{[11]}) & -\det(\mathbf{X}_{[12]}) & \det(\mathbf{X}_{[13]}) \\ -\det(\mathbf{X}_{[21]}) & \det(\mathbf{X}_{[22]}) & -\det(\mathbf{X}_{[23]}) \\ \det(\mathbf{X}_{[31]}) & -\det(\mathbf{X}_{[32]}) & \det(\mathbf{X}_{[33]}) \end{pmatrix}$$

$$= \begin{pmatrix} \begin{vmatrix} 2 & 1 \\ 0 & 2 \end{vmatrix} & -\begin{vmatrix} 3 & 1 \\ 1 & 2 \end{vmatrix} & \begin{vmatrix} 3 & 2 \\ 1 & 0 \end{vmatrix} \\ -\begin{vmatrix} 2 & 1 \\ 0 & 2 \end{vmatrix} & \begin{vmatrix} 1 & 1 \\ 1 & 2 \end{vmatrix} & -\begin{vmatrix} 1 & 2 \\ 1 & 0 \end{vmatrix} \\ \begin{vmatrix} 2 & 1 \\ 2 & 1 \end{vmatrix} & -\begin{vmatrix} 1 & 1 \\ 3 & 1 \end{vmatrix} & \begin{vmatrix} 1 & 2 \\ 3 & 2 \end{vmatrix} \end{pmatrix}$$

$$= \begin{pmatrix} 4 & -5 & -2 \\ -4 & 1 & 2 \\ 0 & 2 & -4 \end{pmatrix}.$$

Since $\det(\mathbf{X}) = -8$, we obtain the inverse as

$$\mathbf{X}^{-1} = -\frac{1}{8}\mathbf{C}_\mathbf{X}^\top$$

$$= -\frac{1}{8}\begin{pmatrix} 4 & -4 & 0 \\ -5 & 1 & 2 \\ -2 & 2 & -4 \end{pmatrix}$$

$$= \begin{pmatrix} -\frac{1}{2} & \frac{1}{2} & 0 \\ \frac{5}{8} & -\frac{1}{8} & -\frac{1}{4} \\ \frac{1}{4} & -\frac{1}{4} & \frac{1}{2} \end{pmatrix}.$$

It can be shown that if the inverse of a square matrix exists, it is unique. In fact, let us assume that a square matrix $\mathbf{A}_n$ is invertible and that there are two distinct inverse matrices $\mathbf{X}$ and $\mathbf{Y}$. In this case, we must have $\mathbf{I} = \mathbf{AX} = \mathbf{AY}$, and thus premultiplying both sides by $\mathbf{X}$, we also have $\mathbf{XAX} = \mathbf{XAY}$, hence $\mathbf{IX} = \mathbf{IY}$, and therefore $\mathbf{X} = \mathbf{Y}$, which is in contradiction with the hypothesis.

21.22 Inverse of a Transformation

In general, if $\mathbf{A}_n$ is a nonsingular square matrix applied on a vector $\mathbf{v}_n$ such that $\mathbf{Av} = \mathbf{u}$, then, applying the inverse $\mathbf{A}^{-1}$ to the transformed vector $\mathbf{u}$, returns the original vector $\mathbf{v}$, since $\mathbf{A}^{-1}\mathbf{u} = \mathbf{v}$. Therefore, the inverse of the matrix antitransforms the transformed vector, converting it into the original vector. This can be verified by studying a generic invertible matrix $\mathbf{A}_{2\times2}$ applied to the vector $\mathbf{v}$.

Defining

$$\mathbf{A} = \begin{pmatrix} a_{11} & a_{12} \\ a_{21} & a_{22} \end{pmatrix}; \ \mathbf{v} = \begin{pmatrix} v_1 \\ v_2 \end{pmatrix},$$

we have:

$$\mathbf{Av} = \begin{pmatrix} a_{11} & a_{12} \\ a_{21} & a_{22} \end{pmatrix}\begin{pmatrix} v_1 \\ v_2 \end{pmatrix}$$

$$= \begin{pmatrix} a_{11}v_1 + a_{12}v_2 \\ a_{21}v_1 + a_{22}v_2 \end{pmatrix} = \mathbf{u}.$$

On the other hand, assuming to have $\det(\mathbf{A}) \neq 0$, the inverse of $\mathbf{A}$ is, by definition,

$$\mathbf{A}^{-1} = \frac{1}{a_{11}a_{22} - a_{12}a_{21}}\begin{pmatrix} a_{22} & -a_{12} \\ -a_{21} & a_{11} \end{pmatrix},$$

so, if we calculate $\mathbf{A}^{-1}\mathbf{u}$, we get:

$$\mathbf{A}^{-1}\mathbf{u} = \frac{1}{a_{11}a_{22} - a_{12}a_{21}} \begin{pmatrix} a_{22} & -a_{12} \\ -a_{21} & a_{11} \end{pmatrix} \begin{pmatrix} a_{11}v_1 + a_{12}v_2 \\ a_{21}v_1 + a_{22}v_2 \end{pmatrix}$$

$$= \frac{1}{a_{11}a_{22} - a_{12}a_{21}} \begin{pmatrix} a_{22}(v_1 a_{11} + v_2 a_{12}) - a_{12}(v_1 a_{21} + v_2 a_{22}) \\ a_{11}(v_1 a_{21} + v_2 a_{22}) - a_{21}(v_1 a_{11} + v_2 a_{12}) \end{pmatrix}$$

$$= \begin{pmatrix} \frac{a_{22}(v_1 a_{11} + v_2 a_{12}) - a_{12}(v_1 a_{21} + v_2 a_{22})}{a_{11}a_{22} - a_{12}a_{21}} \\ \frac{a_{11}(v_1 a_{21} + v_2 a_{22}) - a_{21}(v_1 a_{11} + v_2 a_{12})}{a_{11}a_{22} - a_{12}a_{21}} \end{pmatrix}$$

$$= \begin{pmatrix} \frac{a_{11}a_{22} - a_{12}a_{21}}{a_{11}a_{22} - a_{12}a_{21}} v_1 \\ \frac{a_{11}a_{22} - a_{12}a_{21}}{a_{11}a_{22} - a_{12}a_{21}} v_2 \end{pmatrix}$$

$$= \begin{pmatrix} v_1 \\ v_2 \end{pmatrix} = \mathbf{v},$$

thus, the vector $\mathbf{v}$, since $\frac{a_{11}a_{22} - a_{12}a_{21}}{a_{11}a_{22} - a_{12}a_{21}} = 1$.

To show a simple numerical example, given the transformation $\mathbf{T}_3$ and an arbitrary three-dimensional vector $\mathbf{x}$, respectively defined as

$$\mathbf{T} = \begin{pmatrix} 1 & 2 & 3 \\ 1 & 1 & 2 \\ 2 & 2 & 1 \end{pmatrix}; \quad \mathbf{x} = \begin{pmatrix} 1 \\ 2 \\ 3 \end{pmatrix},$$

we first see that $\mathbf{T}$ is invertible, since $\det(\mathbf{T}) = 3$, and that the inverse is

$$\mathbf{T}^{-1} = \begin{pmatrix} -1 & \frac{4}{3} & \frac{1}{3} \\ 1 & -\frac{5}{3} & \frac{1}{3} \\ 0 & \frac{2}{3} & -\frac{1}{3} \end{pmatrix};$$

hence, with the transformation $\mathbf{T}$ applied to vector $\mathbf{x}$, we obtain the transformed vector $\mathbf{y}$ as follows:

$$\mathbf{Tx} = \begin{pmatrix} 1 & 2 & 3 \\ 1 & 1 & 2 \\ 2 & 2 & 1 \end{pmatrix} \begin{pmatrix} 1 \\ 2 \\ 3 \end{pmatrix} = \begin{pmatrix} 14 \\ 9 \\ 9 \end{pmatrix} = \mathbf{y},$$

while applying the inverse transformation $\mathbf{T}^{-1}$ to the transformed vector $\mathbf{y}$, returns the first vector $\mathbf{x}$:

$$\mathbf{T}^{-1}\mathbf{y} = \begin{pmatrix} -1 & \frac{4}{3} & \frac{1}{3} \\ 1 & -\frac{5}{3} & \frac{1}{3} \\ 0 & \frac{2}{3} & -\frac{1}{3} \end{pmatrix} \begin{pmatrix} 14 \\ 9 \\ 9 \end{pmatrix} = \begin{pmatrix} 1 \\ 2 \\ 3 \end{pmatrix} = \mathbf{x}.$$

21.23 Finding a Transformation

We may deal with a problem like: starting from a vector $\mathbf{x}$ pointing to a given initial position, find the transformation $\mathbf{T}$ needed to let the vector $\mathbf{y}$ pointing to a given final position. For example, if we need to move from position $\mathbf{x}$ to position $\mathbf{y}$, being

$$\mathbf{x} = \begin{pmatrix} 1 \\ 2 \\ 3 \end{pmatrix}; \quad \mathbf{y} = \begin{pmatrix} 3 \\ 2 \\ 1 \end{pmatrix},$$

then we must search for the transformation $\mathbf{T}$ such that

$$\mathbf{Tx} = \mathbf{y}$$

or, in other words

$$\begin{pmatrix} t_{11} & t_{12} & t_{13} \\ t_{21} & t_{22} & t_{23} \\ t_{31} & t_{32} & t_{33} \end{pmatrix} \begin{pmatrix} 1 \\ 2 \\ 3 \end{pmatrix} = \begin{pmatrix} 3 \\ 2 \\ 1 \end{pmatrix}$$

$$= \begin{pmatrix} t_{11} + 2t_{12} + 3t_{13} \\ t_{21} + 2t_{22} + 3t_{23} \\ t_{31} + 2t_{32} + 3t_{33}; \end{pmatrix}$$

thus, we have the system:

$$\begin{cases} t_{11} + 2t_{12} + 3t_{13} = 3 \\ t_{21} + 2t_{22} + 3t_{23} = 2 \\ t_{31} + 2t_{32} + 3t_{33} = 1 \end{cases}$$

which can be solved if we take

$$\mathbf{T} = \begin{pmatrix} 0 & 0 & 1 \\ 0 & 1 & 0 \\ 1 & 0 & 0 \end{pmatrix}$$

so as to have

$$\begin{pmatrix} 0 & 0 & 1 \\ 0 & 1 & 0 \\ 1 & 0 & 0 \end{pmatrix} \begin{pmatrix} 1 \\ 2 \\ 3 \end{pmatrix} = \begin{pmatrix} 0 \times 1 + 0 \times 2 + 1 \times 3 \\ 0 \times 1 + 1 \times 2 + 0 \times 3 \\ 1 \times 1 + 0 \times 2 + 0 \times 3 \end{pmatrix}$$

$$= \begin{pmatrix} 3 \\ 2 \\ 1 \end{pmatrix},$$

and we note that since

$$\mathbf{T}^{-1} = \begin{pmatrix} 0\,0\,1 \\ 0\,1\,0 \\ 1\,0\,0 \end{pmatrix} = \mathbf{T},$$

then also

$$\mathbf{T}^{-1}\mathbf{y} = \begin{pmatrix} 0\,0\,1 \\ 0\,1\,0 \\ 1\,0\,0 \end{pmatrix} \begin{pmatrix} 3 \\ 2 \\ 1 \end{pmatrix}$$

$$= \begin{pmatrix} 0 \times 1 + 0 \times 2 + 1 \times 1 \\ 0 \times 1 + 1 \times 2 + 0 \times 3 \\ 1 \times 3 + 0 \times 2 + 0 \times 3 \end{pmatrix}$$

$$= \begin{pmatrix} 1 \\ 2 \\ 3 \end{pmatrix};$$

thus, **T** and its inverse work as upside down matrices, since they return an upside down vector.

Indeed, this was a simple case, but it can be useful to understand the process needed to find the transformation matrix.

It can be the case of a *robotic arm* (indeed the situation is more complex, but for our purposes, this naïve robotic arm model works well) to be moved in a three-dimensional space from a known initial position to a given target position: let us decide to start from the already defined position **x**, to go to a "resting position" **z** defined by the vector:

$$\mathbf{z} = \begin{pmatrix} 1 \\ 1 \\ 1 \end{pmatrix};$$

in this case we may easily find the transformation:

$$\mathbf{M} = \begin{pmatrix} 0 & 0 & \frac{1}{3} \\ 0 & \frac{1}{2} & 0 \\ 1 & 0 & 0 \end{pmatrix}$$

such that

$$
\begin{pmatrix} 0 & 0 & \frac{1}{3} \\ 0 & \frac{1}{2} & 0 \\ 1 & 0 & 0 \end{pmatrix} \begin{pmatrix} 1 \\ 2 \\ 3 \end{pmatrix} = \begin{pmatrix} 0 \times 1 + 0 \times 2 + \frac{1}{3} \times 3 \\ 0 \times 1 + \frac{1}{2} \times 2 + 0 \times 3 \\ 1 \times 1 + 0 \times 2 + 0 \times 3 \end{pmatrix}
$$

$$
= \begin{pmatrix} 1 \\ 1 \\ 1 \end{pmatrix},
$$

and, again, since

$$
\mathbf{M}^{-1} = \begin{pmatrix} 0 & 0 & 1 \\ 0 & 2 & 0 \\ 3 & 0 & 0 \end{pmatrix},
$$

then

$$
\begin{pmatrix} 0 & 0 & 1 \\ 0 & 2 & 0 \\ 3 & 0 & 0 \end{pmatrix} \begin{pmatrix} 1 \\ 1 \\ 1 \end{pmatrix} = \begin{pmatrix} 0 \times 1 + 0 \times 2 + 1 \times 1 \\ 0 \times 1 + 2 \times 1 + 0 \times 3 \\ 3 \times 1 + 0 \times 2 + 0 \times 3 \end{pmatrix}
$$

$$
= \begin{pmatrix} 1 \\ 2 \\ 3 \end{pmatrix}.
$$

Limiting our considerations only to three-dimensional vectors, we see that to go to any position P_1 starting from any position P_0 in a three-dimensional space, we must find the transformation:

$$
\mathbf{T} = \begin{pmatrix} t_{11} & t_{12} & t_{13} \\ t_{21} & t_{22} & t_{23} \\ t_{31} & t_{32} & t_{33} \end{pmatrix}
$$

such that the vector

$$
\mathbf{u} = \begin{pmatrix} x_0 \\ y_0 \\ z_0 \end{pmatrix}
$$

defining the position P_0 is transformed into the vector

$$\mathbf{v} = \begin{pmatrix} x_1 \\ y_1 \\ z_1 \end{pmatrix}$$

defining the position P_1. Things, in reality, are more complicated, but it was important to present a simple and general description of the problem.

21.24 Orthogonal and Orthonormal Matrices

A square matrix $\mathbf{A}_n$ is said *orthogonal* if $\mathbf{A}^\top \mathbf{A} = \mathrm{diag}(\alpha_1, \ldots, \alpha_n)$, with $\alpha_k \neq 0$.

A square matrix $\mathbf{A}_n$ is said *orthonormal* if $\mathbf{A}\mathbf{A}^\top = \mathbf{A}^\top \mathbf{A} = \mathbf{I}$, which implies $\mathbf{A}^{-1} = \mathbf{A}^\top$. An always cited example of orthonormal matrix is the counterclockwise rotation matrix:

$$\mathbf{R} = \begin{pmatrix} \cos(\theta) & -\sin(\theta) \\ \sin(\theta) & \cos(\theta) \end{pmatrix},$$

where, being $\det(\mathbf{R}) = \cos^2(\theta) + \sin^2(\theta)$, we have

$$\mathbf{R}^{-1} = \begin{pmatrix} \frac{\cos(\theta)}{\cos^2(\theta)+\sin^2(\theta)} & \frac{\sin(\theta)}{\cos^2(\theta)+\sin^2(\theta)} \\ -\frac{\sin(\theta)}{\cos^2(\theta)+\sin^2(\theta)} & \frac{\cos(\theta)}{\cos^2(\theta)+\sin^2(\theta)} \end{pmatrix}$$

$$= \begin{pmatrix} \cos(\theta) & \sin(\theta) \\ -\sin(\theta) & \cos(\theta) \end{pmatrix}$$

and with

$$\mathbf{R}^\top = \begin{pmatrix} \cos(\theta) & \sin(\theta) \\ -\sin(\theta) & \cos(\theta) \end{pmatrix},$$

thus $\mathbf{R}^{-1} = \mathbf{R}^\top$.

The orthonormality holds for the various values of the rotation angles: for example, if

$$\mathbf{R} = \begin{pmatrix} \cos(\frac{\pi}{3}) & -\sin(\frac{\pi}{3}) \\ \sin(\frac{\pi}{3}) & \cos(\frac{\pi}{3}) \end{pmatrix}$$

then

$$\mathbf{R}^\top = \begin{pmatrix} \frac{1}{2} & \frac{1}{2}\sqrt{3} \\ -\frac{1}{2}\sqrt{3} & \frac{1}{2} \end{pmatrix} = \mathbf{R}^{-1}$$

and if

$$\mathbf{R} = \begin{pmatrix} \cos(\frac{7}{9}\pi) & -\sin(\frac{7}{9}\pi) \\ \sin(\frac{7}{9}\pi) & \cos(\frac{7}{9}\pi) \end{pmatrix}$$

then

$$\mathbf{R}^\mathsf{T} = \begin{pmatrix} -\dfrac{\cos\left(\frac{2}{9}\pi\right)}{\cos^2\left(\frac{2}{9}\pi\right)+\sin^2\left(\frac{2}{9}\pi\right)} & \dfrac{\sin\left(\frac{2}{9}\pi\right)}{\cos^2\left(\frac{2}{9}\pi\right)+\sin^2\left(\frac{2}{9}\pi\right)} \\ -\dfrac{\sin\left(\frac{2}{9}\pi\right)}{\cos^2\left(\frac{2}{9}\pi\right)+\sin^2\left(\frac{2}{9}\pi\right)} & -\dfrac{\cos\frac{2}{9}\pi}{\cos^2\left(\frac{2}{9}\pi\right)+\sin^2\left(\frac{2}{9}\pi\right)} \end{pmatrix} = \mathbf{R}^{-1}$$

which, after a little algebra, becomes

$$\mathbf{R}^\mathsf{T} = \begin{pmatrix} -\cos\frac{2}{9}\pi & \sin\frac{2}{9}\pi \\ -\sin\frac{2}{9}\pi & -\cos\frac{2}{9}\pi \end{pmatrix} = \mathbf{R}^{-1}.$$

21.25 Inverse of a Product

Let us consider two generic 2×2 square matrices:

$$\mathbf{A} = \begin{pmatrix} a & b \\ c & d \end{pmatrix}; \quad \mathbf{Z} = \begin{pmatrix} w & x \\ y & z \end{pmatrix}$$

and their inverses

$$\mathbf{A}^{-1} = \frac{1}{ad - bc} \begin{pmatrix} d & -b \\ -c & a \end{pmatrix}; \quad \mathbf{Z}^{-1} = \frac{1}{wz - xy} \begin{pmatrix} z & -x \\ -y & w \end{pmatrix},$$

obviously assuming that $ad - bc \neq 0$ and $wz - xy \neq 0$.

The two matrix products are

$$\mathbf{AZ} = \begin{pmatrix} a & b \\ c & d \end{pmatrix} \begin{pmatrix} w & x \\ y & z \end{pmatrix} = \begin{pmatrix} aw + by & ax + bz \\ cw + dy & cx + dz \end{pmatrix};$$

$$\mathbf{ZA} = \begin{pmatrix} w & x \\ y & z \end{pmatrix} \begin{pmatrix} a & b \\ c & d \end{pmatrix} = \begin{pmatrix} aw + cx & bw + dx \\ ay + cz & by + dz \end{pmatrix},$$

and the inverses of the products are

$$(\mathbf{AZ})^{-1} = \frac{1}{(ad - bc)(wz - xy)} \begin{pmatrix} cx + dz & -(ax + bz) \\ -(cw + dy) & aw + by \end{pmatrix}$$

$$= \frac{1}{\det(\mathbf{A}) \det(\mathbf{Z})} \begin{pmatrix} cx + dz & -(ax + bz) \\ -(cw + dy) & aw + by \end{pmatrix};$$

and

$$(\mathbf{ZA})^{-1} = \frac{1}{(wz - xy)(ad - bc)} \begin{pmatrix} by + dz & -(bw + dx) \\ -(ay + cz) & aw + cx \end{pmatrix}$$

$$= \frac{1}{\det(\mathbf{Z})\det(\mathbf{A})} \begin{pmatrix} by + dz & -(bw + dx) \\ -(ay + cz) & aw + cx \end{pmatrix},$$

whereas the products of the inverses are respectively

$$\mathbf{A}^{-1}\mathbf{Z}^{-1} = \frac{1}{ad - bc} \begin{pmatrix} d & -b \\ -c & a \end{pmatrix} \frac{1}{wz - xy} \begin{pmatrix} z & -x \\ -y & w \end{pmatrix}$$

$$= \frac{1}{(ad - bc)(wz - xy)} \begin{pmatrix} by + dz & -(bw + dx) \\ -(ay + cz) & aw + cx \end{pmatrix}$$

$$= \frac{1}{\det(\mathbf{A})\det(\mathbf{Z})} \begin{pmatrix} by + dz & -(bw + dx) \\ -(ay + cz) & aw + cx \end{pmatrix};$$

and

$$\mathbf{Z}^{-1}\mathbf{A}^{-1} = \frac{1}{wz - xy} \begin{pmatrix} z & -x \\ -y & w \end{pmatrix} \frac{1}{ad - bc} \begin{pmatrix} d & -b \\ -c & a \end{pmatrix}$$

$$= \frac{1}{(wz - xy)(ad - bc)} \begin{pmatrix} cx + dz & -(ax + bz) \\ -(cw + dy) & aw + by \end{pmatrix}$$

$$= \frac{1}{\det(\mathbf{Z})\det(\mathbf{A})} \begin{pmatrix} cx + dz & -(ax + bz) \\ -(cw + dy) & aw + by \end{pmatrix}.$$

Thus, we evolve that $(\mathbf{AZ})^{-1} = \mathbf{Z}^{-1}\mathbf{A}^{-1}$ and that $(\mathbf{ZA})^{-1} = \mathbf{A}^{-1}\mathbf{Z}^{-1}$, e.g., that the inverse matrices of the products $\mathbf{AZ}$ and $\mathbf{ZA}$ are equal to the products of the inverses in reverse order. This is a result valid in general for all the square matrices $n \times n$, and not just for the 2×2 ones.

Therefore, we can write that if $\mathbf{A}_n$ and $\mathbf{Z}_n$ are nonsingular square matrices of the same order n, then $(\mathbf{AZ})^{-1} = \mathbf{Z}^{-1}\mathbf{A}^{-1}$ and $(\mathbf{ZA})^{-1} = \mathbf{A}^{-1}\mathbf{Z}^{-1}$. The demonstration can be obtained observing that

$$(\mathbf{AZ})\mathbf{Z}^{-1}\mathbf{A}^{-1} = \mathbf{AZZ}^{-1}\mathbf{A}^{-1} = \mathbf{AIA}^{-1} = \mathbf{I},$$

and therefore $(\mathbf{AZ})^{-1} = \mathbf{Z}^{-1}\mathbf{A}^{-1}$; the demonstration for $(\mathbf{ZA})^{-1}$ can be carried out using the same procedure since

$$(\mathbf{ZA})\mathbf{A}^{-1}\mathbf{Z}^{-1} = \mathbf{ZAA}^{-1}\mathbf{Z}^{-1} = \mathbf{ZIZ}^{-1} = \mathbf{I}.$$

More generally, from what above, we may demonstrate that

$$(\mathbf{A}_{(1)}\mathbf{A}_{(2)} \cdots \mathbf{A}_{(n-1)}\mathbf{A}_{(n)})^{-1} = \mathbf{A}_{(n)}^{-1}\mathbf{A}_{(n-1)}^{-1} \cdots \mathbf{A}_{(2)}^{-1}\mathbf{A}_{(1)}^{-1}.$$

21.26 Eigenvalues

Given the square matrix $\mathbf{A}_n$, we define *eigenvalues of* $\mathbf{A}$ all the scalars λ such that, given an n-dimensional vector $\mathbf{z}$, defined in turn the *eigenvector*, the equality

$$\mathbf{A}\mathbf{z} = \lambda\mathbf{z} \tag{21.33}$$

holds.

In practice, for a given square matrix of order n, there are some specific vectors, the eigenvectors $\mathbf{z}$, such that the linear transformation $\mathbf{A}\mathbf{z}$ does not change the direction of $\mathbf{z}$, but just can modify its length. Thus $\mathbf{A}\mathbf{z}$ implies a simple multiplication of the modulus of $\mathbf{z}$ times one of the n scalars λ, the eigenvalues.

In other words, the eigenvector $\mathbf{z}$ is that vector whose direction is not changed by the action of the matrix: the only thing that is changed is the modulus, so premultiplying the eigenvector, the matrix exerts the same action as a scalar would, and the premultiplication of the matrix by the eigenvector becomes the simple multiplication by a scalar. To be more precise, the eigenvalue represents the scaling exerted by the matrix on the eigenvector, which does not change direction, but is only lengthened and shortened as a rubber band. The eigenvalue is completely determined for each specific eigenvector.

In particular, we may demonstrate that for each eigenvector $\mathbf{z}$, there exists, net of multiplicity, only one eigenvalue λ of the matrix $\mathbf{A}$. Indeed, if we premultiply by $\mathbf{z}^\top$ both sides of equality $\mathbf{A}\mathbf{z} = \lambda\mathbf{z}$, then we have $\mathbf{z}^\top\mathbf{A}\mathbf{z} = \mathbf{z}^\top\lambda\mathbf{z}$, and since we are dealing with scalars, then

$$\mathbf{z}^\top\mathbf{A}\mathbf{z} = \mathbf{z}^\top\lambda\mathbf{z} = \lambda\mathbf{z}^\top\mathbf{z},$$

and

$$\lambda = \frac{\mathbf{z}^\top\mathbf{A}\mathbf{z}}{\mathbf{z}^\top\mathbf{z}}.$$

Eigenvalues, in general, belong to the field of complex numbers; real eigenvalues can be view as cases where the imaginary part is zero. The set of the eigenvalues of a matrix is called the *spectrum*, while the *spectral radius* $r(\mathbf{A}) = \max(|\lambda_1|, |\lambda_2|, \ldots, |\lambda_n|)$ of a square matrix $\mathbf{A}_n$ is, among the n eigenvalues of $\mathbf{A}_n$, the one with the greatest absolute value.

The calculus of eigenvalues of the matrix $\mathbf{A}$ starts from Eq. (21.33), from which we get

$$\mathbf{0} = \mathbf{A}\mathbf{z} - \lambda\mathbf{z}$$

$$= \mathbf{Az} - \lambda \mathbf{Iz}$$

$$= (\mathbf{A} - \lambda \mathbf{I})\mathbf{z}. \tag{21.34}$$

To verify Eq. (21.34), excluding the trivial case $\mathbf{z} = \mathbf{0}$, it is necessary that $\mathbf{A} - \lambda \mathbf{I}$ is a singular matrix, and therefore we must have

$$\det(\mathbf{A} - \lambda \mathbf{I}) = 0,$$

hence

$$\det \begin{pmatrix} a_{11} - \lambda_1 & a_{12} & \cdots & a_{1n} \\ a_{21} & a_{22} - \lambda_2 & \cdots & a_{2n} \\ \vdots & \vdots & \ddots & \vdots \\ a_{n1} & a_{n2} & \cdots & a_{nn} - \lambda_n \end{pmatrix} = 0,$$

thus the n eigenvalues $\lambda_1, \lambda_2, \ldots, \lambda_n$ are the n roots of the characteristic polynomial in λ (taking into account also their multiplicity).

For example, let us take the 2×2 matrix:

$$\mathbf{A} = \begin{pmatrix} 7 & 4 \\ 3 & 3 \end{pmatrix}; \tag{21.35}$$

to calculate the eigenvalues, we first must obtain the determinant:

$$\det \begin{pmatrix} 7 - \lambda & 4 \\ 3 & 3 - \lambda \end{pmatrix} = (7 - \lambda)(3 - \lambda) - 12$$

$$= \lambda^2 - 10\lambda + 21 - 12$$

$$= \lambda^2 - 10\lambda + 9;$$

then, we must solve the second-degree equation:

$$\lambda^2 - 10\lambda + 9 = 0,$$

from which

$$\lambda_{1,2} = \frac{-b \pm \sqrt{b^2 - 4ac}}{2a} = \frac{10 \pm \sqrt{100 - 4 \times 9}}{2} = \frac{10 \pm \sqrt{64}}{2}$$

$$= \frac{10 \pm 8}{2};$$

hence, the eigenvalues are $\lambda_1 = 9$ and $\lambda_2 = 1$.

As a second example, let us consider the 3×3 matrix:

$$\mathbf{B} = \begin{pmatrix} 0 & 1 & 1 \\ -2 & 1 & 2 \\ 1 & 2 & 1 \end{pmatrix}, \tag{21.36}$$

from which, using the rule of Sarrus:

$$\det \begin{pmatrix} 0-\lambda & 1 & 1 \\ -2 & 1-\lambda & 2 \\ 1 & 2 & 1-\lambda \end{pmatrix} = (-\lambda)(1-\lambda)(1-\lambda) + 2 - 4$$

$$+ 4\lambda + 2(1-\lambda) - 1(1-\lambda)$$

$$= -\lambda(\lambda-1)^2 + 3\lambda - 1$$

$$= -\lambda^3 + 2\lambda^2 + 2\lambda - 1;$$

hence, to obtain the eigenvalues, we must solve the third-degree equation:

$$\lambda^3 - 2\lambda^2 - 2\lambda + 1 = 0.$$

Using the Ruffini rule, we obtain:

$$(\lambda + 1)\left(\lambda^2 - 3\lambda + 1\right) = 0;$$

thus, letting the first factor $\lambda + 1 = 0$, we get the first eigenvalue as $\lambda_1 = -1$, while letting be zero the second factor, we have $\lambda^2 - 3\lambda + 1 = 0$; thus, the solutions are the eigenvalues $\lambda_2 = \frac{3}{2} + \frac{1}{2}\sqrt{5}$, and $\lambda_3 = \frac{3}{2} - \frac{1}{2}\sqrt{5}$.

Notably, we see that the knowledge of the eigenvectors is not necessary to obtain the eigenvalues of a matrix. Moreover, we also see that the determinants of the two matrices (21.35) and (21.36) are respectively equal to 9 and 1 and to $-1, \frac{3}{2} + \frac{1}{2}\sqrt{5}$, and $\lambda_3 = \frac{3}{2} - \frac{1}{2}\sqrt{5}$. Thus, in both cases the determinants are equal to the product of the eigenvalues, since $9 \times 1 = 9$ and $(\frac{3}{2} + \frac{1}{2}\sqrt{5}) \times (\frac{3}{2} - \frac{1}{2}\sqrt{5}) \times (-1) = -1$.

This property holds for all $n \times n$ square matrices, and can be easily verified in the particular case of the 2×2 matrices. Indeed, the characteristic polynomial of a 2×2 matrix is a second-degree equation with unknown λ. In other words, we are dealing with an equation of the type $a\lambda^2 + b\lambda + c = 0$ with $a = 1$, and bearing in mind the properties of the solutions of a second-degree equation with $a = 1$, we may write the characteristic polynomial as

$$\lambda^2 - (\lambda_1 + \lambda_2)\lambda + \lambda_1\lambda_2 = \lambda^2 - s\lambda + p = 0,$$

where $s = \lambda_1 + \lambda_2$, and $p = \lambda_1\lambda_2$, that is to say, the value of the known term of the characteristic polynomial of a 2×2 matrix is always equal to the product of its eigenvalues.

Now, since in any 2×2 square matrix, the characteristic polynomial is

$$(a_{11} - \lambda)(a_{22} - \lambda) - a_{12}a_{21} = 0,$$

it is clear that the known term will be $a_{11}a_{22} - a_{12}a_{21}$, which is not only the product of the eigenvalues but also the determinant of $\mathbf{A}_2$, and therefore, for any square matrix of order 2, we have:

$$\lambda_1 \lambda_2 = a_{11}a_{22} - a_{12}a_{21} = \det(\mathbf{A}).$$

In general, we may demonstrate that the product of the eigenvalues of a $n \times n$ matrix is always equal to its determinant, or, better, if $\mathbf{A}_n$ is a square matrix with eigenvalues $\lambda_1, \lambda_2, \ldots, \lambda_n$, then $\det(\mathbf{A}) = \prod_{k=1}^{n} \lambda_k$.

The proof may be obtained considering that the characteristic polynomial of $\mathbf{A}_n$ may be written as

$$0 = (\lambda_1 - \lambda)(\lambda_2 - \lambda) \cdots (\lambda_n - \lambda) = \prod_{k=1}^{n} (\lambda_k - \lambda),$$

hence

$$\prod_{k=1}^{n} (\lambda_k - \lambda) = (-1)^n \lambda^n + (-1)^{n-1} \lambda^{n-1} \sum_{i=1}^{n} \lambda_i$$

$$+ (-1)^{n-2} \lambda^{n-2} \sum_{i=1}^{C_{n,2}} \left(\prod_{j=1,k=2}^{j=n-1,k=n} \lambda_j \lambda_k \right)$$

$$+ (-1)^{n-3} \lambda^{n-3} \sum_{i=1}^{C_{n,3}} \left(\prod_{j=1,k=2,l=3}^{j=n-2,k=n-1,l=n} \lambda_j \lambda_k \lambda_l \right)$$

$$+ (-1)^{n-4} \lambda^{n-4} \sum_{i=1}^{C_{n,4}} \left(\prod_{j=1,k=2,l=3,m=4}^{j=n-3,k=n-2,l=n-1,m=n} \lambda_j \lambda_k \lambda_l \lambda_m \right)$$

$$+ \cdots + (-1)^0 \prod_{k=1}^{n} \lambda_k;$$

therefore, bearing in mind that the polynomial must be equal to zero, we obtain:

$$\det(\mathbf{A}) = \prod_{k=1}^{n} \lambda_k.$$

A possible shortcut for the proof can be considered knowing that it must be

$$\det(\mathbf{A} - \lambda \mathbf{I}) = (\lambda_1 - \lambda)(\lambda_2 - \lambda) \cdots (\lambda_n - \lambda) = 0,$$

therefore, letting $\lambda = 0$ in both sides of equality, we would have

$$\det(A) = (\lambda_1 - 0)(\lambda_2 - 0) \cdots (\lambda_n - 0)$$

$$= \lambda_1 \lambda_2 \cdots \lambda_n = \prod_{k=1}^{n} \lambda_k.$$

21.27 Trace

The *trace* $\operatorname{tr}(\mathbf{A})$ of a square matrix $\mathbf{A}$ is the sum of its diagonal elements a_{kk}: in other words, given $\mathbf{A}_n$, the trace is

$$\operatorname{tr}(\mathbf{A}_n) = \sum_{k=1}^{n} a_{kk};$$

therefore, the trace is a scalar function with matrix argument.

For example, if

$$\mathbf{A} = \begin{pmatrix} a & 0 & 4 \\ b & 2 & b^2 \\ 3+a & -1 & a-2b \end{pmatrix},$$

then

$$\operatorname{tr}(\mathbf{A}) = 2(a - b + 1).$$

If $\mathbf{A}_n$ and $\mathbf{B}_n$ are square matrices of the same order, then $\operatorname{tr}(\mathbf{A} + \mathbf{B}) = \operatorname{tr}(\mathbf{A}) + \operatorname{tr}(\mathbf{B})$. The statement may be easily verified, since

$$\operatorname{tr}(\mathbf{A} + \mathbf{B}) = \sum_{k=1}^{n} (a_{kk} + b_{kk})$$

$$= (a_{11} + \cdots + a_{nn}) + (b_{11} + \cdots + b_{nn})$$

$$= \sum_{k=1}^{n} a_{kk} + \sum_{k=1}^{n} b_{kk}$$

$$= \operatorname{tr}(\mathbf{A}) + \operatorname{tr}(\mathbf{B}).$$

Moreover, if $\mathbf{A}_n$ and $\mathbf{B}_n$ are square matrices of the same order, then also $\operatorname{tr}(\mathbf{AB}) = \operatorname{tr}(\mathbf{BA})$, as we may easily verify: indeed, from the properties of the product of two matrices, the (j, j)-th element of $\mathbf{AB}$ is $\sum_{k=1}^{n} a_{jk} b_{kj}$, while the (k, k)-th element of $\mathbf{BA}$ is $\sum_{j=1}^{n} b_{kj} a_{jk}$, and therefore

$$\text{tr}(\mathbf{AB}) = \sum_{j=1}^{n} \sum_{k=1}^{n} a_{jk} b_{kj}$$

and

$$\text{tr}(\mathbf{BA}) = \sum_{k=1}^{n} \sum_{j=1}^{n} b_{kj} a_{jk},$$

and being both a_{jk} and b_{kj} scalars, then $a_{jk} b_{kj} = b_{kj} a_{jk}$; hence $\text{tr}(\mathbf{AB}) = \text{tr}(\mathbf{BA})$. Since in a square matrix $\mathbf{A}_2$ the characteristic polynomial is

$$(a_{11} - \lambda)(a_{22} - \lambda) - a_{12} a_{21} = \lambda^2 - (a_{11} + a_{22})\lambda + (a_{11} a_{22} - a_{12} a_{21})$$
$$= \lambda^2 - (\lambda_1 + \lambda_2)\lambda + \lambda_1 \lambda_2$$
$$= 0,$$

then we may also verify that

$$\lambda^2 - \text{tr}(\mathbf{A})\lambda + \det(\mathbf{A}) = 0,$$

e.g., that in a 2×2 square matrix, the trace is equal to the sum of eigenvalues. More generally, given any square matrix $\mathbf{A}_n$, the characteristic polynomial can always be written in the form:

$$(-1)^n \lambda^n + (-1)^{n-1} \text{tr}(\mathbf{A})\lambda^{n-1} + \cdots + \det(\mathbf{A}).$$

In fact, we can write:

$$\prod_{k=1}^{n} (\lambda_k - \lambda) = (-1)^n \lambda^n + \left((-1)^{n-1} \sum_{i=1}^{n} \lambda_i \right) \lambda^{n-1}$$
$$+ \left((-1)^{n-2} \sum_{i=1}^{C_{n,2}} \left(\prod_{j=1,k=2}^{j=n-1,k=n} \lambda_j \lambda_k \right) \right) \lambda^{n-2}$$
$$+ \left((-1)^{n-3} \sum_{i=1}^{C_{n,3}} \left(\prod_{j=1,k=2,l=3}^{j=n-2,k=n-1,l=n} \lambda_j \lambda_k \lambda_l \right) \right) \lambda^{n-3}$$

$$+ \left((-1)^{n-4} \sum_{i=1}^{C_{n,4}} \left(\prod_{j=1,k=2,l=3,m=4}^{j=n-3,k=n-2,l=n-1,m=n} \lambda_j \lambda_k \lambda_l \lambda_m \right) \right) \lambda^{n-4}$$

$$+ \cdots + \left((-1)^0 \prod_{k=1}^{n} \lambda_k \right) \lambda^0,$$

where, observing that numbers $C_{n,k} = \frac{k!}{(n-k)!k!}$ are combinations of n elements chosen k at a time, e.g., they are the values corresponding to the number of subsets with cardinality k which can be extracted from a set of cardinality n ($n \geq k$), and we see that the coefficient of λ^{n-1} is $(-1)^{n-1} \sum_{i=1}^{n} \lambda_i$.

This property can be therefore extended to any square matrix: in fact, in any square matrix, the sum of the diagonal elements is equal to the sum of the eigenvalues, so that, given the matrix $\mathbf{A}_n$ with eigenvalues $\lambda_1, \lambda_2, \ldots, \lambda_n$, it is always $\text{tr}(\mathbf{A}) = \sum_{k=1}^{n} \lambda_k$. The proof may be obtained bearing in mind that the characteristic equation is $(\lambda_1 - \lambda)(\lambda_2 - \lambda) \cdots (\lambda_n - \lambda)$ and that the coefficient of the $(n-1)$-th power of λ is

$$(-1)^{n-1} \sum_{k=1}^{n} \lambda_k = (-1)^{n-1} \sum_{k=1}^{n} a_{kk}$$

$$= (-1)^{n-1} \text{tr}(\mathbf{A});$$

thus, dividing both sides by $(-1)^{n-1}$, we get:

$$\sum_{k=1}^{n} \lambda_k = \text{tr}(\mathbf{A}).$$

21.28 Norm

For any real-valued matrix $\mathbf{A}_{m \times n}$, the norm $\|\mathbf{A}\|$ is the scalar defined as

$$\|\mathbf{A}\| = (\text{tr}(\mathbf{A}^\top \mathbf{A}))^{1/2};$$

hence, using what previously seen in Eq. (21.24), one may write:

$$\|\mathbf{A}\| = (\text{tr}(\mathbf{A}^\top \mathbf{A}))^{1/2}$$

$$= \left(\text{tr} \left(\begin{pmatrix} a_{11} & a_{21} & \cdots & a_{m1} \\ a_{12} & a_{22} & \cdots & a_{mr} \\ \vdots & \vdots & \ddots & \vdots \\ a_{1n} & a_{2n} & \cdots & a_{mn} \end{pmatrix} \begin{pmatrix} a_{11} & a_{12} & \cdots & a_{1n} \\ a_{21} & a_{22} & \cdots & a_{2n} \\ \vdots & \vdots & \ddots & \vdots \\ a_{m1} & a_{m2} & \cdots & a_{mn} \end{pmatrix} \right) \right)^{1/2}$$

$$
= \left(\mathrm{tr} \begin{pmatrix} a_{11}^2 + \ldots + a_{m1}^2 & a_{11}a_{12} + \cdots + a_{m1}a_{m2} & \cdots & a_{11}a_{1n} + \cdots + a_{m1}a_{mn} \\ a_{11}a_{12} + \cdots + a_{m1}a_{m2} & a_{12}^2 + \cdots + a_{m2}^2 & \cdots & a_{12}a_{1n} + \cdots + a_{r2}a_{mn} \\ \vdots & \vdots & \ddots & \vdots \\ a_{11}a_{1n} + \cdots + a_{m1}a_{mn} & a_{12}a_{1n} + \cdots + a_{m2}a_{mn} & \cdots & a_{1n}^2 + \cdots + a_{mn}^2 \end{pmatrix} \right)^{1/2}
$$

$$
= \left(\mathrm{tr} \begin{pmatrix} \sum_{k=1}^m a_{k1}^2 & \sum_{k=1}^m a_{k1}a_{k2} & \cdots & \sum_{k=1}^m a_{k1}a_{kn} \\ \sum_{k=1}^m a_{k1}a_{k2} & \sum_{k=1}^m a_{k2}^2 & \cdots & \sum_{k=1}^m a_{k2}a_{kn} \\ \vdots & \vdots & \ddots & \vdots \\ \sum_{k=1}^m a_{k1}a_{kn} & \sum_{k=1}^m a_{k2}a_{kn} & \cdots & \sum_{k=1}^m a_{kn}^2 \end{pmatrix} \right)^{1/2} .
$$

$$
= \left(\sum_{k=1}^m a_{k1}^2 + \sum_{k=1}^m a_{k2}^2 + \cdots + \sum_{k=1}^m a_{kn}^2 \right)^{1/2}
$$

$$
= \left(\sum_{j=1}^n \sum_{k=1}^m a_{kj}^2 \right)^{1/2} .
$$

In other words,

$$
\|\mathbf{A}\| = \left((a_{11}^2 + \ldots + a_{m1}^2) + \left(a_{12}^2 + \cdots + a_{m2}^2 \right) + \cdots + \left(a_{1c}^2 + \cdots + a_{mn}^2 \right) \right)^{1/2},
$$

therefore, writing the matrix in terms of column vectors, like

$$
\mathbf{A} = \begin{pmatrix} \mathbf{a}_1 & \mathbf{a}_2 & \cdots & \mathbf{a}_n \end{pmatrix}
$$

we find:

$$
\|\mathbf{A}\| = \left(\mathbf{a}_1^\top \mathbf{a}_1 + \mathbf{a}_2^\top \mathbf{a}_2 + \cdots + \mathbf{a}_n^\top \mathbf{a}_n \right)^{1/2} .
$$

Thus, using the matrix

$$
\mathbf{A} = \begin{pmatrix} 2 & 3 & 1 \\ 1 & 2 & 1 \\ 3 & 0 & 2 \\ 2 & -1 & 2 \end{pmatrix},
$$

we get:

$$\|\mathbf{A}\| = (\operatorname{tr}(\mathbf{A}^\top \mathbf{A}))^{1/2} = \left(\operatorname{tr} \begin{pmatrix} 2 & 1 & 3 & 2 \\ 3 & 2 & 0 & -1 \\ 1 & 1 & 2 & 2 \end{pmatrix} \begin{pmatrix} 2 & 3 & 1 \\ 1 & 2 & 1 \\ 3 & 0 & 2 \\ 2 & -1 & 2 \end{pmatrix} \right)^{1/2}$$

$$= \left(\operatorname{tr} \begin{pmatrix} 18 & 6 & 13 \\ 6 & 14 & 3 \\ 13 & 3 & 10 \end{pmatrix} \right)^{1/2}$$

$$= (18 + 14 + 10)^{1/2}$$

$$= \sqrt{42},$$

or even

$$\|\mathbf{A}\| = (\operatorname{tr}(\mathbf{A}^\top \mathbf{A}))^{1/2}$$

$$= \left(\begin{pmatrix} 2 & 3 & 1 & 2 \end{pmatrix} \begin{pmatrix} 2 \\ 3 \\ 1 \\ 2 \end{pmatrix} + \begin{pmatrix} 3 & 2 & 0 & -1 \end{pmatrix} \begin{pmatrix} 3 \\ 2 \\ 0 \\ -1 \end{pmatrix} \right.$$

$$\left. + \begin{pmatrix} 1 & 1 & 2 & 2 \end{pmatrix} \begin{pmatrix} 1 \\ 1 \\ 2 \\ 2 \end{pmatrix} \right)^{1/2}$$

$$= (18 + 14 + 10)^{1/2}$$

$$= \sqrt{42},$$

and thus the concept of the norm of a matrix is a generalization of the concept of the Euclidean norm of a vector.

21.29 Subspaces

If a vector space $\mathbb{V}$ is a subset of $\mathbb{R}^n$, we say that $\mathbb{V}$ is a subspace of $\mathbb{R}^n$ if, and only if, the three following conditions are simultaneously obeyed:

$$\mathbf{0} \in \mathbb{V}$$

$$\mathbf{a}, \mathbf{b} \in \mathbb{V} \implies (\mathbf{a} + \mathbf{b}) \in \mathbb{V}$$

$$\mathbf{a} \in \mathbb{V} \implies \lambda \mathbf{a} \in \mathbb{V}, \quad \lambda \in \mathbb{R}$$

so that we see that the singleton $\{0\}$ is a subspace of $\mathbb{R}$, since: 1) $0 \in \{0\}$; 2) $(0 + 0) \in \{0\}$; 3) $\lambda \in \{0\}$. But even the same $\mathbb{R}$ is a subspace of itself, since $0 \in \mathbb{R}$, $a, b \in \mathbb{R} \Rightarrow (a + b) \in \mathbb{R}$ and $a \in \mathbb{R} \Rightarrow \lambda a \in \mathbb{R}, \forall \lambda \in \mathbb{R}$.

Note that a subspace is not just a subset, but a subset satisfying the above conditions. For example, let us consider the set $\mathbb{R}' = \{x \in \mathbb{R} : x \geq 0\}$: evidently, $0 \in \mathbb{R}'$, and equally evidently $\mathbb{R}'$ is closed under addition, but $\mathbb{R}'$ is not closed under scalar multiplication, because taking $\lambda = -2$, then $\lambda x < 0$, so that $\lambda x \notin \mathbb{R}'$.

As another example, we see that a subset in $\mathbb{R}^3$ is just a collection of vectors in $\mathbb{R}^3$: if we define a space (say, a cube with an edge equal to 1) as

$$S^3 = \{x : 0 \leq x \leq 1; \ y : 0 \leq y \leq 1; \ z : 0 \leq z \leq 1\},$$

then S^3 is not a subspace of $\mathbb{R}^3$: to verify this, one only needs to see that, for

$$\begin{pmatrix} 0.7 \\ 0.2 \\ 0.4 \end{pmatrix} = \mathbf{a} \in S^3, \quad \text{and} \quad \begin{pmatrix} 0.6 \\ 0.9 \\ 0.2 \end{pmatrix} = \mathbf{b} \in S^3,$$

we have

$$\begin{pmatrix} 0.7 \\ 0.2 \\ 0.4 \end{pmatrix} + \begin{pmatrix} 0.6 \\ 0.9 \\ 0.2 \end{pmatrix} = \mathbf{a} + \mathbf{b} = \begin{pmatrix} 1.3 \\ 1.1 \\ 0.6 \end{pmatrix} \notin S^3,$$

and one of the condition is not obeyed. We also see that if

$$\begin{pmatrix} 0.7 \\ 0.2 \\ 0.4 \end{pmatrix} = \mathbf{a} \in S^3, \quad \text{and} \quad \lambda = 6 \in \mathbb{R},$$

then also a second condition is not obeyed, since

$$6 \begin{pmatrix} 0.7 \\ 0.2 \\ 0.4 \end{pmatrix} = \lambda \mathbf{a} = \begin{pmatrix} 4.2 \\ 1.2 \\ 2.4 \end{pmatrix} \notin S^3;$$

hence, only the condition

$$\begin{pmatrix} 0 \\ 0 \\ 0 \end{pmatrix} = \mathbf{0} \in S^3$$

is obeyed.

21.30 Span

Given a set of vectors $\mathbb{V} = \{\mathbf{v}_1, \mathbf{v}_2, \ldots, \mathbf{v}_m\}$ in $\mathbb{R}^n$, we define:

$$\text{Span}(\mathbf{v}_1, \mathbf{v}_2, \ldots, \mathbf{v}_m) = \{a_1\mathbf{v}_1 + a_2\mathbf{v}_2 + \cdots + a_m\mathbf{v}_m\}$$

the set of all the linear combinations among vectors, where the a_k terms indicate any arbitrary real constant. In other words, $\text{Span}(\mathbf{v}_1, \mathbf{v}_2, \ldots, \mathbf{v}_m)$ is a subspace generated by the vectors $\mathbf{v}_k$. In fact, we may verify that

$$0\mathbf{v}_1 + 0\mathbf{v}_2 + \cdots + 0\mathbf{v}_m = \mathbf{0} \in \text{Span}(\mathbf{v}_1, \mathbf{v}_2, \ldots, \mathbf{v}_m)$$

and that, if

$$\{a_1\mathbf{v}_1 + a_2\mathbf{v}_2 + \cdots + a_m\mathbf{v}_m, b_1\mathbf{v}_1 + b_2\mathbf{v}_2 + \cdots + b_m\mathbf{v}_m\} \in \text{Span}(\mathbf{v}_1, \mathbf{v}_2, \ldots, \mathbf{v}_m)$$

then also

$$\{(a_1 + b_1)\mathbf{v}_1 + (a_2 + b_2)\mathbf{v}_2 + \cdots + (a_m + b_m)\mathbf{v}_m\} \in \text{Span}(\mathbf{v}_1, \mathbf{v}_2, \ldots, \mathbf{v}_m).$$

Moreover, if

$$\{a_1\mathbf{v}_1 + a_2\mathbf{v}_2 + \cdots + a_m\mathbf{v}_m\} \in \text{Span}(\mathbf{v}_1, \mathbf{v}_2, \ldots, \mathbf{v}_m)$$

then, given the scalar λ, we have:

$$\{\lambda a_1\mathbf{v}_1 + \lambda a_2\mathbf{v}_2 + \cdots + \lambda a_m\mathbf{v}_m\} \in \text{Span}(\mathbf{v}_1, \mathbf{v}_2, \ldots, \mathbf{v}_m).$$

Here we must bear in mind that a set of vectors $\mathbb{V} = \{\mathbf{v}_1, \ldots, \mathbf{v}_m\}$ is linearly independent if, and only if, the solution to the equation

$$\lambda_1\mathbf{v}_1 + \cdots + \lambda_m\mathbf{v}_m = 0$$

is $\lambda_k = 0, \forall k$.

For example, given the matrix

$$\mathbf{M} = \begin{pmatrix} -2 & 4 & 2 \\ 5 & 5 & 5 \\ 4 & 1 & 2 \end{pmatrix}$$

we see that its columns are not linearly independent, since,

$$-\frac{1}{3}\begin{pmatrix} -2 \\ 5 \\ 4 \end{pmatrix} - \frac{2}{3}\begin{pmatrix} 4 \\ 5 \\ 1 \end{pmatrix} + 1\begin{pmatrix} 2 \\ 5 \\ 2 \end{pmatrix} = \begin{pmatrix} 0 \\ 0 \\ 0 \end{pmatrix}$$

but also

$$\begin{pmatrix} -2 \\ 5 \\ 4 \end{pmatrix} + 2\begin{pmatrix} 4 \\ 5 \\ 1 \end{pmatrix} - 3\begin{pmatrix} 2 \\ 5 \\ 2 \end{pmatrix} = \begin{pmatrix} 0 \\ 0 \\ 0 \end{pmatrix}$$

To calculate whether some vectors are linearly independent, we must take the vectors as columns of a matrix $\mathbf{A}$ and then solve:

$$\mathbf{Ax} = \mathbf{0};$$

in our case, we did

$$\mathbf{A} = \begin{pmatrix} -2 & 4 & 2 \\ 5 & 5 & 5 \\ 4 & 1 & 2 \end{pmatrix} \begin{pmatrix} x_1 \\ x_2 \\ x_3 \end{pmatrix} = \begin{pmatrix} 0 \\ 0 \\ 0 \end{pmatrix},$$

equivalent to

$$\mathbf{A} = x_1 \begin{pmatrix} -2 \\ 5 \\ 4 \end{pmatrix} + x_2 \begin{pmatrix} 4 \\ 5 \\ 1 \end{pmatrix} + x_3 \begin{pmatrix} 2 \\ 5 \\ 2 \end{pmatrix} = \begin{pmatrix} 0 \\ 0 \\ 0 \end{pmatrix},$$

and found (at least) two nontrivial solutions

$$\begin{pmatrix} x_1 \\ x_2 \\ x_3 \end{pmatrix} = \begin{pmatrix} -\frac{1}{3} \\ -\frac{2}{3} \\ 1 \end{pmatrix}, \quad \text{and} \quad \begin{pmatrix} x_1 \\ x_2 \\ x_3 \end{pmatrix} = \begin{pmatrix} 1 \\ 2 \\ -3 \end{pmatrix},$$

so the vectors aren't linearly independent. So, any set of vectors $\mathbb{V}$ spans a space when any vector in that space can be written as a linear combination of $\mathbb{V}$.

21.31 Kernel

Given a matrix $\mathbf{Z}$ in $\mathbb{R}^{m \times n}$ with m and n real, the set of all vectors $\mathbf{x}_i$ in $\mathbb{R}^n$ (e.g., the set of all vectors with n dimensions), such that $\mathbf{Zx} = \mathbf{0}$, defines a subspace of $\mathbb{R}^n$ (e.g., a subspace of vectors with n dimensions), called the *kernel* of $\mathbf{Z}$, or also the *nullspace* of $\mathbf{Z}$. Here we will indicate the kernel of $\mathbf{Z}$ with Ker($\mathbf{Z}$), bearing in mind that some textbooks use the notation Null($\mathbf{Z}$).

Taking a matrix $\mathbf{Z}_{m \times n}$, we have:

$$\mathbf{Zx} = \begin{pmatrix} z_{11} & z_{12} & \cdots & z_{1n} \\ z_{21} & z_{22} & \cdots & z_{2n} \\ \vdots & \vdots & \ddots & \vdots \\ z_{m1} & z_{m2} & \cdots & z_{mn} \end{pmatrix} \begin{pmatrix} x_1 \\ x_2 \\ \vdots \\ x_n \end{pmatrix} = \begin{pmatrix} 0 \\ 0 \\ \vdots \\ 0 \end{pmatrix} = \mathbf{0}_m;$$

thus, we have to solve the following system:

$$\begin{cases} z_{11}x_1 + z_{12}x_2 + \cdots + z_{1n}x_n = 0 \\ z_{21}x_1 + z_{22}x_2 + \cdots + z_{2n}x_n = 0 \\ \qquad\qquad \vdots \\ z_{m1}x_1 + z_{m2}x_2 + \cdots + z_{mn}x_n = 0 \end{cases}$$

so as to obtain all the vectors $\mathbf{x}$, having the solutions $x_1, \ldots, x_n$ as components. We will therefore get $\mathrm{Ker}(\mathbf{Z})$ as the subspace in $\mathbb{R}^n$ containing all the vectors $\mathbf{x}$.

As a practical example, let us take the three matrices:

$$\mathbf{A} = \begin{pmatrix} 1 & 3 & 0 \\ 0 & -2 & 3 \\ 1 & 1 & 2 \end{pmatrix}, \quad \mathbf{B} = \begin{pmatrix} 2 & -1 & -3 \\ -\frac{2}{3} & \frac{1}{3} & 1 \end{pmatrix}, \quad \mathbf{C} = \begin{pmatrix} 1 & 3 \\ 2 & 6 \\ 1 & 1 \end{pmatrix}.$$

To have $\mathbf{Ax} = \mathbf{0}$, it must be

$$\begin{pmatrix} 1 & 3 & 0 \\ 0 & -2 & 3 \\ 1 & 1 & 2 \end{pmatrix} \begin{pmatrix} x_1 \\ x_2 \\ x_3 \end{pmatrix} = \begin{pmatrix} 0 \\ 0 \\ 0 \end{pmatrix};$$

thus, we are dealing with the system:

$$\begin{cases} x_1 + 3x_2 = 0 \\ -2x_2 + 3x_3 = 0 \\ x_1 + x_2 + 2x_3 = 0 \end{cases}$$

having solution

$$\begin{cases} x_1 = 0 \\ x_2 = 0 \\ x_3 = 0 \end{cases}$$

thus; $\mathrm{Ker}(\mathbf{A})$ is a subspace in $\mathbb{R}^3$ containing only the vector $\mathbf{0}_3$; in other words, the nullspace of $\mathbf{A}$ is given only by the point having coordinates $(0, 0, 0)$.

To have $\mathbf{Bx} = \mathbf{0}$, it must be

$$\begin{pmatrix} 2 & -1 & -3 \\ -2/3 & 1/3 & 1 \end{pmatrix} \begin{pmatrix} x_1 \\ x_2 \\ x_3 \end{pmatrix} = \begin{pmatrix} 0 \\ 0 \end{pmatrix};$$

therefore, one must solve the system with two equations and three unknown values:

$$\begin{cases} 2x_1 - x_2 - 3x_3 = 0 \\ -\frac{2}{3}x_1 + \frac{1}{3}x_2 + x_3 = 0 \end{cases},$$

whose solution is $x_1 = \frac{1}{2}x_2 + \frac{3}{2}x_3$; thus, the kernel of $\mathbf{B}$ is a subspace in $\mathbb{R}^3$ given by the plane having equation $x_1 - \frac{1}{2}x_2 - \frac{3}{2}x_3 = 0$, where all linear combinations of the vectors

$$\mathbf{s}_1 = \begin{pmatrix} 1 \\ 2 \\ 1 \\ 0 \end{pmatrix}, \quad \mathbf{s}_2 = \begin{pmatrix} 3 \\ 2 \\ 0 \\ 1 \end{pmatrix};$$

are lying, and these vectors are the *vector basis* of Ker($\mathbf{B}$).

To have $\mathbf{Cx} = \mathbf{0}$, it must be

$$\begin{pmatrix} 1 & 3 \\ 2 & 6 \\ 1 & 3 \end{pmatrix} \begin{pmatrix} x_1 \\ x_2 \end{pmatrix} = \begin{pmatrix} 0 \\ 0 \\ 0 \end{pmatrix},$$

and one must solve the system with three equations and two unknown values:

$$\begin{cases} x_1 + 3x_2 = 0 \\ 2x_1 + 6x_2 = 0 \\ x_1 + 3x_2 = 0 \end{cases},$$

having solutions $x_1 = -3x_2$, and thus the kernel of $\mathbf{C}$ is a subspace in $\mathbb{R}^3$ formed by the plane defined by equation $x_1 + 3x_2 = 0$, where we find all the linear combinations of the vector

$$\mathbf{s} = \begin{pmatrix} -3 \\ 1 \end{pmatrix},$$

and that vector is the basis of Ker($\mathbf{C}$).

By the way, it can be shown that any subspace of $\mathbb{R}^n$ may potentially be the kernel of a given matrix.

21.32 Image

Given a matrix $\mathbf{A}$ in $\mathbb{R}^{m \times n}$ with any m and n, and defined as $\mathbf{A} = (\mathbf{a}_1 \ \mathbf{a}_2 \ \ldots \ \mathbf{a}_n)$, being $\mathbf{a}_i$ the n-dimensional column vectors of the matrix, the subspace $\mathrm{Im}(\mathbf{A})$ in $\mathbb{R}^m$ which contains all the linear combinations of the column vectors $\mathbf{a}_k$ is said the *image* of $\mathbf{A}$ (or also the *range* of $\mathbf{A}$, or—again—the *column space* of $\mathbf{A}$). In other words, given $\mathbf{A} = (\mathbf{a}_1 \ \mathbf{a}_2 \ \ldots \ \mathbf{a}_n)$, we have $\mathrm{Im}(\mathbf{A}) = \mathrm{Span}(\mathbf{a}_1 \ \mathbf{a}_2 \ \ldots \ \mathbf{a}_n)$; moreover, given $\mathbf{A}_{m \times n}$, and recalling the definition of rank, we have $\rho_{\mathrm{col}}(\mathbf{A}) = \dim(\mathrm{Im}(\mathbf{A}))$.

For example, given the matrix

$$\mathbf{A} = \begin{pmatrix} 1 & 3 \\ -1 & 2 \\ 3 & 1 \end{pmatrix},$$

its image $\mathrm{Im}(\mathbf{A})$, using the scalars α_1, α_2, is a plane containing all the vectors

$$\mathbf{x} = \alpha_1 \mathbf{a}_1 + \alpha_2 \mathbf{a}_2$$

$$= \alpha_1 \begin{pmatrix} 1 \\ -1 \\ 3 \end{pmatrix} + \alpha_2 \begin{pmatrix} 3 \\ 2 \\ 1 \end{pmatrix}, \tag{21.37}$$

which are linear combinations of the two column vectors

$$\mathbf{a}_1 = \begin{pmatrix} 1 \\ -1 \\ 3 \end{pmatrix}, \ \mathbf{a}_2 = \begin{pmatrix} 3 \\ 2 \\ 1 \end{pmatrix}$$

which are the *vector basis* of $\mathrm{Im}(\mathbf{A})$. The subspace $\mathrm{Im}(\mathbf{A})$ of the matrix $\mathbf{A}$ is a plane passing through the origin $(0, 0, 0)$, since if we put $\alpha_1, \alpha_2 = 0$ in Eq. (21.37) we have

$$\mathbf{x} = \begin{pmatrix} 0 \\ 0 \\ 0 \end{pmatrix}.$$

21.33 Idempotent Matrices and Their Main Properties

We already met the idempotent matrix $\mathbf{I} - \mathbf{U}/n$, and we said that a square matrix $\mathbf{A}_n$ is idempotent when $\mathbf{A}_n^2 = \mathbf{A}_n$. In the set of real numbers $\mathbb{R}$, the only idempotent elements are 0 and 1, e.g., the neutral element for the sum and the neutral element for the product. The proof is very simple, since a real number n is idempotent if, and only if, $n = n^2$; hence, if

$$n^2 - n = n(n-1) = 0,$$

then, idempotence of real numbers is verified if, and only if, $n = 0$ and $n = 1$.

Among the set of all square matrices in $\mathbb{R}^{n \times n}$ (for any n), the neutral elements for addition $\mathbf{O}_n$ and multiplication $\mathbf{I}_n$ confirm to be idempotent, since it is straightforward to verify that $\mathbf{O}_n = \mathbf{O}_n^2$ and $\mathbf{I}_n = \mathbf{I}_n^2$. However, the idempotence is a property observable in many other matrices different from $\mathbf{O}_n$ and $\mathbf{I}_n$.

Just as an example, considering the set $\mathbb{R}^{2 \times 2}$ of all 2×2 square matrices, we may write for a generic matrix $\mathbf{M}$:

$$\mathbf{M}^2 = \begin{pmatrix} m_{11} & m_{12} \\ m_{21} & m_{22} \end{pmatrix}^2$$

$$= \begin{pmatrix} m_{11}^2 + m_{12}m_{21} & m_{11}m_{12} + m_{12}m_{22} \\ m_{11}m_{21} + m_{21}m_{22} & m_{22}^2 + m_{12}m_{21} \end{pmatrix};$$

thus, to have the case of idempotence $\mathbf{M}^2 = \mathbf{M}$, it must be

$$\begin{cases} m_{11} = m_{11}^2 + m_{12}m_{21} \\ m_{12} = m_{11}m_{12} + m_{12}m_{22} \\ m_{21} = m_{11}m_{21} + m_{21}m_{22} \\ m_{22} = m_{22}^2 + m_{12}m_{21} \end{cases}$$

so that we obtain some possible solutions:

$$\begin{cases} m_{11} = 1 \\ m_{12} = 0 \\ m_{21} = 0 \\ m_{22} = 1 \end{cases} ; \quad \begin{cases} m_{11} = 1 \\ m_{12} = 0 \\ m_{21} = 0 \\ m_{22} = 0 \end{cases} ; \quad \begin{cases} m_{11} = 0 \\ m_{12} = 0 \\ m_{21} = 0 \\ m_{22} = 1 \end{cases} ; \quad \begin{cases} m_{11} = 0 \\ m_{12} = 0 \\ m_{21} = 0 \\ m_{22} = 0 \end{cases} ;$$

$$\begin{cases} m_{11} = 0 \\ m_{12} = r \\ m_{21} = 0 \\ m_{22} = 1 \end{cases} ; \quad \begin{cases} m_{11} = 1 \\ m_{12} = r \\ m_{21} = 0 \\ m_{22} = 0 \end{cases} ; \quad \begin{cases} m_{11} = 1 - r \\ m_{12} = \frac{r - r^2}{s} \\ m_{21} = s \\ m_{22} = r \end{cases} ,$$

where $r, s \in \mathbb{R}$ are arbitrary numbers. Thus, taking into account the set of all 2×2 square matrices with real elements, in addition to the two matrices already known

$$\mathbf{I}_2 = \begin{pmatrix} 1 & 0 \\ 0 & 1 \end{pmatrix}; \quad \mathbf{O}_2 = \begin{pmatrix} 0 & 0 \\ 0 & 0 \end{pmatrix}, \tag{21.38}$$

we see that all the infinite possible matrices having form

$$\mathbf{X} = \begin{pmatrix} 1 & r \\ 0 & 0 \end{pmatrix}; \tag{21.39}$$

$$\mathbf{Y} = \begin{pmatrix} 0 & r \\ 0 & 1 \end{pmatrix}; \tag{21.40}$$

$$\mathbf{Z} = \begin{pmatrix} 1 - r & \frac{r - r^2}{s} \\ s & r \end{pmatrix}; \tag{21.41}$$

are idempotent, for any real number r and $s \neq 0$.

Two particular cases are obtained when $r = 0$ and $r = 1$ in matrices (21.39) and (21.40), where we get

$$\mathbf{X}_{r=0} = \begin{pmatrix} 1 & 0 \\ 0 & 0 \end{pmatrix}; \quad \mathbf{Y}_{r=0} = \begin{pmatrix} 0 & 0 \\ 0 & 1 \end{pmatrix};$$

$$\mathbf{X}_{r=1} = \begin{pmatrix} 1 & 1 \\ 0 & 0 \end{pmatrix}; \quad \mathbf{Y}_{r=1} = \begin{pmatrix} 0 & 1 \\ 0 & 1 \end{pmatrix};$$

two more particular cases are obtained if we let $r = 0, s = 1$, e $r = s = 1$ in the matrix (21.41), from which we have

$$\mathbf{Z}_{r=0, s=1} = \begin{pmatrix} 1 & 0 \\ 1 & 0 \end{pmatrix}; \quad \mathbf{Z}_{r, s=1} = \begin{pmatrix} 0 & 0 \\ 1 & 1 \end{pmatrix}.$$

Finally, in the other particular case $s = r$, the same matrix (21.41) becomes:

$$\mathbf{Z}_{s=r} = \begin{pmatrix} 1 - r & 1 - r \\ r & r \end{pmatrix}.$$

The proof of idempotence of $\mathbf{I}_2$ and $\mathbf{O}_2$ is immediate, while the idempotence of the three matrices $\mathbf{X}$, $\mathbf{Y}$, and $\mathbf{Z}$, may be proven showing that the squared matrices are equal to the original ones.

Thus, we may say that any matrix of the form

$$\mathbf{X} = \begin{pmatrix} 1 & r \\ 0 & 0 \end{pmatrix}$$

is idempotent, for any value of r. The proof is immediate, since by simply using the rules of matrix multiplication, we get

$$\begin{pmatrix} 1 & r \\ 0 & 0 \end{pmatrix}^2 = \begin{pmatrix} 1 & r \\ 0 & 0 \end{pmatrix} \begin{pmatrix} 1 & r \\ 0 & 0 \end{pmatrix}$$

$$= \begin{pmatrix} 1 \times 1 + r \times 0 & 1 \times r + r \times 0 \\ 0 \times 1 + 0 \times 0 & 0 \times r + 0 \times 0 \end{pmatrix}$$

$$= \begin{pmatrix} 1 & r \\ 0 & 0 \end{pmatrix}.$$

Also the matrix

$$\mathbf{Y} = \begin{pmatrix} 0 & r \\ 0 & 1 \end{pmatrix}$$

is idempotent, for any value of r, and also in this case we find the proof just using the rules of matrix multiplication, since

$$\begin{pmatrix} 0 & r \\ 0 & 1 \end{pmatrix}^2 = \begin{pmatrix} 0 & r \\ 0 & 1 \end{pmatrix} \begin{pmatrix} 0 & r \\ 0 & 1 \end{pmatrix}$$

$$= \begin{pmatrix} 0 \times 0 + r \times 0 & 0 \times r + r \times 1 \\ 0 \times 0 + 1 \times 0 & 0 \times r + 1 \times 1 \end{pmatrix}$$

$$= \begin{pmatrix} 0 & r \\ 0 & 1 \end{pmatrix}.$$

Finally, we see that the matrix

$$\mathbf{Z} = \begin{pmatrix} 1 - r & \frac{r - r^2}{s} \\ s & r \end{pmatrix}$$

is idempotent, for any value of r and s, provided $s \neq 0$. Doing the multiplication we have:

$$\begin{pmatrix} 1 - r & \frac{r - r^2}{s} \\ s & r \end{pmatrix}^2 = \begin{pmatrix} 1 - r & \frac{r - r^2}{s} \\ s & r \end{pmatrix} \begin{pmatrix} 1 - r & \frac{r - r^2}{s} \\ s & r \end{pmatrix}$$

$$= \begin{pmatrix} r + (r - 1)^2 - r^2 \frac{r(r - r^2)}{s} & \frac{(r - r^2)(r - 1)}{s} \\ rs - s(r - 1) & r \end{pmatrix}$$

$$= \begin{pmatrix} 1 - r & \frac{r - r^2}{s} \\ s & r \end{pmatrix}.$$

We may extend the search for possible idempotent matrices for any other square matrix $\mathbf{M}_n$ with $n \geq 3$. The starting point is always the same: one must obtain $\mathbf{M}^2$ from $\mathbf{M}$, and then one must impose that elements of $\mathbf{M}^2$ are equal to the respective elements of $\mathbf{M}$. Just for an example, for any 3×3 matrix, we obtain:

$$\mathbf{M}^2 = \begin{pmatrix} m_{11} & m_{12} & m_{13} \\ m_{21} & m_{22} & m_{23} \\ m_{31} & m_{32} & m_{33} \end{pmatrix}^2$$

$$= \begin{pmatrix} M_{11} & M_{12} & M_{13} \\ M_{21} & M_{22} & M_{23} \\ M_{31} & M_{32} & M_{33} \end{pmatrix}$$

where

$$M_{11} = m_{11}^2 + m_{12}m_{21} + m_{13}m_{31}$$

$$M_{12} = m_{11}m_{12} + m_{12}m_{22} + m_{13}m_{32}$$

$$M_{13} = m_{11}m_{13} + m_{12}m_{23} + m_{13}m_{33}$$

$$M_{21} = m_{11}m_{21} + m_{21}m_{22} + m_{31}m_{23}$$

$$M_{22} = m_{22}^2 + m_{12}m_{21} + m_{23}m_{32}$$

$$M_{23} = m_{21}m_{13} + m_{22}m_{23} + m_{23}m_{33}$$

$$M_{31} = m_{11}m_{31} + m_{21}m_{32} + m_{31}m_{33}$$

$$M_{32} = m_{12}m_{31} + m_{22}m_{32} + m_{32}m_{33}$$

$$M_{33} = m_{33}^2 + m_{13}m_{31} + m_{23}m_{32}$$

thus we impose:

$$\begin{cases} m_{11} = m_{11}^2 + m_{12}m_{21} + m_{13}m_{31} \\ m_{12} = m_{11}m_{12} + m_{12}m_{22} + m_{13}m_{32} \\ m_{13} = m_{11}m_{13} + m_{12}m_{23} + m_{13}m_{33} \\ m_{21} = m_{11}m_{21} + m_{21}m_{22} + m_{31}m_{23} \\ m_{22} = m_{22}^2 + m_{12}m_{21} + m_{23}m_{32} \\ m_{23} = m_{21}m_{13} + m_{22}m_{23} + m_{23}m_{33} \\ m_{31} = m_{11}m_{31} + m_{21}m_{32} + m_{31}m_{33} \\ m_{32} = m_{12}m_{31} + m_{22}m_{32} + m_{32}m_{33} \\ m_{33} = m_{33}^2 + m_{13}m_{31} + m_{23}m_{32} \end{cases} .$$

Solving the system, we obtain the generic elements of 3×3 idempotent matrices. Among others, we find

$$\mathbf{I}_3 = \begin{pmatrix} 1 & 0 & 0 \\ 0 & 1 & 0 \\ 0 & 0 & 1 \end{pmatrix}; \quad \mathbf{O}_3 = \begin{pmatrix} 0 & 0 & 0 \\ 0 & 0 & 0 \\ 0 & 0 & 0 \end{pmatrix};$$

and

$$\mathbf{P}_{xy} = \begin{pmatrix} 1 & 0 & 0 \\ 0 & 1 & 0 \\ 0 & 0 & 0 \end{pmatrix}; \quad \mathbf{P}_{xz} = \begin{pmatrix} 1 & 0 & 0 \\ 0 & 0 & 0 \\ 0 & 0 & 1 \end{pmatrix}; \quad \mathbf{P}_{yz} = \begin{pmatrix} 0 & 0 & 0 \\ 0 & 1 & 0 \\ 0 & 0 & 1 \end{pmatrix};$$

and, again,

$$\mathbf{P}_x = \begin{pmatrix} 1 & 0 & 0 \\ 0 & 0 & 0 \\ 0 & 0 & 0 \end{pmatrix}; \quad \mathbf{P}_y = \begin{pmatrix} 0 & 0 & 0 \\ 0 & 1 & 0 \\ 0 & 0 & 0 \end{pmatrix}; \quad \mathbf{P}_z = \begin{pmatrix} 0 & 0 & 0 \\ 0 & 0 & 0 \\ 0 & 0 & 1 \end{pmatrix},$$

Moreover, other notable 3×3 idempotents are

$$\mathbf{M}_{(1)} = \begin{pmatrix} -\frac{ab-a+cd}{a} & -\frac{(b-1)(ab+cd)}{a^2} & -\frac{c(ab+cd)}{a^2} \\ a & b & c \\ d & \frac{d(b-1)}{a} & \frac{a+cd}{a} \end{pmatrix},$$

and

$$\mathbf{M}_{(2)} = \begin{pmatrix} -\frac{ab-a+cd}{a} & -\frac{b(ab-a+cd)}{a^2} & -\frac{c(ab-a+cd)}{a^2} \\ a & b & c \\ d & \frac{bd}{a} & \frac{cd}{a} \end{pmatrix},$$

where a, b, c, and d are arbitrary real numbers (provided $a \neq 0$), such that we may verify that $\mathbf{M}_{(1)}^2 = \mathbf{M}_{(1)}$, and $\mathbf{M}_{(2)}^2 = \mathbf{M}_{(2)}$.

Idempotent matrices show many important and interesting properties: here we simply list some of them, assuming that where the inverse of a matrix is specified, the matrix is indeed invertible, and where a product is specified, it is always computed between conformable matrices.

For first, we see that $\mathbf{A}^2 = \mathbf{A}$ implies $\mathbf{A}^n = \mathbf{A}$ (we may write $\mathbf{A}^2 = \mathbf{A} \Rightarrow \mathbf{A}^n = \mathbf{A}$), for any $n > 2$. The proof may be obtained observing that $\mathbf{A}^n = \mathbf{A}^{n-2}\mathbf{A}^2$; thus, if $\mathbf{A}$ is idempotent, we can write:

$$\mathbf{A}^n = \mathbf{A}^{n-2}\mathbf{A}^2 = \mathbf{A}^{n-2}\mathbf{A} = \mathbf{A}^{n-1}$$

hence,

$$\mathbf{A}^n = \mathbf{A}^{n-1} = \mathbf{A}^{n-3}\mathbf{A}^2 = \mathbf{A}^{n-3}\mathbf{A} = \mathbf{A}^{n-2} = \cdots = \mathbf{A}.$$

Note that the inverse properties is not verified, since choosing $n > 2$, we see that $\mathbf{A}^n = \mathbf{A}$ does not imply $\mathbf{A}^2 = \mathbf{A}$. For example, if we take

$$\mathbf{A} = \begin{pmatrix} 1 & 0 \\ 0 & -1 \end{pmatrix}$$

we see that

$$\mathbf{A}^3 = \begin{pmatrix} 1 & 0 \\ 0 & -1 \end{pmatrix} = \mathbf{A},$$

but also that

$$\mathbf{A}^2 = \begin{pmatrix} 1 & 0 \\ 0 & 1 \end{pmatrix} \neq \mathbf{A};$$

hence, $\mathbf{A}^3 = \mathbf{A}$ and $\mathbf{A}^2 \neq \mathbf{A}$; therefore, $\mathbf{A}^3 = \mathbf{A} \nRightarrow \mathbf{A}^2 = \mathbf{A}$. By the way, the matrices showing this behavior are said *tripotent*.

We also see that, if $\mathbf{A}$ is idempotent, then both $\mathbf{A}^\top$ is also idempotent, since

$$(\mathbf{A}^\top)^2 = (\mathbf{A}^2)^\top = \mathbf{A}^\top.$$

Another interesting fact is that $\mathbf{A}$ can be simultaneously invertible and idempotent if, and only if, $\mathbf{A} = \mathbf{I}$. In fact, assuming to have $\mathbf{A}$ idempotent and invertible, we have $\mathbf{A}^{-1}\mathbf{A} = \mathbf{A}^{-1}\mathbf{A}\mathbf{A}$; thus, $\mathbf{I} = \mathbf{I}\mathbf{A}$, which is verified if, and only if, $\mathbf{A} = \mathbf{I}$.

So, idempotent matrices are always singular and do not have an inverse (with the only exception of the identity matrix). Not possessing the inverse implies not being able to reverse the action of the matrix on the vector obtained from the transformation, i.e., given the transformation $\mathbf{P}\mathbf{v} = \mathbf{u}$, there is no an antitransformation $\mathbf{P}^{-1}\mathbf{u} = \mathbf{v}$, and this means that, in general, the transformation determined by an idempotent matrix (other than $\mathbf{I}$) on a given vector is irreversible.

However, the nonexistence of $\mathbf{P}^{-1}$ does not imply that there is no a matrix $\mathbf{Q} \neq \mathbf{P}$ that is able to transform $\mathbf{u}$ into the vector $\mathbf{v}$, such that $\mathbf{Q}\mathbf{u} = \mathbf{v}$.

We may also verify that, given the real-valued vector $\mathbf{v} \neq \mathbf{0}$, any matrix

$$\mathbf{A} = \frac{\mathbf{v}\mathbf{v}^\top}{\mathbf{v}^\top \mathbf{v}}$$

is idempotent. The proof can be obtained observing that $\mathbf{v}^\top \mathbf{v}$ is a nonzero scalar and therefore

$$\left(\frac{\mathbf{v}\mathbf{v}^\top}{\mathbf{v}^\top \mathbf{v}} \right)^2 = \frac{\mathbf{v}\mathbf{v}^\top}{\mathbf{v}^\top \mathbf{v}} \frac{\mathbf{v}\mathbf{v}^\top}{\mathbf{v}^\top \mathbf{v}} = \frac{\mathbf{v}(\mathbf{v}^\top \mathbf{v})\mathbf{v}^\top}{(\mathbf{v}^\top \mathbf{v})(\mathbf{v}^\top \mathbf{v})}$$

$$= \frac{\mathbf{v}\mathbf{v}^\top}{\mathbf{v}^\top \mathbf{v}}.$$

Notably, if a matrix $\mathbf{A}$ is idempotent, then also $\mathbf{I} - \mathbf{A}$ is idempotent. This can be easily verified, since

$$(\mathbf{I} - \mathbf{A})^2 = \mathbf{I}^2 - \mathbf{IA} - \mathbf{AI} + \mathbf{A}^2 = \mathbf{I} - 2\mathbf{A} + \mathbf{A}$$
$$= \mathbf{I} - \mathbf{A}.$$

From this property we easily infer also that if $\mathbf{A}$ is idempotent, then $\mathbf{A}$ and $\mathbf{I} - \mathbf{A}$ are mutually orthogonal, e.g.,

$$\mathbf{A}(\mathbf{I} - \mathbf{A}) = \mathbf{A} - \mathbf{A}^2 = \mathbf{A} - \mathbf{A} = \mathbf{O},$$

and

$$(\mathbf{I} - \mathbf{A})\mathbf{A} = \mathbf{A} - \mathbf{A}^2 = \mathbf{A} - \mathbf{A} = \mathbf{O}.$$

If $\mathbf{A}$ is idempotent, its possible eigenvalues can be only $\lambda = 0$ or $\lambda = 1$. To verify this property, consider the idempotent matrix $\mathbf{A}$ and the eigenvector $\mathbf{v}$: it must be

$$\lambda\mathbf{v} = \mathbf{A}\mathbf{v} = \mathbf{A}\mathbf{A}\mathbf{v} = \mathbf{A}\lambda\mathbf{v} = \lambda\mathbf{A}\mathbf{v} = \lambda\lambda\mathbf{v} = \lambda^2\mathbf{v}$$

which is verified only when $\lambda = \lambda^2$, and since λ is a scalar, it can be true if, and only if, $\lambda = 0$ or $\lambda = 1$.

Now, since we also know that the trace of a matrix is the sum of its eigenvalues, we argue that, in general, given the idempotent matrix $\mathbf{A}_n$, it must be $\text{tr}(\mathbf{A}_n) \leq n - 1$, with the particular case given by $\mathbf{I}_n$, where, $\text{tr}(\mathbf{I}_n) = n$.

For an idempotent matrix $\mathbf{A}$, the determinant can be only $\det(\mathbf{A}) = 0$, or $\det(\mathbf{A}) = 1$. Indeed, from the Binet theorem, we get:

$$\det(\mathbf{A}) = \det(\mathbf{A}^2) = \det(\mathbf{A})\det(\mathbf{A}) = [\det(\mathbf{A})]^2$$

but the determinant is a scalar; thus, the equivalence $\det(\mathbf{A}) = [\det(\mathbf{A})]^2$ is verified if, and only if, $\det(\mathbf{A}) = 0$ or $\det(\mathbf{A}) = 1$. Note that we can demonstrate this assertion even recalling that for an idempotent matrix with n eigenvalues we can have only $\lambda = 0$ or $\lambda = 1$; therefore, only two cases are possible: in the first case we have:

$$\det(\mathbf{A}_n) = \prod_{k=1}^{n} \lambda_k = 1, \text{ if } \lambda_1 = \cdots = \lambda_n = 1$$

while in the second case it is

$$\det(\mathbf{A}_n) = \prod_{k=1}^{n} \lambda_k = 0, \text{ if, at least one } \lambda_k = 0.$$

In an idempotent matrix, the trace is equal to the rank: in other words,

$$\mathbf{A} = \mathbf{A}^2 \Rightarrow \rho(\mathbf{A}) = r = \mathrm{tr}(\mathbf{A}).$$

In fact, if $\mathbf{A}_n \neq \mathbf{O}_n$ then there must be a matrix $\mathbf{B}_{n \times p}$ and a second matrix $\mathbf{L}_{p \times n}$, such that $\mathbf{A} = \mathbf{BL}$ and $\rho(\mathbf{B}) = \rho(\mathbf{L}) = p$; in this case, $\mathbf{BLBL} = \mathbf{A}^2 = \mathbf{A} = \mathbf{BL}$, and being $\mathbf{BLBL} = \mathbf{B(LB)L}$, we have $\mathbf{LB} = \mathbf{I}_p$, hence

$$\mathrm{tr}(\mathbf{A}) = \mathrm{tr}(\mathbf{BL}) = \mathrm{tr}(\mathbf{I}_p) = p = \rho(\mathbf{A}).$$

A diagonal matrix $\mathbf{D}$ is idempotent if, and only if, its diagonal elements d_k are 0 or 1. The proof of this property is immediate, since to have $\mathbf{D} = \mathbf{D}^2$, it must be $d_k = d_k^2$ for any k-th element of the diagonal, and this can be true if, and only if, $d_k = 0$ or $d_k = 1$.

If $\mathbf{A}$ is idempotent, and $\mathbf{B}$ is nonsingular, then any matrix $\mathbf{BAB}^{-1}$ is idempotent. Also in this case the proof is straightforward since

$$(\mathbf{BAB}^{-1})^2 = \mathbf{BAB}^{-1}\mathbf{BAB}^{-1}$$
$$= \mathbf{BAIAB}^{-1} = \mathbf{BAAB}^{-1}$$
$$= \mathbf{BAB}^{-1};$$

thus, premultiplying and postmultiplying an idempotent matrix by respectively any invertible matrix and its inverse produces a new idempotent matrix. Obviously, given the definition of inverse matrix, we immediately see that, if $\mathbf{BAB}^{-1}$ is idempotent, then $\mathbf{B}^{-1}\mathbf{AB}$ is also idempotent, since

$$(\mathbf{B}^{-1}\mathbf{AB})^2 = \mathbf{B}^{-1}\mathbf{ABB}^{-1}\mathbf{AB}$$
$$= \mathbf{B}^{-1}\mathbf{AIAB} = \mathbf{B}^{-1}\mathbf{AAB}$$
$$= \mathbf{B}^{-1}\mathbf{AB},$$

If $\mathbf{A}$ is a symmetric and idempotent matrix, then $\mathbf{I} - 2\mathbf{A}$ is orthonormal, since from the symmetry of $\mathbf{A}$ we obtain

$$(\mathbf{I} - 2\mathbf{A})^\top = \mathbf{I}^\top - 2\mathbf{A}^\top = \mathbf{I} - 2\mathbf{A},$$

such that

$$(\mathbf{I} - 2\mathbf{A})(\mathbf{I} - 2\mathbf{A})^\top = (\mathbf{I} - 2\mathbf{A})^2 = \mathbf{I}^2 - 2\mathbf{IA} - 2\mathbf{AI} + 4\mathbf{A}^2$$
$$= \mathbf{I} - 4\mathbf{A} + 4\mathbf{A} = \mathbf{I}.$$

We may obviously note that if $\mathbf{A}$ is orthonormal, then $\mathbf{AA}^\top$ is idempotent: indeed, if $\mathbf{A}$ is orthonormal, then $\mathbf{AA}^\top = \mathbf{AA}^{-1} = \mathbf{I}$, which is necessarily idempotent.

We close this brief analysis of the properties of idempotent matrices by stating that any matrix $\mathbf{X(YX)}^{-1}\mathbf{Y}$ is idempotent. The proof is given by observing that

$$(\mathbf{X(YX)}^{-1}\mathbf{Y})^2 = \mathbf{X(YX)}^{-1}\mathbf{YX(YX)}^{-1}\mathbf{Y} = \mathbf{XI(YX)}^{-1}\mathbf{Y}$$
$$= \mathbf{X(YX)}^{-1}\mathbf{Y},$$

from which we obtain as a corollary the very important property regarding the idempotence of $\mathbf{X(X}^\top\mathbf{X)}^{-1}\mathbf{X}^\top$, since it is enough to substitute $\mathbf{Y}$ with $\mathbf{X}^\top$ to get

$$(\mathbf{X(X}^\top\mathbf{X)}^{-1}\mathbf{X}^\top)^2 = \mathbf{X(X}^\top\mathbf{X)}^{-1}\mathbf{X}^\top\mathbf{X(X}^\top\mathbf{X)}^{-1}\mathbf{X}^\top$$
$$= \mathbf{X(X}^\top\mathbf{X)}^{-1}(\mathbf{X}^\top\mathbf{X})(\mathbf{X}^\top\mathbf{X)}^{-1}\mathbf{X}^\top$$
$$= \mathbf{X(X}^\top\mathbf{X)}^{-1}\mathbf{X}^\top \tag{21.42}$$

which is called the *hat matrix*, and shows a very important property in the framework of linear regression, as we will see soon.

21.34   A Matrix as an Exponent

We were previously dealing with expressions like e^a end $e^{f(x)}$; however, we can have a situation in which a basis (e or other) can be raised to a power represented by a matrix, such that

$$e^{\mathbf{A}} = \exp\begin{pmatrix} a_{11} & \cdots & a_{1n} \\ \vdots & \ddots & \vdots \\ a_{n1} & \cdots & a_{nn} \end{pmatrix}. \tag{21.43}$$

In this case, we can recall the Taylor expansion of e^x, which reads

$$e^x = \frac{x^0}{0!} + \frac{x^1}{1!} + \frac{x^2}{2!} + \cdots + \frac{x^n}{n!} + \cdots$$
$$= x^0 + x^1 + \frac{x^2}{2!} + \cdots + \frac{x^n}{n!} + \cdots,$$

so that, for example,

$$e^5 = 5^0 + 5^1 + \frac{5^2}{2} + \frac{5^3}{6} + \frac{5^4}{24} + \frac{5^5}{120} + \frac{5^6}{720} + \cdots;$$

thus, for a square matrix, we may also write:

$$\exp\begin{pmatrix} a_{11} & \cdots & a_{1n} \\ \vdots & \ddots & \vdots \\ a_{n1} & \cdots & a_{nn} \end{pmatrix} = \frac{1}{0!}\begin{pmatrix} a_{11} & \cdots & a_{1n} \\ \vdots & \ddots & \vdots \\ a_{n1} & \cdots & a_{nn} \end{pmatrix}^{0}$$

$$+ \frac{1}{1!}\begin{pmatrix} a_{11} & \cdots & a_{1n} \\ \vdots & \ddots & \vdots \\ a_{n1} & \cdots & a_{nn} \end{pmatrix}^{1}$$

$$+ \frac{1}{2!}\begin{pmatrix} a_{11} & \cdots & a_{1n} \\ \vdots & \ddots & \vdots \\ a_{n1} & \cdots & a_{nn} \end{pmatrix}^{2}$$

$$+ \cdots + \frac{1}{n!}\begin{pmatrix} a_{11} & \cdots & a_{1n} \\ \vdots & \ddots & \vdots \\ a_{n1} & \cdots & a_{nn} \end{pmatrix}^{n} + \cdots.$$

By the way, if we are dealing with an idempotent matrix **B**, we have:

$$\exp\begin{pmatrix} b_{11} & \cdots & b_{1n} \\ \vdots & \ddots & \vdots \\ b_{n1} & \cdots & b_{nn} \end{pmatrix} = \frac{1}{0!}\begin{pmatrix} b_{11} & \cdots & b_{1n} \\ \vdots & \ddots & \vdots \\ b_{n1} & \cdots & b_{nn} \end{pmatrix}^{0} + \frac{1}{1!}\begin{pmatrix} b_{11} & \cdots & b_{1n} \\ \vdots & \ddots & \vdots \\ b_{n1} & \cdots & b_{nn} \end{pmatrix}$$

$$+ \frac{1}{2!}\begin{pmatrix} b_{11} & \cdots & b_{1n} \\ \vdots & \ddots & \vdots \\ b_{n1} & \cdots & b_{nn} \end{pmatrix} + \cdots + \frac{1}{n!}\begin{pmatrix} b_{11} & \cdots & b_{1n} \\ \vdots & \ddots & \vdots \\ b_{n1} & \cdots & b_{nn} \end{pmatrix} + \cdots.$$

21.35 Involutory Matrices

Any square matrix **A** is said *involutory* if $\mathbf{A}^2 = \mathbf{I}$. We immediately see that if **A** is involutory, then it is also tripotent, since

$$\mathbf{A}^3 = \mathbf{AAA} = \mathbf{A}^2\mathbf{A} = \mathbf{IA} = \mathbf{A},$$

and that $\mathbf{A}^{2n+1} = \mathbf{A}$, for any nonnegative integer n, since

$$\mathbf{A}^{2n+1} = \mathbf{A}^{2n}\mathbf{A} = (\mathbf{A}^2)^n\mathbf{A} = \mathbf{I}^n\mathbf{A} = \mathbf{A}.$$

A trivial example of involutory matrix is the identity matrix **I**. However, as previously done, we may construct an involutory 2×2 matrix knowing that it must be

$$\begin{pmatrix} a & b \\ c & d \end{pmatrix} \begin{pmatrix} a & b \\ c & d \end{pmatrix} = \begin{pmatrix} a^2 + bc & ab + bd \\ ac + cd & d^2 + bc \end{pmatrix} = \begin{pmatrix} 1 & 0 \\ 0 & 1; \end{pmatrix}$$

hence, we must solve the system:

$$\begin{cases} a^2 + bc = 1 \\ ab + bd = 0 \\ ac + cd = 0 \\ d^2 + bc = 1 \end{cases}$$

which has a lot of possible solutions (infinite solutions, indeed), for example,

$$\begin{cases} a = -d \\ b = -\frac{1}{c}\left(d^2 - 1\right) \end{cases} ; \quad \begin{cases} a = \pm 1 \\ c = 0 \\ d = \mp 1 \end{cases} ; \quad \begin{cases} a = \pm 1 \\ b = 0 \\ c = 0 \\ d = -1 \end{cases} .$$

Let us take the second solution, allowing to establish that both matrices

$$\mathbf{A} = \begin{pmatrix} 1 & b \\ 0 & -1 \end{pmatrix}; \quad \mathbf{B} = \begin{pmatrix} -1 & b \\ 0 & 1 \end{pmatrix}$$

are involutory, independently of the value of b (e.g., b can be any number). Indeed,

$$\begin{pmatrix} 1 & b \\ 0 & -1 \end{pmatrix} \begin{pmatrix} 1 & b \\ 0 & -1 \end{pmatrix} = \begin{pmatrix} 1^2 + 0 & b - b \\ 0 - 0 & 0 + (-1)^2 \end{pmatrix}$$

$$= \begin{pmatrix} 1 & 0 \\ 0 & 1 \end{pmatrix},$$

and

$$\begin{pmatrix} -1 & b \\ 0 & 1 \end{pmatrix} \begin{pmatrix} -1 & b \\ 0 & 1 \end{pmatrix} = \begin{pmatrix} (-1)^2 + 0 & -b + b \\ 0 - 0 & 0 + 1^2 \end{pmatrix}$$

$$= \begin{pmatrix} 1 & 0 \\ 0 & 1 \end{pmatrix}.$$

21.36 Nilpotent Matrices

A matrix $\mathbf{N}$ is said *nilpotent of degree k* (or also *nilpotent with index k*) if $\mathbf{N}^k = \mathbf{O}$;
note that since $\mathbf{O}^l = \mathbf{O}$, then also $\mathbf{N}^{k+l} = \mathbf{O}$; hence, k must actually be the smallest

positive integer such that $\mathbf{N}^k = \mathbf{O}$. A trivial example of nilpotent matrix of degree 2 is $\mathbf{O}_n$, since evidently $\mathbf{O}_n^2 = \mathbf{O}_n$.

Less trivial examples (looking at 2×2 matrices) can be obtained considering that we must have

$$\begin{pmatrix} a & b \\ c & d \end{pmatrix}^2 = \begin{pmatrix} a & b \\ c & d \end{pmatrix}\begin{pmatrix} a & b \\ c & d \end{pmatrix}$$

$$= \begin{pmatrix} a^2 + bc & ab + bd \\ ac + cd & d^2 + bc \end{pmatrix} = \begin{pmatrix} 0 & 0 \\ 0 & 0 \end{pmatrix},$$

which is true if

$$\begin{cases} a^2 + bc = 0 \\ ab + bd = 0 \\ ac + cd = 0 \\ d^2 + bc = 0 \end{cases}$$

hence if

$$\begin{cases} a^2 = -bc \\ ab = -bd \\ ac = -cd \\ d^2 = -bc \end{cases} \implies \begin{cases} a^2 = -bc \\ a = -d \end{cases}.$$

For example, if

$$\mathbf{N} = \begin{pmatrix} 2 & -4 \\ 1 & -2 \end{pmatrix}$$

then

$$\mathbf{N}^2 = \begin{pmatrix} 2 & -4 \\ 1 & -2 \end{pmatrix}\begin{pmatrix} 2 & -4 \\ 1 & -2 \end{pmatrix}$$

$$= \begin{pmatrix} 2 \times 2 + (-4) \times 1 & 2 \times (-4) + (-4) \times (-2) \\ 1 \times 2 + (-2) \times 1 & 1 \times (-4) + (-2) \times (-2) \end{pmatrix}$$

$$= \begin{pmatrix} 0 & 0 \\ 0 & 0 \end{pmatrix}.$$

Notable nilpotent matrices are the triangular matrices with zero diagonal entries, like

$$\mathbf{N} = \begin{pmatrix} 0 & a & b \\ 0 & 0 & c \\ 0 & 0 & 0 \end{pmatrix},$$

since

$$\mathbf{N}^2 = \begin{pmatrix} 0 & a & b \\ 0 & 0 & c \\ 0 & 0 & 0 \end{pmatrix} \begin{pmatrix} 0 & a & b \\ 0 & 0 & c \\ 0 & 0 & 0 \end{pmatrix} = \begin{pmatrix} 0 & 0 & ac \\ 0 & 0 & 0 \\ 0 & 0 & 0 \end{pmatrix};$$

attention must be paid to what happened to superdiagonal elements after squaring $\mathbf{N}$; then, raising $\mathbf{N}$ to the third power, we get:

$$\mathbf{N}^3 = \begin{pmatrix} 0 & a & b \\ 0 & 0 & c \\ 0 & 0 & 0 \end{pmatrix} \begin{pmatrix} 0 & 0 & ac \\ 0 & 0 & 0 \\ 0 & 0 & 0 \end{pmatrix} = \begin{pmatrix} 0 & 0 & 0 \\ 0 & 0 & 0 \\ 0 & 0 & 0 \end{pmatrix}.$$

Lastly, note that any $n \times n$ matrix of the form

$$\mathbf{N} = \begin{pmatrix} r_1 & r_1 & \cdots & r_1 \\ r_2 & r_2 & \cdots & r_2 \\ \vdots & \vdots & \ddots & \vdots \\ r_{n-1} & r_{n-1} & \cdots & r_{n-1} \\ -(r_1 + \cdots + r_{n-1}) & -(r_1 + \cdots + r_{n-1}) & \cdots & -(r_1 + \cdots + r_{n-1}) \end{pmatrix}$$

is nilpotent. For example, letting $r_1 = 3$ and $r_2 = -2$, such that $-(r1 + r2) = -(3 - 2) = -1$, we have:

$$\mathbf{N} = \begin{pmatrix} 3 & 3 & 3 \\ -2 & -2 & -2 \\ -1 & -1 & -1 \end{pmatrix}$$

hence

$$\mathbf{N}^2 = \begin{pmatrix} 3 & 3 & 3 \\ -2 & -2 & -2 \\ -1 & -1 & -1 \end{pmatrix} \begin{pmatrix} 3 & 3 & 3 \\ -2 & -2 & -2 \\ -1 & -1 & -1 \end{pmatrix} = \begin{pmatrix} 0 & 0 & 0 \\ 0 & 0 & 0 \\ 0 & 0 & 0 \end{pmatrix}.$$

21.37 Projection Matrices

If we think to a vector $\mathbf{v}$ in $\mathbb{R}^3$, with the origin in the point having co-ordinates $(0, 0, 0)$, we may calculate the projections of the vector over the planes defined by the three Cartesian axes X_1, X_2, X_3, transforming $\mathbf{v}$ in another vector by means of some matrices, called *projection matrices*, obtaining

$$\mathbf{Av} = \begin{pmatrix} 1 & 0 & 0 \\ 0 & 1 & 0 \\ 0 & 0 & 0 \end{pmatrix} \begin{pmatrix} v_1 \\ v_2 \\ v_3 \end{pmatrix} = \begin{pmatrix} v_1 \\ v_2 \\ 0 \end{pmatrix} ;$$

$$\mathbf{Bv} = \begin{pmatrix} 1 & 0 & 0 \\ 0 & 0 & 0 \\ 0 & 0 & 1 \end{pmatrix} \begin{pmatrix} v_1 \\ v_2 \\ v_3 \end{pmatrix} = \begin{pmatrix} v_1 \\ 0 \\ v_3 \end{pmatrix} ;$$

$$\mathbf{Cv} = \begin{pmatrix} 0 & 0 & 0 \\ 0 & 1 & 0 \\ 0 & 0 & 1 \end{pmatrix} \begin{pmatrix} v_1 \\ v_2 \\ v_3 \end{pmatrix} = \begin{pmatrix} 0 \\ v_2 \\ v_3 \end{pmatrix} ,$$

where we see that matrices $\mathbf{A}$, $\mathbf{B}$, and $\mathbf{C}$ used to calculate the orthogonal projections of $\mathbf{v}$ are all idempotent. This should not be surprising, since, even intuitively, the projection of a projection must be equal to itself; in practice, it must be always $\mathbf{AAv} = \mathbf{Av}$, $\mathbf{BBv} = \mathbf{Bv}$, and $\mathbf{CCv} = \mathbf{Cv}$.

21.38 Change of Basis

The problem defined by the change of basis is to find a matrix $\mathbf{M}$ allowing the "translation" of a given vector $\mathbf{v}$ having a basis B (this can be the canonical basis) into a vector $\mathbf{w}$ having another basis B'.

Using the canonical basis

$$B = \left\{ \begin{pmatrix} 1 \\ 0 \\ 0 \end{pmatrix} , \begin{pmatrix} 0 \\ 1 \\ 0 \end{pmatrix} , \begin{pmatrix} 0 \\ 0 \\ 1 \end{pmatrix} \right\}$$

and a new arbitrary basis

$$B' = \left\{ \begin{pmatrix} 1 \\ 1 \\ 1 \end{pmatrix} , \begin{pmatrix} 3 \\ 1 \\ 2 \end{pmatrix} , \begin{pmatrix} 0 \\ 2 \\ -1 \end{pmatrix} \right\}$$

we can ask how an arbitrary vector having basis B, say

$$\mathbf{a} = \begin{pmatrix} 3 \\ 4 \\ 5 \end{pmatrix},$$

can be expressed using the new basis B'.

We may solve the linear system:

$$x \begin{pmatrix} 1 \\ 1 \\ 1 \end{pmatrix} + y \begin{pmatrix} 3 \\ 1 \\ 2 \end{pmatrix} + z \begin{pmatrix} 0 \\ 2 \\ -1 \end{pmatrix} = \begin{pmatrix} 3 \\ 4 \\ 5 \end{pmatrix},$$

so that

$$\begin{cases} x + 3y = 3 \\ x + y + 2z = 4 \\ x + 2y - z = 5 \end{cases},$$

with solution

$$\begin{cases} x = \frac{27}{4} \\ y = -\frac{5}{4} \\ z = -\frac{3}{4} \end{cases},$$

but we can also search for the components of the canonical basis B with respect to the new basis B'; in other words, we can search for a matrix governing the change of basis.

Let us assume to have, in the same n-dimensional vector space $\mathbb{V}$, two basis defined as

$$B = \{e_1, e_2, \ldots, e_n\},$$
$$B' = \{\varepsilon_1, \varepsilon_2, \ldots, \varepsilon_n\};$$

in this case we can use the matrix for the change of basis to get from the vector components given for the basis B, the components for the basis B'. If $\mathbf{x}$ is the vector with basis B, then $\mathbf{Px}$ will be the same vector with basis B' and $\mathbf{QPx}$ will be the transformation giving back the vector $\mathbf{x}$. Obviously, if $\mathbf{QPx} = \mathbf{x}$, then $\mathbf{QP} = \mathbf{I}$, so that $\mathbf{Q} = \mathbf{P}^{-1}$.

21.39 Prevalence of a Chronic Disease

Matrices are also good tools for the study of people immigration and emigration, and in general for population dynamics. For this aim, we try to analyze the distribution of a given chronic disease (say, diabetes) among the population of a city. To be simple, no immigration and emigration processes are involved, and we assume that population will be constant, without births and deaths.

Thus, let us assume that at year $y = 0$, the healthy subjects are 85% of the city population, so that diabetics are 15% (the data are of pure invention and do not refer to any screening for this disease, nor to any epidemiological data), and we may describe this diabetes prevalence at year zero with the vector:

$$\mathbf{d}_{y=0} = \begin{pmatrix} 0.85 \\ 0.15 \end{pmatrix}.$$

Let us now assume that, on an annual basis, 5% of healthy individuals become diabetic, and 2% of diabetic individuals can recover and become healthy (again, the data are of pure invention). This may be represented by a "diabetes dynamics matrix" as follows:

$$\mathbf{D} = \begin{pmatrix} 0.95 & 0.02 \\ 0.05 & 0.98 \end{pmatrix}$$

and we assume that in our very simple simulation, disease dynamics data do not change along time; thus, the frequency of the new ill subjects and those of recovered ones remains constant.

With these premises, we expect that at year $y = 1$ the prevalence of disease will be as follows.

$$\mathbf{D}\mathbf{d}_{y=0} = \begin{pmatrix} 0.95 & 0.02 \\ 0.05 & 0.98 \end{pmatrix} \begin{pmatrix} 0.85 \\ 0.15 \end{pmatrix}$$

$$= \begin{pmatrix} 0.811 \\ 0.190 \end{pmatrix} = \mathbf{d}_{y=1}$$

so, the prevalence of diabetes arises from 15% to about 19%, and in the following year, we will have as follows.

$$\mathbf{D}\mathbf{d}_{y=1} = \begin{pmatrix} 0.95 & 0.02 \\ 0.05 & 0.98 \end{pmatrix} \begin{pmatrix} 0.811 \\ 0.190 \end{pmatrix}$$

$$= \begin{pmatrix} 0.774 \\ 0.226 \end{pmatrix} = \mathbf{d}_{y=2}$$

and the prevalence of ill subjects increases from about 19% to about 22.6%. Note that if we calculate the prevalence after 2 years, using $\mathbf{D}^2$ we get the following.

$$\mathbf{D}^2\mathbf{d}_{y=0} = \begin{pmatrix} 0.95 & 0.02 \\ 0.05 & 0.98 \end{pmatrix}^2 \begin{pmatrix} 0.85 \\ 0.15 \end{pmatrix}$$

$$= \begin{pmatrix} 0.774 \\ 0.226 \end{pmatrix} = \mathbf{d}_{y=2},$$

thus obtaining the same result. Hence, for example, we may guess the prevalence after 4 years as follows.

$$\mathbf{D}^4\mathbf{d}_{y=0} = \begin{pmatrix} 0.95 & 0.02 \\ 0.05 & 0.98 \end{pmatrix}^4 \begin{pmatrix} 0.85 \\ 0.15 \end{pmatrix}$$

$$= \begin{pmatrix} 0.708 \\ 0.292 \end{pmatrix} = \mathbf{d}_{y=4},$$

with a diabetes prevalence of more than 29%. Therefore, in general, after n years we will have

$$\mathbf{D}^n\mathbf{d}_{y=0} = \mathbf{d}_{y=n}$$

where $\mathbf{D}$ is the matrix reporting the disease dynamics, here assumed to be constant (but working with a variable matrix will be equally simple), $\mathbf{d}_{y=0}$ and $\mathbf{d}_{y=n}$ are the vectors giving the prevalence at year zero and after n years, respectively.

This kind of modeling has very general purposes: it can describe the individual interrelationships in many situations changing over time, like the evolution of wealth, the dynamics of the social classes of citizens, the processes of immigration and emigration, and many other types of analysis, involving social, economical, and epidemiological developments.

References

1. Banerjee S, Roy A. Linear algebra and matrix analysis for statistics. Boca Raton: CRC Press; 2014.
2. Brown WC. Matrices and vector spaces. New York: Marcel Dekker, Inc.; 1991.

Matrix Differentiation

22

Matrix differentiation deals with the differential calculus involving matrices and vectors (which are $n \times 1$ matrices). The differentiation of the functions with vector or matrix argument will be of great importance when treating some matrix calculus issues dealing with regression and other statistical methods. When needed, we will tacitly assume that vectors and matrices combined in the various products to be differentiated are conformable.

We already met vector functions $\vec{f}$ of a real variable, which can be also indicated by $\mathbf{f}(x)$, or by $\mathbf{f}_n(x)$ when if it is necessary to specify that the vector function has n dimensions. A matrix function $\mathbf{F}_{m \times n}(x)$ is a matrix of functions $f_{jk}(x)$ of a real variable arranged in m rows and n columns. A vector and a matrix function of a real variable x can be given respectively as

$$
\mathbf{f}(x) = \begin{pmatrix} f_1(x) \\ f_2(x) \\ \vdots \\ f_n(x) \end{pmatrix} ; \quad \mathbf{F}(x) = \begin{pmatrix} f_{11}(x) & f_{12}(x) & \cdots & f_{1n}(x) \\ f_{21}(x) & f_{22}(x) & \cdots & f_{2n}(x) \\ \vdots & \vdots & \ddots & \vdots \\ f_{m1}(x) & f_{m2}(x) & \cdots & f_{mn}(x) \end{pmatrix} .
$$

First, we define the derivative of an m-dimensional vector $\mathbf{y}$ with respect to an n-dimensional vector $\mathbf{x}$ as the $m \times n$ matrix:

$$
\frac{\partial \mathbf{y}}{\partial \mathbf{x}} = \begin{pmatrix} \partial_{x_1} y_1 & \partial_{x_2} y_2 & \cdots & \partial_{x_n} y_m \\ \partial_{x_1} y_2 & \partial_{x_2} y_2 & \cdots & \partial_{x_n} y_m \\ \vdots & \vdots & \ddots & \vdots \\ \partial_{x_1} y_m & \partial_{x_2} y_m & \cdots & \partial_{x_n} y_m \end{pmatrix} \tag{22.1}
$$

By the way, we note that in the case of scalar y, then $\frac{\partial y}{\partial \mathbf{x}}$ would become an m-dimensional row vector, while in the case of scalar x, then $\frac{\partial \mathbf{y}}{\partial x}$ would become an

© The Author(s), under exclusive license to Springer Nature Switzerland AG 2025
M. Nichelatti, *Mathematical Tools for Telemedicine*, TELe-Health,
https://doi.org/10.1007/978-3-031-81709-0_22

n-dimensional column vector. Clearly, with both y and x scalars, $\frac{\partial y}{\partial x}$ will become the usual derivative $\frac{\partial y}{\partial x}$.

For example, let us take the linear system:

$$\begin{cases} y_1 = 2x_1^3 - 4 \\ y_2 = -x_1^2 + 3x_2 \\ y_3 = x_1 - 5x_2^3 \end{cases} \tag{22.2}$$

where the function $\mathbf{y}$ is a three-dimensional vector, whose values are defined by means of the elements of a two-dimensional vector $\mathbf{x}$. According to definition (22.1), the derivative will be the 3×2 matrix:

$$\frac{\partial \mathbf{y}}{\partial \mathbf{x}} = \begin{pmatrix} \partial_{x_1} y_1 & \partial_{x_2} y_1 \\ \partial_{x_1} y_2 & \partial_{x_2} y_2 \\ \partial_{x_1} y_3 & \partial_{x_2} y_3 \end{pmatrix}$$

$$= \begin{pmatrix} \partial_{x_1}(2x_1^3 - 4) & \partial_{x_2}(2x_1^3 - 4) \\ \partial_{x_1}(-x_1^2 + 3x_2) & \partial_{x_2}(-x_1^2 + 3x_2) \\ \partial_{x_1}(x_1 - 5x_2^3) & \partial_{x_2}(x_1 - 5x_2^3) \end{pmatrix}$$

$$= \begin{pmatrix} 6x^2 & 0 \\ -2x_1 & 3 \\ 1 & -15x_2^2 \end{pmatrix}.$$

The $m \times n$ matrix in (22.1) is called the *Jacobian*, which could be better defined, for a vector function:

$$\mathbf{y} = \mathbf{f}(\mathbf{x}) = \begin{pmatrix} f_1(\mathbf{x}) \\ f_2(\mathbf{x}) \\ \vdots \\ f_m(\mathbf{x}) \end{pmatrix}$$

using the notation

$$\mathbf{J} = \frac{\partial \mathbf{f}(\mathbf{x})}{\partial \mathbf{x}} = \begin{pmatrix} \partial_{x_1} f_1(\mathbf{x}) & \partial_{x_2} f_1(\mathbf{x}) & \cdots & \partial_{x_n} f_1(\mathbf{x}) \\ \partial_{x_1} f_2(\mathbf{x}) & \partial_{x_2} f_2(\mathbf{x}) & \cdots & \partial_{x_n} f_2(\mathbf{x}) \\ \vdots & \vdots & \ddots & \vdots \\ \partial_{x_1} f_m(\mathbf{x}) & \partial_{x_2} f_m(\mathbf{x}) & \cdots & \partial_{x_n} f_m(\mathbf{x}) \end{pmatrix}$$

$$= \nabla \mathbf{f}(\mathbf{x}),$$

where ∇ is the nabla operator. In a square matrix, e.g., if $\mathbf{f}$ and $\mathbf{x}$ have the same dimensions, the determinant of the Jacobian is an important tool for the change of basis in a vector space.

Now, a precisation is needed. A great amount of textbooks uses the present definition, such that with a scalar $\mathbf{y}$, $\frac{\partial y}{\partial \mathbf{x}}$ is a row vector, but an equivalent amount uses the opposite definition, such that, if $\mathbf{y}$ is a scalar, then $\frac{\partial y}{\partial \mathbf{x}}$ would be a column vector: let us call the first kind of assumption, the *numerator layout* (nl), and the second the *denominator layout* (dl) [1, 2]. There are some reasons to prefer either the first or the second notation: here we will use the numerator, since it seems more natural, having to deal with a system of equations, to list the y_k as a column, like we did in the example (22.2).

Anyway, for completeness, we give the definition also according to the denominator layout as follows:

$$\left.\frac{\partial \mathbf{y}}{\partial \mathbf{x}}\right|_{dl} = \begin{pmatrix} \partial_{x_1} y_1 & \partial_{x_1} y_2 & \cdots & \partial_{x_1} y_m \\ \partial_{x_2} y_1 & \partial_{x_2} y_2 & \cdots & \partial_{x_n} y_m \\ \vdots & \vdots & \ddots & \vdots \\ \partial_{x_n} y_1 & \partial_{x_n} y_2 & \cdots & \partial_{x_n} y_m \end{pmatrix}$$

where we see that the matrix is the transpose of (22.1). To see what this can mean in terms of results, we again use the system (22.2), to obtain the 2×3 matrix:

$$\left.\frac{\partial \mathbf{y}}{\partial \mathbf{x}}\right|_{dl} = \begin{pmatrix} \partial_{x_1}(2x_1^3 - 4) & \partial_{x_1}(-x_1^2 + 3x_2) & \partial_{x_1}(x_1 - 5x_2^3) \\ \partial_{x_2}(2x_1^3 - 4) & \partial_{x_2}(-x_1^2 + 3x_2) & \partial_{x_2}(x_1 - 5x_2^3) \end{pmatrix}$$

$$= \begin{pmatrix} 6x_1^2 & -2x_1 & 1 \\ 0 & 3 & -15x_2^2 \end{pmatrix},$$

which, as expected, is the transpose of the matrix obtained using the numerator layout.

The second definition is the derivative of a scalar y with respect to a vector $\mathbf{x}$, given as follows:

$$\frac{\partial y}{\partial \mathbf{x}} = \begin{pmatrix} \partial_{x_1} y & \partial_{x_2} y & \cdots & \partial_{x_n} y \end{pmatrix}, \tag{22.3}$$

thus as a row vector having components $\partial_{x_k} y$, e.g., the derivatives of the scalar with respect to the single components of $\mathbf{x}$. This form is coherent with the definition of the matrix (22.1), since it has the same form of a row vector of that matrix. Here also the definition found in some textbooks may be in the form of column vector.

Generalizing equation (22.3), we may define the derivative of a scalar with respect to a $m \times n$ matrix as follows:

$$\frac{\partial y}{\partial \mathbf{X}} = \begin{pmatrix} \partial_{x_{11}} y & \partial_{x_{12}} y & \cdots & \partial_{x_{1n}} y \\ \partial_{x_{21}} y & \partial_{x_{22}} y & \cdots & \partial_{x_{2n}} y \\ \vdots & \vdots & \ddots & \vdots \\ \partial_{x_{m1}} y & \partial_{x_{m2}} y & \cdots & \partial_{x_{mn}} y \end{pmatrix} \tag{22.4}$$

We can now define the derivative of a vector $\mathbf{y}$ with respect to a scalar x, which, again according to (22.1), must be written as

$$\frac{\partial \mathbf{y}}{\partial x} = \begin{pmatrix} \partial_x y_1 \\ \partial_x y_2 \\ \vdots \\ \partial_x y_m \end{pmatrix}, \tag{22.5}$$

which is again coherent with the definition since it is in the form of a column vector of the matrix (22.1). However, one always must bear in mind that in some textbooks this would be given as a row vector.

The generalization of Eq. (22.5) leads to the definition of the derivative of a $m \times n$ matrix with respect to a scalar in the form:

$$\frac{\partial \mathbf{A}}{\partial x} = \begin{pmatrix} \partial_x \alpha_{11} & \partial_x \alpha_{12} & \cdots & \partial_x \alpha_{1n} \\ \partial_x \alpha_{21} & \partial_x \alpha_{22} & \cdots & \partial_x \alpha_{2n} \\ \vdots & \vdots & \ddots & \vdots \\ \partial_x \alpha_{m1} & \partial_x \alpha_{m2} & \cdots & \partial_x \alpha_{mn} \end{pmatrix}, \tag{22.6}$$

always considering that some textbooks will define this derivative using the denominator layout.

In general, using the matrix $\mathbf{M}_{m \times n}$ as the definition of one of the above differentiation with the numerator layout (again, considering that a vector is a $m \times 1$ matrix), the corresponding matrix with the denominator layout will be $\mathbf{M}_{n \times m}^{\top} = \mathbf{M}_{m \times n}$.

In most cases, the derivative with the denominator layout is the transpose of the derivative with the numerator layout; indeed, as we will soon verify, using the numerator layout, we have:

$$\frac{\partial (\mathbf{y}^{\top} \mathbf{x})}{\partial \mathbf{x}} = \mathbf{y}^{\top},$$

while with the denominator layout the result is

$$\frac{\partial (\mathbf{y}^{\top} \mathbf{x})}{\partial \mathbf{x}} \bigg|_{\text{dl}} = \mathbf{y}.$$

Sometimes the result would be a bit different, since with the numerator layout the derivative of a quadratic form is

$$\frac{\partial(\mathbf{x}^\top \mathbf{M} \mathbf{x})}{\partial \mathbf{x}} = \mathbf{x}^\top (\mathbf{M} + \mathbf{M}^\top)$$

while in the denominator layout, we read the result from left:

$$\left.\frac{\partial(\mathbf{x}^\top \mathbf{M} \mathbf{x})}{\partial \mathbf{x}}\right|_{\mathrm{dl}} = (\mathbf{M} + \mathbf{M}^\top)\mathbf{x}^\top ;$$

the same inverted reading we find when dealing with the chain rule: in the numerator layout, it is

$$\frac{\partial \mathbf{f}(\mathbf{g}(\mathbf{y}))}{\partial \mathbf{x}} = \frac{\partial \mathbf{f}(\mathbf{g})}{\partial \mathbf{g}} \frac{\partial \mathbf{g}(\mathbf{y})}{\partial \mathbf{y}} \frac{\partial \mathbf{y}}{\partial \mathbf{x}},$$

whereas, in the denominator layout, we have:

$$\left.\frac{\partial \mathbf{f}(\mathbf{g}(\mathbf{y}))}{\partial \mathbf{x}}\right|_{\mathrm{dl}} = \frac{\partial \mathbf{y}}{\partial \mathbf{x}} \frac{\partial \mathbf{g}(\mathbf{y})}{\partial \mathbf{y}} \frac{\partial \mathbf{f}(\mathbf{g})}{\partial \mathbf{g}} ;$$

thus, a lot of attention must be paid using the different layouts. In particular, the same layout must always be maintained along all the calculus.

22.1 Differentiation of a Linear Form

As first example, we consider the linear form $\mathbf{y}^\top \mathbf{x}$, and take the derivative with respect to the vector $\mathbf{x}$. Since it is the derivative of a scalar, so we invoke definition (22.3) to obtain

$$
\begin{aligned}
\frac{\partial(\mathbf{y}^\top \mathbf{x})}{\partial \mathbf{x}} &= \left(\partial_{x_1}\left(\textstyle\sum_{k=1}^n y_k x_k\right) \cdots \partial_{x_n}\left(\textstyle\sum_{k=1}^n y_k x_k\right)\right) \\
&= \left(\partial_{x_1}(y_1 x_1 + \cdots + y_n x_n) \cdots \partial_{x_n}(y_1 x_1 + \cdots + y_n x_n)\right) \\
&= \left(\partial_{x_1}(y_1 x_1) + \cdots + \partial_{x_1}(y_n x_n) \cdots \partial_{x_n}(y_1 x_1) + \cdots + \partial_{x_n}(y_n x_n)\right) \\
&= \left(y_1 + 0 + \cdots + 0\ 0 + y_2 + \cdots + 0 \cdots 0 + 0 + \cdots + y_n\right) \\
&= \left(y_1\ y_2 \cdots y_n\right) \\
&= \mathbf{y}^\top .
\end{aligned}
\tag{22.7}
$$

Moreover, since $\mathbf{y}^\top \mathbf{x}$ is a scalar, it is $\mathbf{y}^\top \mathbf{x} = (\mathbf{y}^\top \mathbf{x})^\top = \mathbf{y}^\top \mathbf{x}$; thus:

$$\frac{\partial (\mathbf{x}^\top \mathbf{y})}{\partial \mathbf{x}} = \frac{\partial (\mathbf{y}^\top \mathbf{x})}{\partial \mathbf{x}} = \mathbf{y}^\top, \tag{22.8}$$

as expected.

By the way, we see that assuming to use the denominator layout, the result would be

$$\frac{\partial (\mathbf{y}^\top \mathbf{x})}{\partial \mathbf{x}} = \begin{pmatrix} \partial_{x_1} (y_1 x_1 + y_2 x_2 + \cdots + y_n x_n) \\ \vdots \\ \partial_{x_n} (y_1 x_1 + y_2 x_2 + \cdots + y_n x_n) \end{pmatrix}$$

$$= \begin{pmatrix} \partial_{x_1} (y_1 x_1) + \partial_{x_1} (y_2 x_2) + \cdots + \partial_{x_1} (y_n x_n) \\ \vdots \\ \partial_{x_n} (y_1 x_1) + \partial_{xn} (y_2 x_2) + \cdots + \partial_{x_n} (y_n x_n) \end{pmatrix}$$

$$= \begin{pmatrix} y_1 + 0 + \cdots + 0 \\ 0 + y_2 + \cdots + 0 \\ \vdots \\ 0 + 0 + \cdots + y_n \end{pmatrix} = \begin{pmatrix} y_1 \\ y_2 \\ \vdots \\ y_n \end{pmatrix}$$

$$= \mathbf{y};$$

hence, the result is actually the transpose of the result obtained with the numerator layout.

We also note that

$$\frac{\partial (\mathbf{x}^\top \mathbf{x})}{\partial \mathbf{x}} = \left(\partial_{x_1} \left(\sum_{k=1}^n x_k^2 \right) \cdots \partial_{x_n} \left(\sum_{k=1}^n x_k^2 \right) \right)$$

$$= \left(\partial_{x_1} (x_1^2 + \cdots + x_n^2) \cdots \partial_{x_n} (x_1^2 + \cdots + x_n^2) \right)$$

$$= \left(\partial_{x_1} x_1^2 + \cdots + \partial_{x_1} x_n^2 \cdots \partial_{x_n} x_1^2 + \cdots + \partial_{x_n} x_n^2 \right)$$

$$= \left(2x_1 + 0 + \cdots + 0 \; 0 + 2x_2^2 + \cdots + 0 \cdots 0 + 0 + \cdots + 2x_n^2 \right)$$

$$= \left(2x_1 \; 2x_2 \cdots 2x_n \right)$$

$$= 2\mathbf{x}^\top, \tag{22.9}$$

and using the denominator layout

$$\frac{\partial(\mathbf{x}^\top \mathbf{x})}{\partial \mathbf{x}} = \begin{pmatrix} \partial_{x_1}\left(\sum_{k=1}^n x_k^2\right) \\ \vdots \\ \partial_{x_n}\left(\sum_{k=1}^n x_k^2\right) \end{pmatrix}$$

$$= \begin{pmatrix} \partial_{x_1}x_1^2 + \cdots + \partial_{x_1}x_n^2 \\ \vdots \\ \partial_{x_n}x_1^2 + \cdots + \partial_{x_n}x_n^2) \end{pmatrix}$$

$$= \begin{pmatrix} 2x_1 + 0 + \cdots + 0 \\ 0 + 2x_2 + \cdots + 0 \\ \vdots \\ 0 + 0 + \cdots + 2x_n^2 \end{pmatrix}$$

$$= \begin{pmatrix} 2x_1 \\ 2x_2 \\ \vdots \\ 2x_n \end{pmatrix}$$

$$= 2\mathbf{x}.$$

If, on the other hand, we have both $\mathbf{x}$ and $\mathbf{y}$ functions of another vector $\mathbf{z}$, the derivative of the linear form with respect to $\mathbf{z}$ is

$$\frac{\partial(\mathbf{x}^\top \mathbf{y})}{\partial \mathbf{z}} = \partial_{\mathbf{z}}\left(\sum_{k=1}^n x_k y_k\right)$$

$$= \partial_{\mathbf{z}}(x_1 y_1 + \cdots + x_n y_n)$$

$$= \left(\partial_{z_1}(x_1 y_1 + \cdots + x_n y_n) \cdots \partial_{z_n}(x_1 y_1 + x_2 y_2 + \cdots + x_n y_n)\right)$$

$$= \left(\partial_{z_1}(x_1 y_1) + \cdots + \partial_{z_1}(x_n y_n) \cdots \partial_{z_n}(x_1 y_1) + \cdots + \partial_{z_n}(x_n y_n)\right)$$

$$= \left(x_1 \partial_{z_1} y_1 + y_1 \partial_{z_1} x_1 + \cdots + x_n \partial_{z_1} y_n + y_n \partial_{z_1} x_n \cdots x_1 \partial_{z_n} y_1\right)$$

$$= \left(x_1 \partial_{z_1} y_1 + y_1 \partial_{z_1} x_1 + \cdots + x_n \partial_{z_1} y_n + y_n \partial_{z_1} x_n \cdots x_1 \partial_{z_n} y_1\right.$$

$$\left. + y_1 \partial_{z_n} x_1 + \cdots + x_n \partial_{z_n} y_n + y_n \partial_{z_n} x_n\right)$$

$$= \left(\sum_{k=1}^n \left(x_k \partial_{z_1} y_k + y_k \partial_{z_1} x_k\right) \cdots \sum_{k=1}^n \left(x_k \partial_{z_n} y_k + y_k \partial_{z_n} x_k\right)\right)$$

$$= \left(\sum_{k=1}^n x_k \partial_{z_1} y_k + \sum_{k=1}^n y_k \partial_{z_1} x_k \cdots \sum_{k=1}^n x_k \partial_{z_n} y_k + \sum_{k=1}^n y_k \partial_{z_n} x_k\right)$$

$$= \left(x_1 \cdots x_n\right)\begin{pmatrix} \partial_{z_1} y_1 & \cdots & \partial_{z_n} y_1 \\ \vdots & \ddots & \vdots \\ \partial_{z_1} y_n & \cdots & \partial_{z_n} y_n \end{pmatrix} + \left(y_1 \cdots y_n\right)\begin{pmatrix} \partial_{z_1} x_1 & \cdots & \partial_{z_n} x_1 \\ \vdots & \ddots & \vdots \\ \partial_{z_1} x_n & \cdots & \partial_{z_n} x_n \end{pmatrix}$$

hence

$$\frac{\partial \left(\mathbf{x}^\top \mathbf{y}\right)}{\partial \mathbf{z}} = \mathbf{x}^\top \frac{\partial \mathbf{y}}{\partial \mathbf{z}} + \mathbf{y}^\top \frac{\partial \mathbf{x}}{\partial \mathbf{z}}, \qquad (22.10)$$

and if $\mathbf{x} = \mathbf{y}$, then

$$\frac{\partial \left(\mathbf{x}^\top \mathbf{x}\right)}{\partial \mathbf{z}} = \mathbf{x}^\top \frac{\partial \mathbf{x}}{\partial \mathbf{z}} + \mathbf{x}^\top \frac{\partial \mathbf{x}}{\partial \mathbf{z}}$$

$$= 2\mathbf{x}^\top \frac{\partial \mathbf{x}}{\partial \mathbf{z}}. \qquad (22.11)$$

22.2   Differentiation of a Linear Transformation

The derivative of the linear transformation $\mathbf{y}_m = \mathbf{A}_{m \times n} \mathbf{x}_n$ with respect to $\mathbf{x}$, assuming that $\mathbf{A}$ is not a function of $\mathbf{x}$, can be obtained using the generic element:

$$y_j = \sum_{k=1}^{n} a_{jk} x_k, \qquad (22.12)$$

of the transformed vector $\mathbf{y}$, so as to have

$$\frac{\partial \left(\mathbf{A}\mathbf{x}\right)}{\partial \mathbf{x}} = \begin{pmatrix} \partial_\mathbf{x} \left(\sum_{k=1}^{n} a_{jk} x_k\right) \\ \partial_\mathbf{x} \left(\sum_{k=1}^{n} a_{jk} x_k\right) \\ \vdots \\ \partial_\mathbf{x} \left(\sum_{k=1}^{n} a_{jk} x_k\right) \end{pmatrix}$$

$$= \begin{pmatrix} \partial_\mathbf{x} \left(a_{11} x_1 + \cdots + a_{1n} x_n\right) \\ \partial_\mathbf{x} \left(a_{21} x_1 + \cdots + a_{2n} x_n\right) \\ \vdots \\ \partial_\mathbf{x} \left(a_{m1} x_1 + \cdots + a_{mn} x_n\right) \end{pmatrix}$$

$$= \begin{pmatrix} \partial_{x_1} \left(a_{11} x_1 + \cdots + a_{1n} x_n\right) & \cdots & \partial_{x_n} \left(a_{11} x_1 + \cdots + a_{1n} x_n\right) \\ \partial_{x_1} \left(a_{21} x_1 + \cdots + a_{2n} x_n\right) & \cdots & \partial_{x_n} \left(a_{21} x_1 + \cdots + a_{2n} x_n\right) \\ \vdots & \ddots & \vdots \\ \partial_{x_1} \left(a_{m1} x_1 + \cdots + a_{mn} x_n\right) & \cdots & \partial_{x_n} \left(a_{m1} x_1 + \cdots + a_{mn} x_n\right) \end{pmatrix}$$

$$= \begin{pmatrix} a_{11} + 0 + \cdots + 0 & \cdots & 0 + 0 + \cdots + a_{1n} \\ a_{21} + 0 + \cdots + 0 & \cdots & 0 + 0 + \cdots + a_{2n} \\ \vdots & \ddots & \vdots \\ a_{m1} + 0 + \cdots + 0 & \cdots & 0 + 0 + \cdots + a_{mn} \end{pmatrix}$$

$$= \begin{pmatrix} a_{11} & a_{12} & \cdots & a_{1n} \\ a_{21} & a_{22} & \cdots & a_{2n} \\ \vdots & \vdots & \ddots & \vdots \\ a_{m1} & a_{m2} & \cdots & a_{mn} \end{pmatrix},$$

hence

$$\frac{\partial (\mathbf{A}\mathbf{v})}{\partial \mathbf{x}} = \mathbf{A}.$$

The derivative of $\mathbf{y}_m = \mathbf{A}_{m \times n}\mathbf{x}_n$ with respect to a vector $\mathbf{w}_n$, if $\mathbf{x}$ is a function of $\mathbf{w}$, again using (22.12), can be obtained as

$$\frac{\partial (\mathbf{A}\mathbf{x})}{\partial \mathbf{w}} = \begin{pmatrix} \partial_{\mathbf{w}} (a_{11}x_1 + \cdots + a_{1n}x_n) \\ \partial_{\mathbf{w}} (a_{21}x_1 + \cdots + a_{2n}x_n) \\ \vdots \\ \partial_{\mathbf{w}} (a_{m1}x_1 + \cdots + a_{mn}x_n) \end{pmatrix}$$

$$= \begin{pmatrix} \partial_{w_1} (a_{11}x_1 + \cdots + a_{1n}x_n) & \cdots & \partial_{w_n} (a_{11}x_1 + \cdots + a_{1n}x_n) \\ \partial_{w_1} (a_{21}x_1 + \cdots + a_{2n}x_n) & \cdots & \partial_{w_n} (a_{21}x_1 + \cdots + a_{2n}x_n) \\ \vdots & \ddots & \vdots \\ \partial_{w_1} (a_{m1}x_1 + \cdots + a_{mn}x_n) & \cdots & \partial_{w_n} (a_{m1}x_1 + \cdots + a_{mn}x_n) \end{pmatrix}$$

$$= \begin{pmatrix} a_{11}\partial_{w_1}x_1 + \cdots + a_{1n}\partial_{w_1}x_n & \cdots & a_{11}\partial_{w_n}x_1 + \cdots + a_{mn}\partial_{w_n}x_m \\ a_{21}\partial_{w_1}x_1 + \cdots + a_{2n}\partial_{w_1}x_n & \cdots & a_{21}\partial_{w_n}x_1 + \cdots + a_{mn}\partial_{w_n}x_m \\ \vdots & \ddots & \vdots \\ a_{m1}\partial_{w_1}x_1 + \cdots + a_{mn}\partial_{w_1}x_n & \cdots & a_{m1}\partial_{w_n}x_1 + \cdots + a_{mn}\partial_{w_n}x_m \end{pmatrix}$$

$$= \begin{pmatrix} a_{11} & a_{12} & \cdots & a_{1n} \\ a_{21} & a_{22} & \cdots & a_{2n} \\ \vdots & \vdots & \ddots & \vdots \\ a_{m1} & a_{m2} & \cdots & a_{mn} \end{pmatrix} \begin{pmatrix} \partial_{w_1}x_1 & \partial_{w_2}x_1 & \cdots & \partial_{w_n}x_1 \\ \partial_{w_1}x_2 & \partial_{w_2}x_2 & \cdots & \partial_{w_n}x_2 \\ \vdots & \vdots & \ddots & \vdots \\ \partial_{w_1}x_n & \partial_{w_2}x_n & \cdots & \partial_{w_n}x_n \end{pmatrix},$$

hence

$$\frac{\partial (\mathbf{A}\mathbf{x})}{\partial \mathbf{w}} = \mathbf{A}\frac{\partial \mathbf{x}}{\partial \mathbf{w}}.$$

22.3   Differentiation of Bilinear and Quadratic Forms

The derivative of the bilinear form $\mathbf{x}_{1 \times m}^{\top} \mathbf{A}_{m \times n} \mathbf{y}_{n \times 1}$ with respect to $\mathbf{y}$, assuming that $\mathbf{A}$ is not a function of $\mathbf{y}$, may be obtained bearing in mind that

$$
\mathbf{x}^{\top} \mathbf{A} \mathbf{y} = \begin{pmatrix} x_1 & x_2 & \cdots & x_m \end{pmatrix} \begin{pmatrix} a_{11} & a_{12} & \cdots & a_{1n} \\ a_{21} & a_{22} & \cdots & a_{2n} \\ \vdots & \vdots & \ddots & \vdots \\ a_{m1} & a_{m2} & \cdots & a_{mn} \end{pmatrix} \begin{pmatrix} y_1 \\ y_2 \\ \vdots \\ y_n \end{pmatrix}
$$

$$
= \sum_{k=1}^{n} \left(\sum_{j=1}^{n} a_{jk} x_j \right) y_k,
$$

from which

$$
\frac{\partial (\mathbf{x}^{\top} \mathbf{A} \mathbf{y})}{\partial \mathbf{y}} = \partial_{\mathbf{y}} \left(\sum_{k=1}^{n} \left(\sum_{j=1}^{n} a_{jk} x_j \right) y_k \right)
$$

$$
= \partial_{\mathbf{y}} y_1 \left(x_1 a_{11} + \cdots + x_m a_{m1} \right) + \partial_{\mathbf{y}} y_2 \left(x_1 a_{12} + \cdots + x_m a_{m2} \right)
$$

$$
+ \cdots + \partial_{\mathbf{y}} y_n \left(x_1 a_{1n} + \cdots + x_m a_{mn} \right)
$$

$$
= \left(\partial_{y_1} \left(x_1 a_{11} + \cdots + x_m a_{m1} \right) y_1 \cdots \partial_{y_n} \left(x_1 a_{11} + \cdots + x_m a_{m1} \right) y_1 \right)
$$

$$
+ \left(\partial_{y_1} \left(x_1 a_{12} + \cdots + x_m a_{m2} \right) y_2 \cdots \partial_{y_n} \left(x_1 a_{12} + \cdots + x_m a_{m2} \right) y_2 \right)
$$

$$
+ \cdots + \left(\partial_{y_1} \left(x_1 a_{1n} + \cdots + x_m a_{mn} \right) y_n \cdots \partial_{y_n} \left(x_1 a_{1n} + \cdots + x_m a_{mn} \right) y_n \right)
$$

$$
= \left(\left(x_1 a_{11} + \cdots + x_m a_{m1} \right) 0 \cdots 0 \right)
$$

$$
+ \left(0 \left(x_1 a_{12} + \cdots + x_m a_{m2} \right) \cdots 0 \right)
$$

$$
+ \cdots + \left(0 \; 0 \cdots \left(x_1 a_{1n} + \cdots + x_m a_{mn} \right) \right)
$$

$$
= \begin{pmatrix} x_1 & x_2 & \cdots & x_m \end{pmatrix} \begin{pmatrix} a_{11} & a_{12} & \cdots & a_{1n} \\ a_{21} & a_{22} & \cdots & a_{2n} \\ \vdots & \vdots & \ddots & \vdots \\ a_{m1} & a_{m2} & \cdots & a_{mn} \end{pmatrix}
$$

hence

$$
\frac{\partial \left(\mathbf{x}^{\top} \mathbf{A} \mathbf{y} \right)}{\partial \mathbf{y}} = \mathbf{x}^{\top} \mathbf{A}, \tag{22.13}
$$

and since we are dealing with a scalar, and also since

$$\mathbf{x}_{1\times m}^\top \mathbf{A}_{m\times n} \mathbf{y}_{n\times 1} = (\mathbf{x}^\top \mathbf{A}\mathbf{y})^\top = \mathbf{y}_{1\times n}^\top \mathbf{A}_{n\times m}^\top \mathbf{x}_{m\times 1};$$

thus, from (22.13), we must have

$$\frac{\partial \left(\mathbf{y}^\top \mathbf{A}^\top \mathbf{x}\right)}{\partial \mathbf{x}} = \mathbf{y}^\top \mathbf{A}^\top. \tag{22.14}$$

The derivative of a quadratic form $\mathbf{x}_{1\times n}^\top \mathbf{A}_{n\times n} \mathbf{x}_{n\times 1}$ with respect to $\mathbf{x}$, assuming $\mathbf{A}$ (which in a quadratic form is always a square matrix) not being a function of $\mathbf{x}$, can be obtained from

$$\mathbf{x}^\top \mathbf{A}\mathbf{x} = \begin{pmatrix} x_1 & x_2 & \cdots & x_n \end{pmatrix} \begin{pmatrix} a_{11} & a_{12} & \cdots & a_{1n} \\ a_{21} & a_{22} & \cdots & a_{2n} \\ \vdots & \vdots & \ddots & \vdots \\ a_{n1} & a_{n2} & \cdots & a_{nn} \end{pmatrix} \begin{pmatrix} x_1 \\ x_2 \\ \vdots \\ x_n \end{pmatrix}$$

$$= \sum_{j=1}^{n} \left(\sum_{k=1}^{n} a_{kj} v_k \right) v_j,$$

thus

$$\frac{\partial (\mathbf{x}^\top \mathbf{A}\mathbf{x})}{\partial \mathbf{x}} = \partial_\mathbf{x} \left(\sum_{k=1}^{n} \left(\sum_{j=1}^{n} a_{jk} x_j \right) x_k \right)$$

$$= \partial_\mathbf{x} (a_{11}x_1 + a_{21}x_2 + \cdots + a_{n1}x_n) x_1 + \partial_\mathbf{x} (a_{12}x_1 + a_{22}x_2 + \cdots + a_{n2}x_n) x_2$$

$$+ \cdots + \partial_\mathbf{x} (a_{1n}x_1 + a_{2n}x_2 + \cdots + a_{nn}x_n) x_n$$

$$= \left(\partial_{x_1} (a_{11}x_1^2 + a_{21}x_2 + \cdots + a_{n1}x_1x_n) \cdots \partial_{x_n} (a_{11}x_1^2 + a_{21}x_2 + \cdots + a_{n1}x_1x_n) \right)$$

$$+ \left(\partial_{x_1} (a_{12}x_1x_2 + a_{22}x_2^2 + \cdots + a_{n2}x_2x_n) \cdots \partial_{x_n} (a_{12}x_1x_2 + a_{22}x_2^2 + \cdots + a_{n2}x_2x_n) \right)$$

$$+ \cdots + \left(\partial_{x_1} (a_{1n}x_1x_n + a_{2n}x_2x_n + \cdots + a_{nn}x_n^2) \cdots \partial_{x_n} (a_{1n}x_1x_n + a_{2n}x_2x_n + \cdots + a_{nn}x_n^2) \right)$$

$$= \left(2a_{11}x_1 + a_{21}x_2 + \cdots + a_{n1}x_n \ x_1 a_{21} \cdots a_{n1}x_1 \right)$$

$$+ \left(a_{12}x_2 \ a_{12}x_1 + 2a_{22}x_2 + \cdots + a_{n2}x_n \cdots a_{n2}x_2 \right)$$

$$+ \cdots + \left(a_{1n}x_n \ a_{2n}x_n \cdots a_{1n}x_1 + a_{2n}x_2 + \cdots + 2a_{nn}x_n \right)$$

$$= \left(a_{11}x_1 + \cdots + a_{n1}x_n \ a_{12}x_1 + \cdots + a_{n2}x_n \cdots a_{1n}x_1 + \cdots + a_{nn}x_n \right)$$

$$+ \left(a_{11}x_1 + \cdots + a_{1n}x_n \ a_{21}x_1 + \cdots + a_{2n}x_n \cdots a_{n1}x_1 + \cdots + a_{nn}x_n \right)$$

$$= \begin{pmatrix} x_1 & x_2 & \cdots & x_n \end{pmatrix} \begin{pmatrix} a_{11} & a_{12} & \cdots & a_{1n} \\ a_{21} & a_{22} & \cdots & a_{2n} \\ \vdots & \vdots & \ddots & \vdots \\ a_{n1} & a_{n2} & \cdots & a_{nn} \end{pmatrix}$$

$$+ \begin{pmatrix} x_1 & x_2 & \cdots & x_n \end{pmatrix} \begin{pmatrix} a_{11} & a_{21} & \cdots & a_{n1} \\ a_{12} & a_{22} & \cdots & a_{n2} \\ \vdots & \vdots & \ddots & \vdots \\ a_{1n} & a_{2n} & \cdots & a_{nn} \end{pmatrix}$$

hence

$$\frac{\partial (\mathbf{x}^\top \mathbf{A} \mathbf{x})}{\partial \mathbf{x}} = \mathbf{x}^\top \mathbf{A} + \mathbf{x}^\top \mathbf{A}^\top$$

$$= \mathbf{x}^\top (\mathbf{A} + \mathbf{A}^\top). \tag{22.15}$$

In the particular case of symmetric $\mathbf{A}$ the result (22.15) becomes:

$$\frac{\partial \left(\mathbf{x}^\top \mathbf{A} \mathbf{x}\right)}{\partial \mathbf{x}} = \mathbf{x}^\top \mathbf{A} + \mathbf{x}^\top \mathbf{A}$$

$$= 2\mathbf{x}^\top \mathbf{A}, \tag{22.16}$$

and since $\mathbf{A}^\top \mathbf{A}$ is symmetric by definition, then

$$\frac{\partial \left(\mathbf{x}^\top \mathbf{A}^\top \mathbf{A} \mathbf{x}\right)}{\partial \mathbf{x}} = 2\mathbf{x}^\top \mathbf{A}^\top \mathbf{A}. \tag{22.17}$$

22.4 Derivatives in the Regression Analysis and the *hat* Matrices

For the n subjects composing the sample we are studying, equations are written as follows:

$$y_1 = b_0 + b_1 x_{11} + b_2 x_{12} + \cdots + b_p x_{1p} + \epsilon_1$$

$$y_2 = b_0 + b_1 x_{21} + b_2 x_{22} + \cdots + b_p x_{2p} + \epsilon_2$$

$$\vdots = \qquad\qquad \vdots$$

$$y_i = b_0 + b_1 x_{i1} + b_2 x_{i2} + \cdots + b_p x_{ip} + \epsilon_i$$

$$\vdots = \qquad\qquad \vdots$$

$$y_n = b_0 + b_1 x_{n1} + b_2 x_{n2} + \cdots + b_p x_{np} + \epsilon_n$$

hence we can use the matrix form of the equation as follows:

$$
\begin{pmatrix} y_1 \\ y_2 \\ \vdots \\ y_n \end{pmatrix} = \begin{pmatrix} 1 & x_{11} & x_{12} & \cdots & x_{1p} \\ 1 & x_{21} & x_{22} & \cdots & x_{2p} \\ \vdots & \vdots & \vdots & \ddots & \vdots \\ 1 & x_{n1} & x_{n2} & \cdots & x_{np} \end{pmatrix} \begin{pmatrix} b_0 \\ b_1 \\ \vdots \\ b_p \end{pmatrix} + \begin{pmatrix} \epsilon_1 \\ \epsilon_2 \\ \vdots \\ \epsilon_n \end{pmatrix}.
$$

hence, putting

$$
\mathbf{y} = \begin{pmatrix} y_1 \\ y_2 \\ \vdots \\ y_n \end{pmatrix} ; \ \mathbf{X} = \begin{pmatrix} 1 & x_{11} & x_{12} & \cdots & x_{1p} \\ 1 & x_{21} & x_{22} & \cdots & x_{2p} \\ \vdots & \vdots & \vdots & \ddots & \vdots \\ 1 & x_{n1} & x_{n2} & \cdots & x_{np} \end{pmatrix} ; \ \mathbf{b} = \begin{pmatrix} b_0 \\ b_1 \\ \vdots \\ b_p \end{pmatrix} ; \ \boldsymbol{\epsilon} = \begin{pmatrix} \epsilon_1 \\ \epsilon_2 \\ \vdots \\ \epsilon_n \end{pmatrix},
$$

we write in a syntetic form

$$
\mathbf{y} = \mathbf{Xb} + \boldsymbol{\epsilon} \tag{22.18}
$$

in which $\mathbf{X}$ is a matrix of n rows (as many as the subjects) and $p + 1$ columns (as many as the number of unknown parameters), which in some textbooks is called *design matrix*. The assumptions for the model, in matrix form, are $E(\boldsymbol{\epsilon}) = \mathbf{0}$ and $\mathrm{cov}(\boldsymbol{\epsilon}) = \sigma^2 \mathbf{I}$.

If we call $\mathbf{X_d}$ the data matrix, we will be able to write the design matrix $\mathbf{X}$ in the form of a partitioned matrix:

$$
\mathbf{X} = \left(\mathbf{1} \mid \mathbf{X_d} \right)
$$

in which the first column is formed by the vector $\mathbf{1}$ having all n entries equal to 1, while the second column is the data matrix. The vector $\mathbf{b}$ of the unknown variables is, in turn, formed by $p + 1$ rows, e.g., by the number of unknowns incremented by one.

From Eq. (22.18) we write the error as

$$
\boldsymbol{\epsilon} = \mathbf{y} - \mathbf{Xb}, \tag{22.19}
$$

and since the sum of squares of all residuals can be written as the scalar $\boldsymbol{\epsilon}^\top \boldsymbol{\epsilon}$, then we may obtain $\hat{\mathbf{b}}$ (whose elements are the estimates $\hat{b}_k$ of single parameters), using the equation:

$$
\begin{aligned}
\boldsymbol{\epsilon}^\top \boldsymbol{\epsilon} &= (\mathbf{y} - \mathbf{Xb})^\top (\mathbf{y} - \mathbf{Xb}) \\
&= (\mathbf{y}^\top - \mathbf{b}^\top \mathbf{X}^\top)(\mathbf{y} - \mathbf{Xb}) \\
&= \mathbf{y}^\top \mathbf{y} - \mathbf{y}^\top \mathbf{Xb} - \mathbf{b}^\top \mathbf{X}^\top \mathbf{y} + \mathbf{b}^\top \mathbf{X}^\top \mathbf{Xb}.
\end{aligned} \tag{22.20}
$$

Note that in (22.20), both $\mathbf{y}^\top\mathbf{Xb}$ and $\mathbf{b}^\top\mathbf{X}^\top\mathbf{y}$ must be scalars. In the first case, we have the transpose $1 \times n$ of a vector which multiplies a matrix $n \times (p+1)$ which, in turn, multiplies a vector $(p+1) \times 1$; thus, the result is a scalar (a 1×1 vector). In the second case, we have a transposed $1 \times (p+1)$ vector multiplying a transpose matrix $(p+1) \times n$ which, in turn, multiplies a vector $n \times 1$; hence, we again obtain a scalar.

Therefore, dealing with two scalars, it must be

$$\mathbf{y}^\top\mathbf{Xb} = \mathbf{b}^\top\mathbf{X}^\top\mathbf{y};$$

thus, from (22.20) we obtain:

$$\boldsymbol{\epsilon}^\top\boldsymbol{\epsilon} = \mathbf{y}^\top\mathbf{y} - 2\mathbf{b}^\top\mathbf{X}^\top\mathbf{y} + \mathbf{b}^\top\mathbf{X}^\top\mathbf{Xb}. \qquad (22.21)$$

Now, we must find the values of $\mathbf{b}$ minimizing the error $\boldsymbol{\epsilon}^\top\boldsymbol{\epsilon}$; thus, as we do when dealing with scalars, we must derive equation (22.21) and then let it equal to zero. The derivative with respect to $\mathbf{b}$ is

$$\frac{\partial(\boldsymbol{\epsilon}^\top\boldsymbol{\epsilon})}{\partial\mathbf{b}} = \frac{\partial(\mathbf{y}^\top\mathbf{y})}{\partial\mathbf{b}} - 2\frac{\partial(\mathbf{b}^\top\mathbf{X}^\top\mathbf{y})}{\partial\mathbf{b}} + \frac{\partial(\mathbf{b}^\top\mathbf{X}^\top\mathbf{X}\beta)}{\partial\mathbf{b}}, \qquad (22.22)$$

where we see that on the r.h.s., starting from left, we find the derivative of a linear form, the derivative of a bilinear form, and the derivative of a quadratic form. Since $\mathbf{y}^\top\mathbf{y}$ does not depend on $\mathbf{b}$, we get:

$$\frac{\partial(\mathbf{y}^\top\mathbf{y})}{\partial\mathbf{b}} = 0, \qquad (22.23)$$

while both the linear form $\mathbf{b}^\top\mathbf{X}^\top\mathbf{y}$ and the quadratic form $\mathbf{b}^\top\mathbf{X}^\top\mathbf{Xb}$ are evidently functions of $\mathbf{b}$, and therefore, for what obtained in the section devoted to matrix derivatives, we have:

$$\frac{\partial(\mathbf{b}^\top\mathbf{X}^\top\mathbf{y})}{\partial\mathbf{b}} = \mathbf{X}^\top\mathbf{y} \qquad (22.24)$$

and

$$\frac{\partial(\mathbf{b}^\top\mathbf{X}^\top\mathbf{Xb})}{\partial\mathbf{b}} = 2\mathbf{X}^\top\mathbf{Xb}, \qquad (22.25)$$

since $\mathbf{X}^\top\mathbf{X}$ is evidently a symmetric matrix.

Substituting equations (22.23), (22.24), and (22.25) into (22.22), we get:

$$\frac{\partial(\boldsymbol{\epsilon}^\top\boldsymbol{\epsilon})}{\partial\mathbf{b}} = 0 - 2\mathbf{X}^\top\mathbf{y} + 2\mathbf{X}^\top\mathbf{Xb}$$

$$= 2(\mathbf{X}^\top\mathbf{Xb} - \mathbf{X}^\top\mathbf{y})$$

thus, to have $\partial(\boldsymbol{\epsilon}^\top\boldsymbol{\epsilon})/\partial\mathbf{b} = 0$, it must be

$$\mathbf{X}^\top\mathbf{X}\mathbf{b} - \mathbf{X}^\top\mathbf{y} = 0,$$

hence

$$\mathbf{X}^\top\mathbf{X}\mathbf{b} = \mathbf{X}^\top\mathbf{y}. \tag{22.26}$$

Premultiplying both sides of the above equation by $(\mathbf{X}^\top\mathbf{X})^{-1}$, we obtain:

$$(\mathbf{X}^\top\mathbf{X})^{-1}\mathbf{X}^\top\mathbf{X}\mathbf{b} = (\mathbf{X}^\top\mathbf{X})^{-1}\mathbf{X}^\top\mathbf{y}$$

and therefore

$$\mathbf{I}\mathbf{b} = (\mathbf{X}^\top\mathbf{X})^{-1}\mathbf{X}^\top\mathbf{y},$$

so that the estimator $\hat{\mathbf{b}}$ of $\mathbf{b}$ is

$$\hat{\mathbf{b}} = (\mathbf{X}^\top\mathbf{X})^{-1}\mathbf{X}^\top\mathbf{y}. \tag{22.27}$$

It is very easy to verify that $\hat{\mathbf{b}}$ is an unbiased estimator of $\mathbf{b}$, since using Eq. (22.26) we immediately see that the expected value $E(\hat{\mathbf{b}})$ is

$$\begin{aligned}
E(\hat{\mathbf{b}}) &= E((\mathbf{X}^\top\mathbf{X})^{-1}\mathbf{X}^\top\mathbf{y}) \\
&= (\mathbf{X}^\top\mathbf{X})^{-1}\mathbf{X}^\top\mathbf{X}\mathbf{b} \\
&= (\mathbf{X}^\top\mathbf{X})^{-1}(\mathbf{X}^\top\mathbf{X})\mathbf{b} \\
&= \mathbf{b},
\end{aligned}$$

and we can therefore define the *hat matrix* $\hat{\mathbf{H}}$ for the least squares regression

$$\hat{\mathbf{H}} = \mathbf{X}(\mathbf{X}^\top\mathbf{X})^{-1}\mathbf{X}^\top.$$

The hat matrix has a version also for the logistic regression: in this case, the hat matrix cannot be defined unless one uses the linear approximation:

$$\begin{aligned}
\mathbf{y} &= \mathbf{X}\mathbf{W}^{1/2}\beta + \epsilon \\
&= \mathbf{Z}\beta + \epsilon;
\end{aligned}$$

thus, the hat matrix for the logistic regression reads:

$$\hat{\mathbf{H}}_{\text{log}} = \mathbf{Z}(\mathbf{Z}^\top \mathbf{Z})^{-1} \mathbf{Z}^\top$$
$$= \mathbf{W}^{1/2} \mathbf{X}(\mathbf{X}^\top \mathbf{W}^{1/2} \mathbf{W}^{1/2} \mathbf{X})^{-1} \mathbf{X}^\top \mathbf{W}^{1/2}$$
$$= \mathbf{W}^{1/2} \mathbf{X}(\mathbf{X}^\top \mathbf{W} \mathbf{X})^{-1} \mathbf{X}^\top \mathbf{W}^{1/2}$$

being $\mathbf{W}$ a diagonal matrix whose diagonal entries are

$$w_i = g_i \pi(x_i)[1 - \pi(x_i)],$$

in which g_i denotes the subjects with the same value of the covariate $x = x_i$. With these premises, the i-th diagonal element of the hat matrix is

$$h_i = g_i \pi(x_i)[1 - \pi(x_i)]\mathbf{x}_i^\top (\mathbf{X}^\top \mathbf{W} \mathbf{X})^{-1} \mathbf{x}_i^\top$$

so that $\sum_i h_i$ is the number of parameters.

References

1. Dhrymes PJ. Mathematics for econometrics. New York: Springer; 2013.
2. Deisenroth MP, Faisal AA, Ong CS. Mathematics for machine learning. Cambridge: Cambridge University Press; 2020.

Differential Equations

23

A differential equation is an equation in which there is one or more derivatives involved: for example,

$$y'(x) = y, \tag{23.1}$$

where we are searching for an unknown function of x, such that its derivative is the function itself. Clearly, the solution should be $y = e^x$ since we already know that the derivative of e^x is e^x. However, this is not "the solution," but just one of the possible solutions. Indeed, if we take $y = 2e^x$, we see that

$$\frac{d(2e^x)}{dx} = 2e^x$$

and therefore also $y = 2e^x$ is a solution of (23.1), as well as any solution of the form $y = ke^x$, being k a real constant. Thus, how to obtain this "solution" for (23.1)? Let's first write it in the form:

$$\frac{y'(x)}{y} = \frac{1}{y}\frac{dy}{dx} = 1,$$

and then let's take the integral on both sides w.r.t. x, so as to have

$$\int \frac{1}{y}\frac{dy}{dx}dx = \int \frac{1}{y}dy = \int 1dx,$$

giving

$$\log(y) = x + C$$

thus passing to the exponentials

$$e^{\log(y)} = e^{x+C}$$

and since, by definition, $e^{\log(y)} = y$, then

$$y = e^C e^x$$
$$= Ce^x,$$

since $e^C \rightarrow C$ is a constant.

In some case the solution is easy: let us consider the differential equation:

$$\frac{d^2 y}{dx^2} - 3 = 0;$$

which is immediately changed in

$$\frac{d^2 y}{dx^2} = 3$$

such that we may integrate both sides obtaining

$$\int \frac{d^2 y}{dx^2} dx = \int 3 \, dx$$

thus

$$\frac{dy}{dx} = 3x + C_1$$

hence, integrating a second time we get

$$\int \frac{dy}{dx} dx = \int dy = \int (3x + C_1) dx$$

and therefore

$$y = \frac{3}{2} x^2 + C_1 x + C_2.$$

We can check the result by differentiating y twice, to get

$$y' = \frac{6}{2} x + C_1 = 3x + C_1$$

and

$$y'' = 3.$$

A differential equation can have solutions and also can have not solution; some are easy and immediate, and some others are very hard to be solved; in any case, a differential equation is one of the most reliable tools to investigate the evolution of a system, as we will see.

23.1 A Preamble: Linearity and Nonlinearity

The understanding of the concept of linearity, and therefore also the concept of nonlinearity, is of paramount importance for the study of differential equations. In general, when things sum up, we will deal with linearity, and when things do not exactly add, but there is some more or some less than an algebraic sum of the effects, or even if the effects are periodic in time, then we will deal with nonlinearity. The world is largely or (better) generally nonlinear, so that we can well say that linearity is just a particular case of the more general case of nonlinearity.

Pretend we are doing an experiment. We want to see if a system we are studying is able to respond to a given stimulus, and which kind of response we will be dealing with. A system, at present, can be everything: a vending machine, an electrical circuit, a living tissue, a population composed by many individuals, and so on. If we submit a stimulus (a signal, an input) x to our system, then we expect that the response (the output) y we will record will be somehow a function of x, so as to hypothesize a relation like $y = f(x)$. Now, let us send a first input x_1 to the system, so as to get the response $f(x_1)$, and then let us send a second input x_2, so as to get a second response $f(x_2)$. What will we have to expect if we will send a new input $x_3 = x_1 + x_2$? Will we observe a response $f(x_3) = f(x_1 + x_2) = f(x_1) + f(x_2)$, or maybe, should we expect a response $f(x_3)$ totally independent of $f(x_1)$ and $f(x_2)$? And, what will we have to expect sending another input $2x_1$, e.g., an input which is the exact double of the first one? Will we observe a response $f(2x_1) = 2f(x_1)$ which is exactly the double of the response $f(x_1)$?

It depends on the linearity or nonlinearity of our system. More precisely, being α a real constant, and being $f(x)$ continuous, if both equations

$$f(x_1) + f(x_2) = f(x_1 + x_2) \tag{23.2}$$

and

$$f(\alpha x_1) = \alpha f(x_1) \tag{23.3}$$

are simultaneously obeyed, then the system we are investigating is a *linear system*; note that conditions for linearity may be expressed by the unique relation:

$$\alpha f(x_1) \pm \beta f(x_2) = f(\alpha x_1 \pm \beta x_2), \tag{23.4}$$

being β also a real constant.

If, otherwise, we see that

$$f(x_1) + f(x_2) \neq f(x_1 + x_2)$$

or

$$f(\alpha x_1) \neq \alpha f(x_1),$$

then we are dealing with a *nonlinear system*.

The condition reported in Eq. (23.2) is called the *superposition condition*, while condition in Eq. (23.3) is called the *homogeneity condition*. We note that superposition implies homogeneity for any $f(x)$ when α is rational, while this implication holds also for α real, but only when $f(x)$ is continuous. The implication is instead not more valid when α is a complex number.

Any mathematical function $y = f(x)$ behaves somehow like a vending machine, which takes an input x and gives back an output y which depends on (or which is a function of) the input. For example, writing $y = 3x$, we acknowledge that we are dealing with a system which is able to give us an output equal to three times the input, so that doubling the input from x to $2x$ we will expect an output equal to $y = 3 \times (2x) = 6x$, and hence that system is a linear one. In other words, linearity means that adding two or more inputs $x_1 + x_2 + \cdots + x_n$ will always and everywhere produce an output equal to the sum of the elementary outputs $y_1 + y_2 + \cdots + y_n$, such that the behavior of a linear system, if the input is given by only one variable, is representable with a straight line on a x, y plane.

Nonlinearity is in general given by everything is not linear: we may write $\sin(2x) = 2\sin(x)$, but this equation is valid if and only if $x = \pi n$ (with $n \in \mathbb{N}$), and is not valid always, for any value of x, so that in general the inequality $\sin(2x) \neq 2\sin(x)$ holds. We also note that using the trigonometric "product to sum" formula, we have:

$$\sin(2x) = 2\sin(x)\cos(x);$$

thus, we also may infer $\sin(2x) = 2\sin(x)$, which would be true only in the particular case $\cos(x) = 1$, e.g., again, when $x = \pi n$; in any case, we can be sure that $\sin(x)$ is not linear, since a linear behavior observed only when $x = \pi n$ is like a broken clock that tells the exact time twice a day. Nonetheless, it is also true that $\sin(x) \approx x$ when x is very small. Thus, it would be possible, in some circumstances, to substitute $\sin(x)$ with x (we will see such a situation when dealing with the model of simple pendulum in one of the following sections), and to linearize the equations governing the system.

This is a generalized need for a scientist: indeed, it is much easier to deal with a linear system, so that the possibility of a linearization would render an easier approach to the analysis. However, this is not always a simple task, and requires a very accurate approach for any specific problem, because, if a linearization in possible, it cannot be equally usable in all the possible situations encompassed in an equation.

23.2   A First Experiment

Pretend we are doing an experiment: in a Petri dish with nutrient, a biologist places a strain of bacteria, so that its initial (at day zero, e.g., at $t = 0$) diameter is $y_0 = 1.2$ mm. Day by day, the biologist checks the diameter of the circular area (we assume the bacteria grow identically in all directions, so that the surface area they fill in the dish is an almost perfect circle) covered by the growing colony, measuring $y_1 = 2.4$ mm at day 1 ($t = 1$), $y_2 = 3.6$ mm at day 2 ($t = 2$), $y_3 = 4.8$ mm at day 3 ($t = 3$), $y_4 = 6.0$ mm at day 4 ($t = 4$), and $y_5 = 7.2$ mm at day 5 ($t = 5$).

Clearly, the biologist measures a constant growth of the diameter of the area occupied by the colony, corresponding to a 1.2-mm increase per day. Then, taking $n = \{1, 2, 3, 4, 5\}$, it is possible for him to write something like

$$\frac{y_n - y_{n-1}}{t_n - t_{n-1}} = 1.2 \text{ mm}$$

or also:

$$\frac{\Delta y}{\Delta t} = 1.2,$$

but since the rate of change of the diameter is constant, so it must be also the derivative; in particular, we recall that the general equation of a straight line reads:

$$y = mx + q = \frac{dy}{dx}x + q;$$

hence, we are allowed to write a relation like

$$\frac{dy}{dt} = 1.2, \tag{23.5}$$

that is, a *first order, linear differential equation* (the meanings of these terms will be clarified very soon), which can be solved by direct integration of both sides, since

$$dy = 1.2 \, dt$$

thus

$$\int dy = 1.2 \int dt$$

and, after integrating both sides,

$$y + C_1 = 1.2\,t + C_2$$

from which, defining $C = C_2 - C_1$ as a new constant given by the difference between the two constants of integration, we have the *general solution* of the differential equation in the form

$$y = 1.2\,t + C$$

which is a bundle of parallel lines. We may however be more specific, asking which must be the value of C, e.g., which straight line corresponds to the behavior of the system we are studying. This can be done by recalling that at $t = 0$, the biologist measured $y = 1.2$, so that our equation becomes

$$1.2 = 1.2 \times 0 + C\,;$$

hence, we see that the value satisfying the *initial conditions* is $C = 1.2$, and the equation describing the time evolution of the diameter of the bacteria strain is

$$y = 1.2\,t + 1.2 = 1.2(t + 1)\,,$$

e.g., the *particular solution* of the differential equation, that is, the solution arising taking into account the initial conditions, given by the (known) value of y when $t = 0$.

23.3   What Is a Differential Equation

A differential equation is an equation in which the unknown is not a variable, but a function of one or more variables [1–4]. The unknown function is obtained as the solution (if the solution exists) of this equation, which must contain at least one term in which the unknown function is expressed in form of derivative of any order $n > 0$, since with $n = 0$, we would have an algebraic or transcendental equation.

The *solution of a differential equation* does not necessarily exist and, if it actually exists, can be not unique. However, dealing, for example, with an unknown function of only one variable, we can obtain the solution of a differential equation of order n, if, and only if, in a given interval $t \in]t_1, t_2[$, there is at least one $y(t)$, derivable n times, and satisfying the differential equation in a *nontrivial* manner.

In a differential equation, the unknown function is often designed by y, while t is often normally used as independent variable, or as one of the independent variables. This convention has some practical implications, because, in most cases, the differential equations are used to analyze the evolution in time of a given system. It is important, at least in the very first steps of the study of the differential equation, to specify the variable dependence, for example, by writing $y'(t)$ instead of a simple y', even if the dependence can be evolved from the framework of a problem.

To define a derivative in a differential equation, there are several notations: in the scientific literature, a second derivative of the function y with respect to an independent variable t can be indifferently written as $\ddot{y}$ (the notation used by

Newton), $y''(t)$, y_{tt}, y_t^2, $\partial_{tt}\,y$, or even in more ways other than the usual Leibniz notation $\frac{d^2 y}{dt^2}$.

It is required that a differential equation is satisfied in a nontrivial manner, since one must distinguish an equation from an identity containing derivatives, which is commonly satisfied by any derivable function. For example,

$$\left(\frac{dy(t)}{dt}\right)^2 - 4 = \left(\frac{dy(t)}{dt} + 2\right)\left(\frac{dy(t)}{dt} - 2\right)$$

is not a differential equation, since it is an equality of the kind $a^2 - b^2 = (a+b)(a-b)$, satisfied by any $y(t)$, provided $y(t)$ continuous and derivable, and so, if it were a differential equation, any function $y(t)$ would be its solution, and this is not what should be expected from a differential equation.

An *ordinary differential equation* (ODE) having y as unknown function and t as independent variable (the ODEs have only one independent variable) takes the general form:

$$\xi\left(y, t, \frac{dy}{dt}, \frac{d^2 y}{dt^2}, \ldots, \frac{d^n y}{dt^n}\right) = 0,$$

while for a *partial differential equation* where y is the function and $t_1, \cdots, t_n$ the independent variables (they must be two, at least), the general form is

$$\zeta\left(y, t_1, \ldots, t_n, \frac{\partial y}{\partial t_1}, \ldots, \frac{\partial y}{\partial t_n}, \ldots, \frac{\partial^2 y}{\partial t_1^2}, \ldots, \frac{\partial^2 y}{\partial t_1 \partial t_2}, \ldots, \frac{\partial^n y}{\partial t_1 \cdots \partial t_n}\right) = 0.$$

23.4   More About $y'(t) = y$

We already saw how to deal with the simple differential equation:

$$\frac{dy(t)}{dt} = y(t);$$

obtaining a general solution

$$y(t) = e^t e^C$$

and being $e^C = k$ a constant, we can also write that solution in the form:

$$y(t) = ke^t,$$

and we will immediately see that would have been written as

$$y(t) = y(0)e^t .$$

Indeed, we may infer that e^t multiplied by any real number k (but also by any imaginary number) must be a solution; hence, to encompass all the infinite possible solutions, we write the *general solution* as $y(t) = ke^t$, being k a real constant, and this means whichever real constant, while $y(t) = e^t$, $y(t) = 3e^t$, and $y(t) = -5e^t$ are only three due to the different values assumed by k, respectively, $k = 1$, $k = 3$, and $k = -5$.

However, we may have a situation in which, say,

$$y(t) = 3e^t \tag{23.6}$$

is not a solution, but "the solution." It will be needed to define the *initial conditions* for the equation, or—in other words—the value of $y(0) = y_0$, e.g., the value of y at the beginning of the whole history, so that $y(t) = 3e^t$ will be the only solution compatible with the initial condition. In our case, if we put $y_0 = 3$, then we are saying $y_0 = 3e^0 = 3 \times 1 = 3$. In this case (differential equation, plus initial condition), we are facing the *Cauchy problem*, also called the , and we must not solve the differential equation alone, but the system

$$\begin{cases} \dfrac{dy(t)}{dt} = y(t) \\ y(0) = 3 \end{cases} .$$

Thus, we find:

$$y(0) = ke^0 = 3$$

or

$$y(0) = k = 3;$$

hence, for this differential equation, the constant k is the initial value y_0.

This differential equation is widely used in biology, in particular, it can be used to describe the growth of a population of individuals having unlimited resources in terms of food and territory (we are dealing with the so-called Malthus model), at least in its earliest stages, since after a given time passed from $t = 0$, this model becomes unrealistic.

We have briefly explored the role of the possible values assumed by k constant; we did not consider the case $k = 0$, where we obtain the trivial result $y(t) = 0e^t = 0$, which corresponds to an initial condition $y_0 = 0$.

We may now consider a slightly different situation, in which the differential equation is

$$\frac{\mathrm{d}y(t)}{\mathrm{d}t} = ny(t);$$

being n a real number. The general solution is very easy to obtain, since by integrating both sides we find

$$y(t) = ke^{nt}$$

so that the solution is strongly influenced by the value of n: if $n > 0$, the solution is an increasing exponential function, while, if $n < 0$, the solution is a decreasing exponential function. Of course, if $n = 0$, the solution is $y = k$, e.g., a constant function (a straight line parallel to the abscissa) indicating a population at a steady state.

23.5   A Basic Classification Scheme

There are many way to categorize the differential equations: for the moment, we cite some of the most used, like:

- **Ordinary differential equations vs. partial differential equations**. One calls *ordinary differential equation* (ODE) the differential equation in which the unknown function y and its derivatives depend only by a single independent variable t, while one calls *partial differential equation* (PDE) the differential equation in which the unknown function and its derivatives depend on two or more independent variables $t_1, t_2, \ldots, t_n$.
- **Linear vs. nonlinear differential equations**. An ordinary differential equation is *linear*: (1) if y and all its derivatives appear not raised at any power $n > 1$; (2) if the y is not the argument of any other function; (3) if the equation itself does not contain any term given as the product of y by any of its derivatives; if all of these requirements are not all simultaneously obeyed, then the equation is said *nonlinear*. For the partial differential equations, the classifications include linear, quasilinear, and nonlinear differential equations:
- **Autonomous vs. nonautonomous differential equations**. A differential equation is *autonomous* if the independent variable t does not appear explicitly, while, instead, the equation is said *nonautonomous*.
- **Homogeneous vs. nonhomogeneous differential equations**. A differential equation is *homogeneous* if all the terms are multiplied by y or by one of its derivatives, while, instead, the equation is said *nonhomogeneous*.
- **Order of a differential equation**. A differential equation is of n-th order (or of order n) if the highest derivative of y appearing in the equation is a n-th derivative.

We can do the following examples:

- Ordinary, linear, nonautonomous, second-order, nonhomogeneous differential equation

$$\frac{1}{t^3 + 2t - 1} \frac{d^2 y(t)}{dt^2} + \sin t \frac{dy(t)}{dt} - 2y(t) = t^2$$

  is an *ordinary* differential equation (y is a function of t only), *linear* (no y, nor its derivatives are multiplied between them, nor they are argument of a function, nor are raised to any power), *non autonomous* (two coefficients, $1/(t^3 + 2t - 1)$, and $\sin t$ are functions of t), of *second-order* (the highest derivative is a second derivative), *nonhomogeneous* (the term t^2 on the r.h.s. is not multiplied by y, nor by a derivative of y).

- Ordinary, linear, autonomous, fourth-order, homogeneous differential equation

$$\frac{d^4 y(t)}{dt^4} = y(t)$$

  is an *ordinary* differential equation (y is function of t only), *linear* (no y, nor its derivatives are multiplied between them, nor they are argument of a function, nor are raised to any power), *autonomous* (none of the coefficients of y or of y derivatives are function of t), of *fourth-order* (the highest derivative is a fourth derivative), *homogeneous* (all terms contain y or a derivative of y).

- Ordinary, nonlinear, nonautonomous, first-order, homogeneous differential equation

$$t(1 - t)y \frac{dy(t)}{dt} = 0$$

  is an *ordinary* differential equation (y is a function of t only), *nonlinear* (y is multiplied by one of its derivatives), *nonautonomous* (the coefficient $t(1-t)y$ of the derivative depends on t, other than y), of *first order* (the highest derivative is a first derivative), *homogeneous* (all terms contain y or a derivative of y).

- Ordinary, nonlinear, nonautonomous, first-order, nonhomogeneous differential equation

$$\left(\frac{dy(t)}{dt}\right)^2 = t + 1$$

  is an *ordinary* differential equation (y is a function of t only), *nonlinear* (the derivative of $y(t)$ is raised at second power), *nonautonomous* (the term $t + 1$ on the r.h.s. is a function of t), of *first-order* (the highest derivative is a first derivative), *nonhomogeneous* (the term $t + 1$ is not multiplied by y, nor by a derivative of y).

- Ordinary, nonlinear, autonomous, third-order, nonhomogeneous differential equation

$$\frac{k}{k-1}\frac{\mathrm{d}^3 y(t)}{\mathrm{d}t^3} + (3-k)^2 \frac{\mathrm{d}^2 y(t)}{\mathrm{d}t^2} - y(t)^2 + 1 = 0$$

is an *ordinary* differential equation (y is a function of t only), *nonlinear* ($y(t)$ is raised at second power compared in the third term), *autonomous* (all coefficients are constant, or they depend on the parameter k, which is not a function of t, nor of y), of *third- order* (the highest derivative is a third derivative), *nonhomogeneous* (the constant term 1 is not multiplied by y, nor by a derivative of y).
- Linear, autonomous, first-order in t, second order in x, partial differential equation

$$\frac{\partial y(x,t)}{\partial t} = \frac{\partial^2 y(x,t)}{\partial x^2}$$

is a *partial* differential equation, *linear*, *autonomous*, of *first order* in t and of *second order* in x (y is derived once with respect to t, and twice with respect to x).

A special emphasis must be assigned to difference between linear and nonlinear differential equations. From what we saw above, when a nonlinear differential equation must be used to describe the future evolution of a given system, we might face a situation in which the evolution depends on the solution itself, so that the solution can become a very hard goal. This can be the case we will encounter once we found a differential equation describing the future of a single individual, as well as the evolution of the whole mankind: in these cases, the future depends also on the individual itself, or on the mankind itself, and this would mean that it would be possibly unpredictable from an analytical point of view.

A simple rule to distinguish a linear ordinary differential equation of n-th degree from a nonlinear one is that a linear equation may be always written in the form:

$$a_n(t)\frac{\mathrm{d}^n y(t)}{\mathrm{d}t^n} + a_{n-1}(t)\frac{\mathrm{d}^{n-1} y(t)}{\mathrm{d}t^{n-1}} + \ldots + a_1(t)\frac{\mathrm{d}y(t)}{\mathrm{d}t} + a_0(t)y(t) = b(t),$$

the linearity of the ODE being totally independent of the form of the various $a_k(t)$ functions, which can either be linear (e.g., $a_j(t) = 3t + 1$) or nonlinear (say, $e^{\cos t}$); the only requirement is that at least for one of the $a_j(t)$ the condition $a_j(t) \neq 0$ is obeyed. Indeed, if an ODE can't be written in this form, then it can't be linear.

In a more compact form, we can also write:

$$\sum_{\alpha=0}^{n} a_k(t)\frac{d^\alpha y(t)}{dt^\alpha} = b(t);$$

and in the same way, we also may write a linear ordinary homogeneous differential equation of n-th degree in the form:

$$a_n(t)\frac{d^n y(t)}{dt^n} + a_{n-1}(t)\frac{d^{n-1} y(t)}{dt^{n-1}} + \ldots + a_1(t)\frac{dy(t)}{dt} + a_0(t)y(t) = 0$$

and hence

$$\sum_{k=0}^{n} a_k(t)\frac{d^k y(t)}{dt^k} = 0,$$

while a linear autonomous equation of n-th degree may be written as

$$a_n\frac{d^n y(t)}{dt^n} + a_{n-1}\frac{d^{n-1} y(t)}{dt^{n-1}} + \ldots + a_1\frac{dy(t)}{dt} + a_0 y(t) = 0$$

since the a_j are constant coefficients, and not more functions of t, so that its compact form is

$$\sum_{k=0}^{n} a_k\frac{d^k y(t)}{dt^k} = 0.$$

In the case of a linear equation of first degree, we also must bear in mind that there is another, quite different meaning of the term *homogeneous* differential equation, since a linear ODE is defined homogeneous also if it can be written as

$$\frac{dy(t)}{dt} = \Psi\left(\frac{y}{t}\right),$$

or, equivalently, as

$$P(y,t)\frac{dy(t)}{dt} + Q(y,t) = 0,$$

where $P(y,t)$ and $Q(y,t)$ are *homogeneous functions* of the same degree k, such that, for any $a \in \mathbb{R}$, it must be $P(ay,at) = a^k P(y,t)$ and $Q(ay,at) = a^k Q(y,t)$, and therefore we have:

$$\frac{P(ay,at)}{Q(ay,at)} = \frac{P(1,y/t)}{Q(1,y/t)} = \Psi\left(\frac{y}{t}\right).$$

Let us take the differential equation:

$$\frac{dy(t)}{dt} = y(t) \, ; \tag{23.7}$$

which we already encountered before. This equation tells that we must search for the unknown function which is equal to its first derivative. To find the solution, we first divide both sides by $y(t)$, to get

$$\frac{1}{y(t)} \frac{dy(t)}{dt} = 1$$

hence, integrating results

$$\int \frac{1}{y(t)} \frac{dy(t)}{dt} \, dt = \int 1 \, dt$$

$$\int \frac{y'(t)}{y(t)} \, dt = t + A \, , \tag{23.8}$$

where A is the integration constant.

The l.h.s. of above equation may be easily obtained integrating by substitution. Indeed, defining the new variable $u = y(t)$, such that $y'(t) = \frac{du}{dt}$, and $du = y'(t) \, dt$, we rewrite the l.h.s. integral as

$$\int \frac{y'(t)}{y(t)} \, dt = \int \frac{1}{u} y'(t) \, dt$$

$$= \int \frac{1}{u} \, du$$

$$= \log u + B$$

$$= \log(y(t)) + B, \tag{23.9}$$

B being a second integration constant. Using this result in the (23.8), we get:

$$\log(y(t)) + B = t + A$$

thus

$$y(t) = e^{-B} e^{t+A} = e^{A-B} e^t = C e^t$$

where $C = e^{A-B}$ is obviously a constant.

23.6   The Cauchy Problem

The *Cauchy problem*, which we may call also the *initial value problem* (IVP), is the search of the solutions of an ODE such that these solutions may satisfy the initial conditions. We already encountered the specification of initial conditions in a previous section, when dealing with Eq. (23.6). Moreover, as we anticipated in the section devoted to second Newton's law, if we are dealing with an ODE of order n, we would have to define n initial conditions, relative to a time that we arbitrarily define $t = 0$ for the value from $y(0)$, up to $y^{(n-1)}(0)$.

In practice, given the differential equation

$$\xi\left(y, t, \frac{dy}{dt}, \frac{d^2 y}{dt^2}, \ldots, \frac{d^n y}{dt^n}\right) = 0,$$

one must search for the solutions given by

$$y_0 = y(0)$$

$$y_0' = y'(0) = \left.\frac{dy(t)}{dt}\right|_{t=0}$$

$$y_0'' = y''(0) = \left.\frac{d^2 y(t)}{dt^2}\right|_{t=0}$$

until

$$y_0^{(n-1)} = y^{(n-1)}(0) = \left.\frac{d^{n-1} y(t)}{dt^{n-1}}\right|_{t=0}.$$

In general, one calls *Dirichlet condition* the initial condition to be attributed to y, and *Neumann condition* the condition to be attributed to a derivative $y^{(n)}$ of order n of y.

The *existence and uniqueness theorem* for a Cauchy problem says that the solution exists and this solution is also locally unique if f meets some opportune requirements.

Dealing with a Cauchy problem usually means to study the shape of the frontier of the domain of the equation, and to find a solution that may satisfy the Cauchy boundary conditions. In a second-order ODE, to get a particular solution, one must specify the value of the unknown function and its derivative at a given point at initial or the frontier of the domain of definition of the equation.

When studying a differential equation, an initial value problem is an ordinary differential equation together with a specific value of the unknown function at some point in the solution domain, called the initial condition. In the various fields of applied mathematics, many modeling techniques in physics, biology, or other sciences often require solving a problem at initial values. In this context, the differential equation is the description of the time evolution of a given event, depending on its initial conditions.

Assume we are dealing with a differential equation:

$$y'(t) = f(t, y(t))$$

with $f : \mathbb{R}^2 \to \mathbb{R}$, and to which corresponds a point in the domain of f

$$(t_0, y_0) \in \mathbb{R}^2$$

e.g., its initial condition.

A solution of an initial value problem is a function y that is the solution of the differential equation and that also satisfies the condition $y(t_0) = y_0$.

Dealing with higher-order problems, y can be a vector, with its derivatives from second to higher order. In other words, the unknown function y can take values in infinite-dimensional spaces, such as Banach spaces.

23.7   Linear Ordinary Differential Equations

We already saw that an ordinary differential equation is linear if, and only if, it can be written in the form:

$$a_n(t)\frac{\mathrm{d}^n y(t)}{\mathrm{d}t^n} + a_{n-1}(t)\frac{\mathrm{d}^{n-1} y(t)}{\mathrm{d}t^{n-1}} + \ldots + a_1(t)\frac{\mathrm{d}y(t)}{\mathrm{d}t} + a_0(t)y(t) = b(t) \qquad (23.10)$$

or in the more compact form

$$\sum_{k=0}^{n} a_k(t)\frac{\mathrm{d}^k y(t)}{\mathrm{d}t^k} = b(t)$$

where the various terms $a_k(t)$ can be some functions of t, or also some constants (also zero-valued), provided that at least one $a_n(t)$ and $a_1(t)$ is not a constant; otherwise (23.10) is not more a differential equation, but rather an algebraic or a transcendental equation. It is very important to know that if one of the $a_k(t)$ is a function of t, it can be either a linear or nonlinear one: the linearity or nonlinearity of the functions $a_k(t)$ does not affect the linearity of the differential equation, since this last depends only on the $y^{(k)}(t)$ appearing in the equation. In other words, if all the a_k functions depend on t only, or are constants, then the differential equation is linear, but if at least one of the a_k depends on y (only on y, or also on y), then the differential equation is nonlinear. In the case of first-order linear ODE, Eq. (23.10) reduces to the simpler form:

$$a_1(t)\frac{dy(t)}{dt} + a_0(t)y(t) = b(t) \tag{23.11}$$

in which it is required to have $a_1(t) \neq 0$ and that at least one of the conditions $a_1(t) \neq 0$ and $b(t) \neq 0$ are verified.

23.8   Solving a Linear First-Order ODE

Using the general form of an ordinary linear differential equation given in (23.10), we can write the form of a linear equation of order one as

$$\frac{dy(t)}{dt} + a(t)y(t) = b(t) \tag{23.12}$$

where, multiplying both members by a function $\phi(t)$, we have

$$\phi(t)\frac{dy(t)}{dt} + \phi(t)a(t)y(t) = \phi(t)b(t).$$

Now, imposing the condition

$$\phi(t)a(t) = \frac{d\phi(t)}{dt}, \tag{23.13}$$

so as to have also

$$a(t) = \frac{1}{\phi(t)}\frac{d\phi(t)}{dt} = \frac{\phi'(t)}{\phi(t)}, \tag{23.14}$$

we get:

$$\phi(t)\frac{dy(t)}{dt} + y(t)\frac{d\phi(t)}{dt} = \phi(t)b(t). \tag{23.15}$$

Bearing in mind the rule to be used to calculate the derivative of a product of two functions (here, $\phi(t)$ and $b(t)$), we also have:

$$\phi(t)\frac{dy(t)}{dt} + y(t)\frac{d\phi(t)}{dt} = \frac{d(\phi(t)y(t))}{dt}; \tag{23.16}$$

therefore, equating the r.h. sides of Eqs. (23.15) and (23.16), one gets:

$$\phi(t)b(t) = \frac{d(\phi(t)y(t))}{dt}$$

in other words

$$\int \phi(t)b(t)\,\mathrm{d}t = \int \frac{\mathrm{d}(\phi(t)y(t))}{\mathrm{d}t}\,\mathrm{d}t$$

$$= \phi(t)y(t) + c_1 \tag{23.17}$$

where c_1 is the integration constant.

From Eq. (23.17) we have:

$$y(t) = \frac{1}{\phi(t)}\left(k + \int \phi(t)b(t)\,\mathrm{d}t\right) \tag{23.18}$$

where $k = -c_1$ is the new integration constant.

On the basis of the assumption imposed, we immediately evolve:

$$a(t) = \frac{\mathrm{d}(\log \phi(t))}{\mathrm{d}t} \tag{23.19}$$

where, integrating both members, we obtain

$$\int a(t)\,\mathrm{d}t = \int \frac{\mathrm{d}(\log \phi(t))}{\mathrm{d}t}\,\mathrm{d}t$$

hence

$$\int a(t)\,\mathrm{d}t = \log \phi(t) + c_3$$

that is

$$\log \phi(t) = \int a(t)\,\mathrm{d}t - c_3$$

and, with the new integration constant $c_4 = -c_3$

$$\phi(t) = \exp\left(\int a(t)\,\mathrm{d}t + c_4\right)$$

$$= e^{c_4}\exp\left(\int a(t)\,\mathrm{d}t\right)$$

$$= \alpha \exp\left(\int a(t)\,\mathrm{d}t\right) \tag{23.20}$$

where, again, $\alpha = e^{c_4}$ is a constant.

At this point, using the value of $\phi(t)$ found with Eq. (23.20), and inserting it into (23.19), we obtain the solution $y(t)$ of the linear differential equation of order one (23.12):

$$
y(t) = \frac{\displaystyle\int \left(\alpha \exp \left(\int a(t)\,dt \right) b(t) \right) dt + k}{\displaystyle \alpha \exp \left(\int a(t)\,dt \right)}
$$

$$
= \frac{\displaystyle \alpha \int \left(\exp \left(\int a(t)\,dt \right) b(t) \right) dt + k}{\displaystyle \alpha \exp \left(\int a(t)\,dt \right)}
$$

$$
= \frac{\displaystyle\int \left(\exp \left(\int a(t)\,dt \right) b(t) \right) dt + C}{\displaystyle \exp \left(\int a(t)\,dt \right)} \tag{23.21}
$$

where $C = k/\alpha$ is the new integration constant.

23.9   Directly Integrable ODEs

A first-order directly integrable ODE reads:

$$
g'(t) = f(t)
$$

so that, recalling the fundamental theorem of calculus, we have

$$
g(t) = \int f(t)\,dt + C
$$

as the general solution.

If an initial condition is given, say $g(t_0) = g_0$, then we may also give the solution as the definite integral:

$$
g(t) = g(t_0) + \int_{t_0}^{t} f(\tau)\,d\tau.
$$

For example, assume to have

$$
g'(t) = t^2 - 2t + 1;
$$

we get:

$$g(t) = \int (t^2 - 2t + 1)dt$$

$$= \int t^2 dt - \int 2t dt + \int 1 dt$$

$$= \frac{1}{3}t^3 + C_1 - t^2 + C_2 + t + C_3$$

$$= \frac{1}{3}t^3 - t^2 + t + C,$$

being $C = C_1 + C_2 + C_3$, and applying the initial conditions $g(0) = 2$, we obtain:

$$2 = \frac{1}{3}2^3 - 2^2 + 2 + C$$

thus

$$C = \frac{4}{3}$$

so that, since $g(0) = 2$,

$$g(t) = \int (t^2 - 2t + 1)dt$$

$$= \frac{1}{3}t^3 - t^2 + t + \frac{4}{3}.$$

Alternatively, by definite integration

$$g(t) = g(0) + \int_2^t (\tau^2 - 2\tau + 1)d\tau$$

$$= 2 + \int_2^t \tau^2 d\tau - \int_2^t 2\tau d\tau + \int_2^t 1 d\tau$$

$$= 2 + \left(\frac{1}{3}t^3 - \frac{8}{3} - t^2 + 4 + t - 2 \right)$$

$$= \frac{1}{3}t^3 - t^2 + t + \frac{4}{3},$$

giving the same result obtained with the indefinite integration technique.

23.10 Superposition Principle for Homogeneous Equations

The *superposition principle* has been already introduced in a previous section, when we saw that in a linear homogeneous differential equation, any linear combination of the solutions is a solution, too. This superposition principle is the same one encountered defining the linearity of a response $f(x)$, when the condition $\alpha f(x_1) + \beta f(x_2) = f(\alpha x_1 + \beta x_2)$ are obeyed, being α and β two arbitrary constants.

The proof of the superposition principle for an ordinary differential equation of degree one is quite simple: let us assume that both $y_1(t)$ and $y_2(t)$ are solutions of the homogeneous equation:

$$\frac{dy(t)}{dt} = a(t)y(t) \tag{23.22}$$

so that we must have

$$\frac{dy_1(t)}{dt} = a(t)y_1(t)\,, \tag{23.23}$$

and

$$\frac{dy_2(t)}{dt} = a(t)y_2(t)\,. \tag{23.24}$$

Now, using the real-valued constants A_1 and A_2, let us try to verify if also the linear combination $A_1 y_1(t) + A_2 y_2(t)$ is a solution of Eq. (23.22), by checking validity of the relation:

$$\frac{d(A_1 y_1(t) + A_2 y_2(t))}{dt} = a(t)(A_1 y_1(t) + A_2 y_2(t))\,,$$

where we see that, from Eqs. (23.23) and (23.24), we have

$$\frac{d(A_1 y_1(t) + A_2 y_2(t))}{dt} = A_1 \frac{dy_1(t)}{dt} + A_2 \frac{dy_2(t)}{dt}$$

$$= A_1 a(t)y_1(t) + A_2 a(t)y_2(t)$$

$$= a(t)(A_1 y_1(t) + A_2 y_2(t))\,,$$

that is, the superposition principle for a homogeneous linear differential equation of first order is verified.

It is quite simple to apply the same procedure in the case of $n > 2$ solutions; at least, one may also assume that both $y_1(t)$ and $y_2(t)$ are linear combinations of other solutions.

The same reasoning may be applied to homogeneous equations of any order. For example, considering the linear homogeneous equation of order two

$$\frac{\mathrm{d}^2 y(t)}{\mathrm{d}t^2} = a_1(t)\frac{\mathrm{d}y(t)}{\mathrm{d}t} + a_2(t)y(t), \tag{23.25}$$

we still may assume that $y_1(t)$ and $y_2(t)$ are the solutions, so as to have

$$\frac{\mathrm{d}^2 y_1(t)}{\mathrm{d}t^2} = a_1(t)\frac{\mathrm{d}y_1(t)}{\mathrm{d}t} + a_2(t)y_1(t) \tag{23.26}$$

and

$$\frac{\mathrm{d}^2 y_2(t)}{\mathrm{d}t^2} = a_1(t)\frac{\mathrm{d}y_2(t)}{\mathrm{d}t} + a_2(t)y_2(t); \tag{23.27}$$

hence, we may verify if the linear combination $A_1 y_1(t) + A_2 y_2(t)$ (where, again, A_1 and A_2 are some constants) is a solution: in this case the equation

$$\frac{\mathrm{d}^2(A_1 y_1(t) + A_2 y_2(t))}{\mathrm{d}t^2} = a_1(t)\frac{\mathrm{d}(A_1 y_1(t) + A_2 y_2(t))}{\mathrm{d}t}$$
$$+ a_2(t)(A_1 y_1(t) + A_2 y_2(t)), \tag{23.28}$$

must be true.

Inserting (23.26) and (23.27) into (23.28), one obtains:

$$\frac{\mathrm{d}^2(A_1 y_1(t) + A_2 y_2(t))}{\mathrm{d}t^2} = A_1 \frac{\mathrm{d}^2 y_1(t)}{\mathrm{d}t^2} + A_2 \frac{\mathrm{d}^2 y_2(t)}{\mathrm{d}t^2}$$

$$= A_1 \left(a_1(t)\frac{\mathrm{d}y_1(t)}{\mathrm{d}t} + a_2(t)y_1(t) \right)$$

$$+ A_2 \left(a_1(t)\frac{\mathrm{d}y_2(t)}{\mathrm{d}t} + a_2(t)y_2(t) \right)$$

$$= A_1 a_1(t)\frac{\mathrm{d}y_1(t)}{\mathrm{d}t} + A_1 a_2(t)y_1(t)$$

$$+ A_2 a_1(t)\frac{\mathrm{d}y_2(t)}{\mathrm{d}t} + A_2 a_2(t)y_2(t)$$

$$= a_1(t)\left(A_1 \frac{\mathrm{d}y_1(t)}{\mathrm{d}t} + A_2 \frac{\mathrm{d}y_2}{\mathrm{d}t} \right)$$

$$+ a_2(t)(A_1 y_1(t) + A_2 y_2(t))$$

$$= a_1(t) \frac{d(A_1 y_1(t) + A_2 y_2(t))}{dt}$$

$$+ a_2(t)(A_1 y_1(t) + A_2 y_2(t)), \qquad (23.29)$$

which allows us to verify that the superposition principle is true also for the linear homogeneous equations of order two. The proof may be extended to homogeneous equations of whichever order.

23.11 First-Order Nonlinear ODEs

The first-order nonlinear equation most useful for further application is possibly the *Riccati equation* (after the Italian mathematician Jacopo Riccati), which is written as

$$\frac{dy(t)}{dt} = a(t)y(t) + b(t)y^2(t) + c(t), \qquad (23.30)$$

where $y^2(t)$ here stands for $[y(t)]^2$, and where we assume $a(t)$ and $b(t)$ be continuous, and $c(t)$ nonzero at least somewhere in the $\mathbb{R}$ subset in which the equation holds. Clearly, we are facing a nonlinear ODE, due to $y^2(t)$ term, but we may transform it to let it become a linear one. First, assume we know a particular solution $y_p(t)$ of the equation, so that we may write the general solution as $y(t) = y_p + z(t)$. Now, the Riccati equation reads:

$$\frac{d(y_p + z)}{dt} = \frac{dy_p(t)}{dt} + \frac{dz(t)}{dt} = a(t)(y_p + z) + b(t)(y_p + z)^2 + c(t)$$

$$= a(t)y_p(t) + a(t)z(t) + b(t)y_p^2(t)$$

$$+ b(t)z^2(t) + 2b(t)y_p(t)z(t) + c(t), \qquad (23.31)$$

from which we can cancel the terms not containing $z(t)$ and the (23.31) becomes a new differential equation called the *Bernoulli equation*

$$\frac{dz(t)}{dt} = b(t)z^2(t) + a(t)z(t) + 2b(t)y_p(t)z(t)$$

$$= b(t)z^2(t) + [a(t) + 2b(t)y_p(t)]z(t), \qquad (23.32)$$

which can be conveniently linearized by using the transformation $\frac{1}{x(t)} \leftarrow z(t)$, so that Eq. (23.32) becomes

$$\frac{d\left(\dfrac{1}{x(t)}\right)}{dt} = \frac{b(t)}{x^2(t)} + \frac{a(t) + 2b(t)y_p(t)}{x(t)}. \tag{23.33}$$

23.12 Exact ODEs

When a first-order nonlinear equation can be written in the form:

$$\frac{dy}{dt} = -\frac{P(t, y(t))}{Q(t, y(t))} \tag{23.34}$$

and therefore

$$Q(t, y(t))\, dy + P(t, y(t))\, dt = 0, \tag{23.35}$$

and if also there exists a function $Z(t, y(t))$ such that

$$Q(t, y) = \frac{\partial Z(t, y)}{\partial y};$$

$$P(t, y) = \frac{\partial Z(t, y)}{\partial t}$$

then we may rewrite (23.35) as

$$\frac{\partial Z(t, y)}{\partial y}\, dy + \frac{\partial Z(t, y)}{\partial t}\, dt = 0$$

from which, using the definition of total derivative, we deduce $dZ = 0$, or—in other words—that Z must be a constant, and (23.34) is defined an *exact differential equation*.

Thus, a candidate to be an exact ODE should be written as

$$P(t, y) + Q(t, y)\frac{dy}{dt} = 0,$$

where we realize that the equation is nonlinear, since the derivative of y is multiplied by a function of y.

Equation can be written as

$$Q(t, y)\frac{dy}{dt} = -P(t, y)$$

and

$$\frac{dy}{dt} = -\frac{P(t, y)}{Q(t, y)}.$$

Now, the unknown function $Z(t, y(t))$ must be chosen such that

$$\frac{\partial Z(t, y)}{\partial t} = P(t, y)$$

and

$$\frac{\partial Z(t, y)}{\partial y} = Q(t, y),$$

so that our equation can be written as

$$\frac{\partial Z(t, y)}{\partial t} + \frac{\partial Q(t, y)}{\partial y}\frac{dy(t)}{dt} = 0.$$

For example, consider the following ODE:

$$6ty + y^2 + (3t^2 + 2ty - 3)\frac{dy}{dt} = 0;$$

clearly, here we have:

$$P(t, y) = 6ty + y^2,$$

and

$$Q(t, y) = 3t^2 + 2ty - 3.$$

If we take

$$Z_1 = 3t^2y + ty^2,$$

then

$$\frac{\partial Z_1(t, y)}{\partial t} = 6ty + y^2 = P(t, y),$$

and if we take

$$Z_2 = 3t^2y + ty^2 - 3y,$$

then

$$\frac{\partial Z_2(t, y)}{\partial y} = 3t^2 + 2ty - 3 = Q(t, y).$$

However, in this case, we have $Z_1 \neq Z_2$, but our choice of Z must be aimed to find a function such that $Z = Z_1 = Z_2$; in other words, we have to take

$$Z(t, y) = 3t^2 y + ty^2 - 3y,$$

in order to get

$$\frac{\partial Z(t, y)}{\partial t} = 6ty + y^2;$$

$$\frac{\partial Z(t, y)}{\partial y} = 3t^2 + 2ty - 3.$$

At this point, invoking the total derivative of Z, we have:

$$\frac{\partial Z(t, y)}{\partial y} \, dy + \frac{\partial Z(t, y)}{\partial t} \, dt = d(3t^2 y + ty^2 - 3y) = 0$$

which means Z being equal to a constant C, e.g.,

$$3t^2 y + ty^2 - 3y = C,$$

from which we obtain a second-degree algebraic equation in the unknown y

$$ty^2 + (3t^2 - 3)y - C = 0,$$

so that we get the general solution using the well-known formula

$$y = \frac{-b \pm \sqrt{b^2 - 4ac}}{2a},$$

as

$$y(t) = \frac{-(3t^2 - 3) \pm \sqrt{(3t^2 - 3)^2 - 4tC}}{2t}$$

$$= \frac{3(1 - t^2) \pm \sqrt{9(t^4 - 2t^2 + 1) - 4tC}}{2t}$$

from which we may obtain the desired particular solutions on the basis of the choice of the initial conditions.

23.13 Infectious Disease Transmission

Pretend we are studying a region with N inhabitants, of which $S(t)$ are healthy and susceptible to being infected by a certain transmissible disease. We are not interested, at present, in which vector could be responsible for transmission, but we will assume that each encounter between vector and a susceptible individual is effective in determining the infection of that individual, but none of the infected inhabitants $I(t)$ will die because of the disease, so that we may take N as a constant, assuming that births and deaths balance and—since no immigration nor emigration processes are to be expected—thus no variations will occur in the number of inhabitants.

Under these somewhat unrealistic assumptions, we may write:

$$N = S(t) + I(t),$$

at any $t \geq 0$: in particular, at $t = 0$, we assume to have $I(0) = 1$, thus

$$N = S(0) + I(0) = S(0) + 1.$$

It is reasonable to hypothesize that at any given time t, the increase in the number of infected people $\frac{dI(t)}{dt}$ will depend somehow on the actual number of infected $I(t)$ (people able to spread the disease) as well as on the number of still susceptible subjects $S(t)$ (the number of potential disease recipients); hence, we can write the first-order nonlinear differential equation governing the epidemics as follows:

$$\frac{dI(t)}{dt} = \zeta S(t)I(t)$$
$$= \zeta(N - I(t))I(t), \tag{23.36}$$

ζ being some real proportional factor.

We may obtain the solution by writing

$$\frac{1}{(N - I(t))I(t)} \frac{dI(t)}{dt} = \zeta$$

and then integrating both sides

$$\int \frac{1}{(N - I(t))I(t)} \frac{dI(t)}{dt} \, dt = \int \zeta \, dt$$

to get

$$\frac{\log(I(t))}{N} - \frac{\log(I(t) - N)}{N} = \zeta t + C$$

being C the integration constant, and hence we obtain the general solution for $I(t)$ as

$$I(t) = \frac{Ne^{N(\zeta t + C)}}{e^{N(\zeta t + C)} - 1}.$$ (23.37)

This kind of model (called the SIS model) is used to model infectious diseases where individuals can be infected many times since there is not immunity (at least, no long-term immunity) after healing.

A somewhat more complicate situation would have been observed letting $N = N(t)$, e.g., don't assuming N as a constant value, but a function of time. In this case, Eq. (23.36) reads:

$$\frac{dI(t)}{dt} = \zeta(N(t) - I(t))I(t),$$ (23.38)

from which

$$-\frac{1}{I(t)^2}\frac{dI(t)}{dt} + \frac{\zeta N(t)}{I(t)} = \zeta;$$

thus, with the substitution $u(t) = \frac{1}{I(t)^2}$, we have:

$$\frac{du(t)}{dt} + \zeta N(t)u(t) = \zeta.$$

23.14 More About Infectious Diseases: The SIR Model

The SIR model is possibly the most known among the simplest mathematical models used in epidemiology to describe the spread of infectious diseases within a population of N individuals. With the SIR model, we are dealing with three compartments in which a population is divided at a given time t: (1) susceptible individuals $S(t)$; (2) infected individuals $I(t)$; and (3) recovered individuals $R(t)$. We assume that at $t = 0$, it must be $S(0) + I(0) + R(0) = N$, and $S(0), I(0), R(0) \geq 0$.

In this model, any individual can move from one compartment to another one, but we assume that to go from susceptibles to recovered compartment, an individual must pass through the infected compartment.

Susceptibles are all the subjects which have not yet been infected: the rate at which individuals become infected depends on the transmission rate, but also on the number of already infected people. As one would expect, the more the infected individuals, the higher the probability to be infected for a healthy subject at any encounter with another subject.

Infected are all individuals who are currently sick. The rate of infection depends on the transmission rate, as well as on the number of susceptible people. Assuming that people do not die for the disease, we evolve that all infected ones will become healthy at a rate depending on the recovery rate.

Recovered individuals recover from the disease and also acquire permanent immunity, at least for a significant period of time, which is sufficient to say—in terms of outbreak considered by the model. Thus, the compartment of recovered people is a state of no return.

The SIR model can be represented by a system of differential equations:

$$\frac{dS(t)}{dt} = -\frac{b}{N}S(t)I(t) \tag{23.39}$$

$$\frac{dI(t)}{dt} = \frac{b}{N}S(t)I(t) - I(t) \tag{23.40}$$

$$\frac{dR(t)}{dt} = rI(t) \tag{23.41}$$

where b is the disease transmission rate, e.g., the rate at which susceptible individuals are infected, and r is the recovery rate, e.g., the rate at which infected individuals become healthy again. Note that it must be

$$\frac{dS(t)}{dt} + \frac{dI(t)}{dt} + \frac{dR(t)}{dt} = 0$$

This model was due to Kermack and McKendrick and Carvalho and Goncalves have found an analytical solution for that model [5], so that we may write:

$$S(t) = S(0)\exp\left(-\frac{b}{N}\int_0^t I(t)dt\right)$$

$$I(t) = N - S(t) - R(t)$$

$$R(t) = R(0) + b\int_0^t I(t)dt.$$

In this model we also define the basic reproduction number R_0 as

$$R_0 = \frac{b}{r},$$

representing the number of new infections expected caused by a single infection when all individuals are susceptible. Indeed, since we find that the time elapsed between two encounters is approximated as

$$t_c = \frac{1}{b}$$

and that whereas the time needed for removing a subject from the infected pool is until removal is

$$t_r = \frac{1}{r},$$

then

$$\frac{t_r}{t_c} = \frac{\dfrac{1}{r}}{\dfrac{1}{b}} = \frac{b}{r} = R_0.$$

In the case $R_0 > 1$, we infer that an epidemic is actually underway, whereas, when $R_0 \leq 1$, no epidemic is underway.

We may note that from Eqs. (23.39), (23.40), and (23.41), we get:

$$\frac{dI(t)}{dS(t)} = \left(-\frac{b}{N}SI\right)^{-1}\left(\frac{\beta}{N}S(t) - r\right)I = \frac{Nr}{bS} - 1$$

thus

$$\int dI = \int\left(\frac{Nr}{b}\frac{1}{S} - 1\right)dS = \frac{Nr}{b}\int\frac{1}{S}dS - \int dS$$

and therefore, calculating the integrals, and bearing in mind that $I(0) = 1$ and $S(0) = N - 1$, we have:

$$S(t) + I(t) = N + \frac{Nr}{b}(\log(S(t)) - \log(N - 1)),$$

from which, since we expect that on the long run the number of infected will approach zero, passing to the limit $\Delta t \to +\infty$ we get

$$S_{+\infty} - N = \frac{Nr}{b}\log\frac{S_{+\infty}}{N - 1}$$

where $S_{+\infty} = S(t)|_{t \to +\infty}$.

23.15 Second-Order Linear ODEs

Consider the second-order homogeneous and autonomous differential equation:

$$y''(t) = y(t),$$

which is to say, we are in search for a function $y(t)$ equal to its second derivative. It is immediate to realize that the only two functions with this property are e^t and e^{-t}, so that (as the equation is homogeneous) the general solution is any linear combination of the two possible solutions, and hence, with the integration constants c_1 and c_2, we will have

$$y(t) = c_1 e^t + c_2 e^{-t} \, .$$

Let us now take a slightly more difficult second-order differential equation:

$$y''(t) = -y(t) \, ; \tag{23.42}$$

here we see that, again, two functions, respectively, e^{jt} and e^{-jt} have the property to be equal to their second derivative taken with the minus sign, since

$$\frac{\mathrm{d}}{\mathrm{d}t} \left(\frac{\mathrm{d}e^{jt}}{\mathrm{d}t} \right) = \frac{\mathrm{d}(j\, e^{jt})}{\mathrm{d}t} = -e^{jt} \, ,$$

and

$$\frac{\mathrm{d}}{\mathrm{d}t} \left(\frac{\mathrm{d}e^{-jt}}{\mathrm{d}t} \right) = \frac{\mathrm{d}(-j\, e^{-jt})}{\mathrm{d}t} = -e^{-jt} \, .$$

On the other hand, bearing in mind the Euler identity

$$e^{\pm jt} = \cos(t) \pm j \, \sin(t) \, ,$$

and using k_1 and k_2 as integration constants, the general solution is

$$
\begin{aligned}
y(t) &= k_1 e^{jt} + k_2 e^{-jt} \\
&= k_1 [\cos(t) + j \, \sin(t)] + k_2 [\cos(t) - j \, \sin(t)] \\
&= (k_1 + k_2) \cos(t) + j(k_1 - k_2) \sin(t)
\end{aligned}
$$

thus letting $c_1 = k_1 + k_2$ and $c_2 = j(k_1 - k_2)$, we may rewrite the general solution as

$$y(t) = c_1 \cos(t) + c_2 \sin(t) \, . \tag{23.43}$$

The approach we have seen is a general one with the second-order linear differential equation: to guess (to assume) a solution of the form $e^{\lambda t}$ and then to obtain the values of the constant λ to get the actual solution, in terms of exponentials or trigonometric functions.

23.16 Mass-Spring Systems and RLC Circuits

Consider a system done by a mass m and a spring with spring constant K connected in series with a wall, and at rest. If an external force $F_E(t)$ is applied to the mass, and a constant friction ξ is exerted on the whole system, then we can write the second-order nonhomogeneous linear differential equation:

$$m \frac{d^2 y(t)}{dt^2} + \xi \frac{dy(t)}{dt} + Ky(t) = F_E(t) \tag{23.44}$$

which is a general-purpose model of the *forced spring-mass system* (forced, since $F_E(t)$ is nonzero). There are, however, special cases of (23.44), where we can distinguish an *unforced system*, when $F_E(t) = 0$ for any t, where (23.44) becomes the homogeneous equation

$$m \frac{d^2 y(t)}{dt^2} + \xi \frac{dy(t)}{dt} + Ky(t) = 0, \tag{23.45}$$

while if the friction ξ is zero, then we are dealing with an *undamped system*, given by equation

$$m \frac{d^2 y(t)}{dt^2} + Ky(t) = F_E(t), \tag{23.46}$$

whereas if both $F(t) = \xi = 0$, then the system is both undamped and unforced, and governed by the homogeneous equation

$$m \frac{d^2 y(t)}{dt^2} + Ky(t) = 0. \tag{23.47}$$

The situation described by the mass-spring system has a general validity in many other cases, like an *electrical RLC circuit* having in series a resistance R, an inductance L, and a capacitance C, with a battery giving a voltage $v(t)$.

In this case, the current $i(t)$ (here $i(t)$ is the current intensity: nothing to do with $i = \sqrt{-1}$) passing through the circuit is given by the inhomogeneous differential equation

$$L \frac{d^2 i(t)}{dt^2} + R \frac{di(t)}{dt} + \frac{1}{C} i(t) = \frac{dv(t)}{dt} \tag{23.48}$$

which is evolved by differentiating with respect to t the well-known equation giving the total voltage $v(t)$ in a RLC circuit:

$$L \frac{di(t)}{dt} + Ri(t) + \frac{q(t)}{C} = v(t)$$

in which $q(t)$ is the electric charge, bound to the current by the well-known relation

$$i(t) = \frac{dq(t)}{dt}.$$

23.17 The Harmonic Oscillator

Let us take the homogeneous autonomous Eq. (23.47), and let us define:

$$\omega^2 = \frac{K}{m},$$

so as to write

$$\frac{d^2 y(t)}{dt^2} + \omega^2 y(t) = 0, \qquad\qquad (23.49)$$

which is known as the *harmonic oscillator*, where we implicitly assume $\omega^2 = 1$.

To solve (23.49), as seen before, we assume that a solution is $e^{\lambda t}$, for some constant λ, so as to rewrite our equation in the form

$$\frac{d^2 e^{\lambda t}}{dt^2} + \omega^2 e^{\lambda t} = 0;$$

thus, calculating the second derivative, we have:

$$\lambda^2 e^{\lambda t} + \omega^2 e^{\lambda t} = 0$$

and eliminating $e^{\lambda t}$

$$\lambda^2 = -\omega^2,$$

from which we obtain the values of λ

$$\lambda_1 = i\omega$$
$$\lambda_2 = -i\omega$$

then inserting the values found for λ, we get the general solution as the linear combination of the two solutions as follows:

$$y(t) = k_1 e^{i\omega t} + k_2 e^{-i\omega t}$$

which, using again the Euler identity, becomes

$$y(t) = k_1[\cos(\omega t) + i \sin(\omega t)] + k_2[\cos(\omega t) - i \sin(\omega t)]$$

thus

$$y(t) = (k_1 + k_2)\cos(\omega t) + i(k_1 - k_2)\sin(\omega t)$$

hence, using $A = k_1 + k_2$ and $B = i(k_1 - k_2)$, we write the general solution of the harmonic oscillator in the form:

$$y(t) = A\cos(\omega t) + B\sin(\omega t)\,, \tag{23.50}$$

where $\sqrt{A^2 + B^2}$ is the *amplitude* and

$$\omega = 2\pi\nu = \frac{2\pi}{T}$$

is the pulsation, ν being the frequency, and T the period.

Moreover, defining the new constants

$$Z_1 = \frac{A}{\cos(\phi)} = -\frac{B}{\sin(\phi)}\,,$$

$$Z_2 = \frac{A}{\sin(\phi + \pi/2)} = \frac{B}{\cos(\phi + \pi/2)}$$

we can rewrite (23.50) in the two equivalent forms:

$$y(t) = Z_1\cos(\omega t + \phi)$$
$$= Z_2\sin(\omega t + \phi + \pi/2)$$

where ϕ is the *phase* of the oscillator.

In the case of an electrical circuit, from (23.48) we easily evolve the equation of the harmonic oscillator in the form:

$$\frac{d^2 i(t)}{dt^2} + \frac{1}{LC}i(t) = 0\,,$$

where, again, using

$$\omega^2 = \frac{1}{LC}\,,$$

we get

$$\frac{d^2 i(t)}{dt^2} + \omega^2 i(t) = 0\,. \tag{23.51}$$

23.18 Homogeneous ODEs with Constant Coefficients

A second-order homogeneous linear ODE with constant coefficients takes (or can be reduced to) the form:

$$\frac{d^2 y(t)}{dt^2} + a\frac{dy(t)}{dt} + by(t) = 0 \tag{23.52}$$

and in general its solutions depend on e^t. This is indeed the more practical starting point to solve these equations: *to guess* a solution in the form $e^{\lambda t}$, being λ a scalar, so as to have, respectively

$$\frac{d^2 y(t)}{dt^2} = \lambda^2 e^{\lambda t}; \quad \frac{dy(t)}{dt} = \lambda e^{\lambda t}; \quad y(t) = e^{\lambda t}$$

thus (23.52) becomes

$$\lambda^2 e^{\lambda t} + a\lambda e^{\lambda t} + be^{\lambda t} = 0 \tag{23.53}$$

hence, eliminating the common factor $e^{\lambda t}$

$$\lambda^2 + a\lambda + b = 0 \tag{23.54}$$

and

$$\lambda_{1,2} = \frac{-a \pm \sqrt{a^2 - 4b}}{2} \tag{23.55}$$

or, in a more convenient form, like

$$\lambda_{1,2} = -\frac{a}{2} \pm \sqrt{\frac{a^2}{4} - b^2} \tag{23.56}$$

from which one may get the general solution $y(t)$ using the values found for λ, e.g.,

$$y(t) = C_1 e^{-a/2 + \sqrt{a^2/4 - b^2}} + C_2 e^{-a/2 - \sqrt{a^2/4 - b^2}} \tag{23.57}$$

where we used the fact that in a homogeneous DE with more distinct solutions, then also their sum is a solution.

As one may easily infer from (23.55) or, still better, from (23.56), the λ value depends on the difference $\Delta = a^24 - b^2$, according to the three possible cases: $\Delta < 0$, or $\Delta = 0$, or $\Delta > 0$, which are respectively realized when $a^2/4 < b^2$ (e.g., $a^2 < 4b^2$), $a^2/4 = b^2$ (e.g., $a^2 = 4b^2$) and $a^2/4 > b^2$ (e.g., $a^2 > 4b^2$):

- **Case 1:** $\Delta < 0$. When Δ is negative, then we have $\lambda_{1,2} = -a/2 \pm \omega i$, where $\omega = \sqrt{b^2 - a^2/4}$.
- **Case 2:** $\Delta = 0$. When $\Delta = 0$, we have two coincident solutions $\lambda_{1,2} = -\frac{a}{2}$.
- **Case 3:** $\Delta > 0$. When Δ is positive, then we have $\lambda_{1,2} = -a/2 \pm \omega$.

23.19 The Simple Pendulum

An oscillating pendulum of length l and mass m is suspended at a given point O: at maximum displacement, reached at the point M, it forms an angle μ with the vertical position OV, while during the oscillations (all dissipations are neglected), the angle formed with the vertical is $\theta(t)$.

When the pendulum is in vertical position (at point V), its potential energy is zero, and its kinetic energy reaches its maximum, and when the pendulum is in M, its potential energy reaches its maximum, while the kinetic energy is zero, since the instantaneous speed of oscillation in M is zero. Since in M the vertical distance is $l \cos \mu$, and in any other position the vertical distance is $l \cos \theta$, and since the velocity of oscillation is $l \frac{d\theta}{dt}$ then, in the absence of dissipation, we may invoke the correspondent differential equation by writing

$$\frac{1}{2}ml^2 \left(\frac{d\theta(t)}{dt} \right)^2 - mg(l \cos(\theta) - l \cos(\mu)) = 0, \tag{23.58}$$

where g is the acceleration of gravity.

Now, eliminating $m \neq 0$ and $l \neq 0$ in both sides, (23.58) reads:

$$\frac{1}{2}l \left(\frac{d\theta(t)}{dt} \right)^2 - g(\cos(\theta) - \cos(\mu)) = 0, \tag{23.59}$$

and taking the derivatives with respect to t of both sides, recalling the chain rule, for which

$$\left(\frac{d\theta(t)}{dt} \right)^2 = \frac{d \left(\frac{d\theta(t)}{dt} \right)^2}{d \left(\frac{d\theta(t)}{dt} \right)} \frac{d \left(\frac{d\theta(t)}{dt} \right)}{dt} = 2 \frac{d\theta(t)}{dt} \frac{d^2\theta(t)}{dt^2},$$

and

$$\frac{d \cos \theta}{dt} = \frac{d \cos \theta}{d\theta} \frac{d\theta(t)}{dt} = -\sin \theta \frac{d\theta(t)}{dt},$$

then

$$l \frac{d\theta(t)}{dt} \frac{d^2\theta(t)}{dt^2} + g \sin(\theta(t)) \frac{d\theta(t)}{dt} = 0 \qquad (23.60)$$

and hence

$$\frac{d^2\theta(t)}{dt^2} + \frac{g}{l} \sin(\theta(t)) = 0 \qquad (23.61)$$

which is a second-order nonlinear differential equation (because of the $\sin(\theta)$ term), but in the case of small oscillations, we can assume $\sin(\theta) \approx \theta$. Since the Taylor expansion for $\sin(\theta)$ is

$$\sin(\theta) = t - \frac{\theta^3}{3!} + \frac{\theta^5}{5!} - \frac{\theta^7}{7!} + \frac{\theta^9}{9!} + \cdots,$$

then we may say that for very small θ, we have:

$$\lim_{\theta \to 0} \frac{\theta^n}{n!} = 0$$

so, they rapidly decrease to zero, hence, we may (almost) correctly assume $\sin(\theta) \approx \theta$ with an error of order $O(\theta^3)$, for $|\theta| < \frac{\pi}{12}$, e.g., less than about 0.25 radians.

Thus, let us use

$$\frac{d^2\theta(t)}{dt^2} + \frac{g}{l} \theta(t) = 0 \qquad (23.62)$$

which is now a second-order linear differential equation; it can be solved assuming the solution be proportional to $e^{\lambda t}$, so that, substituting this value into Eq. (23.61), we get

$$\lambda^2 e^{\lambda t} + \frac{g}{l} e^{\lambda t} = \left(\lambda^2 + \frac{g}{l}\right) e^{\lambda t} = 0$$

thus, since $e^{\lambda t} \neq 0$, for all $\lambda \neq 0$, $t \neq 0$, then it must be

$$\lambda^2 + \frac{g}{l} = 0; \qquad (23.63)$$

hence, being g/l always greater than zero, we get:

$$\lambda_{1,2} = \pm i \sqrt{\frac{g}{l}}$$

where, as $\lambda_{1,2}$ is complex, we immediately verify the oscillatory nature of the solution thus, using the constants of integration k_1 and k_2, the general solution of the linearized simple pendulum is

$$\theta(t) = k_1 e^{-j\sqrt{g/l}t} + k_2 e^{j\sqrt{g/l}t}$$

$$= k_1 \left(\cos\left(\sqrt{\frac{g}{l}}t\right) - j\sin\left(\sqrt{\frac{g}{l}}t\right) \right)$$

$$+ k_2 \left(\cos\left(\sqrt{\frac{g}{l}}t\right) + j\sin\left(\sqrt{\frac{g}{l}}t\right) \right)$$

$$= k_1 \cos\left(\sqrt{\frac{g}{l}}t\right) - jk_1 \sin\left(\sqrt{\frac{g}{l}}t\right)$$

$$+ k_2 \cos\left(\sqrt{\frac{g}{l}}t\right) + k_2 j \sin\left(\sqrt{\frac{g}{l}}t\right)$$

$$= (k_1 + k_2) \cos\left(\sqrt{\frac{g}{l}}t\right) - j(k_1 - k_2)\sin\left(\sqrt{\frac{g}{l}}t\right)$$

$$= c_1 \cos\left(\sqrt{\frac{g}{l}}t\right) + c_2 \sin\left(\sqrt{\frac{g}{l}}t\right), \qquad (23.64)$$

where, as usual, $c_1 = k_1 + k_2$ and $c_2 = -i(k_1 - k_2)$ are the new constants of integration; moreover, we note that if, having used in Eq. (23.62) the substitution $\frac{g}{l} = \omega^2$, then (23.64) for the simple linearized pendulum would have the more familiar form:

$$\theta(t) = c_1 \cos(\omega t) + c_2 \sin(\omega t), \qquad (23.65)$$

in which we appreciate how the substitution $\frac{g}{l} = \omega^2$ may render less heavier the mathematical notation.

We may now assume the initial conditions for the linearized pendulum to get a specific particular solution: for example, letting $\theta(0) = \theta_0$ and $\theta'(0) = 0$, after a little algebra, we have:

$$\theta(t) = Z\cos(\omega t + \phi),$$

where, in analogy with the harmonic oscillator, $Z = \sqrt{c_1 + c_2}$ is the amplitude and ϕ the phase of oscillations.

23.20 A Linear Homogeneous Equation

As the first example of the solution of a linear ordinary differential equation, we use:

$$\frac{d^4 y(t)}{dt^4} = y(t) \tag{23.66}$$

e.g., a homogeneous differential equation in which the unknown function $y(t)$ is equal to its fourth derivative. We may start the search of the solution by asking ourselves which functions are known to be equal to their fourth derivative.

Indeed, there are some functions showing this behavior, and we may begin to look at first of them, e.g., $\sin(t)$, having the first derivative given by

$$\frac{d \sin(t)}{dt} = \cos(t) . \tag{23.67}$$

The last equation is itself a differential equation, which can be solved by integrating both members, to get

$$\int \frac{d \sin(t)}{dt} \, dt = \int \cos(t) \, dt$$

that is

$$\int \frac{d \sin(t)}{dt} \, dt = \sin(t) + C;$$

hence, we understand that some differential equations are immediately solvable, starting from the knowledge of the fundamental derivatives.

Indeed, using the formula for the cosine of a sum

$$\cos(t + \Delta t) = \cos(t) \cos(\Delta t) - \sin(t) \sin(\Delta t)$$

and the Taylor expansions, we easily see that the derivative of $\cos t$ is

$$\frac{d \cos t}{dt} = - \sin t. \tag{23.68}$$

thus, from (23.67) and (23.68), we deduce

$$\frac{d^4 \sin(t)}{dt^4} = \frac{d^3 \cos(t)}{dt^3} \tag{23.69}$$

$$= -\frac{d^2 \sin(t)}{dt^2} \tag{23.70}$$

$$= -\frac{d\cos(t)}{dt} = \sin(t), \tag{23.71}$$

and

$$\frac{d^4\cos(t)}{dt^4} = -\frac{d^3\sin(t)}{dt^3} \tag{23.72}$$

$$= -\frac{d^2\cos(t)}{dt^2} \tag{23.73}$$

$$= \frac{d\sin(t)}{dt} = \cos(t). \tag{23.74}$$

Therefore, given our differential equation (23.66), we see immediately from (23.69) and from (23.72) that one of its possible solutions is $\sin(t)$ and another one is $\cos(t)$, since also in this case we are dealing with a function equal to its fourth derivative. Moreover, one must point out that we would have found $\sin(t)$ and $\cos(t)$ among the possible solutions of the differential equation:

$$\frac{d^3 y(t)}{dt^3} = -\frac{dy(t)}{dy}, \tag{23.75}$$

or

$$\frac{d^4 y(t)}{dt^4} = -\frac{d^2 y(t)}{dy^2}, \tag{23.76}$$

or, even

$$\frac{d^2 y(t)}{dt^2} = -y(t). \tag{23.77}$$

At the same time, from calculus, we know that

$$\frac{d e^t}{dt} = e^t$$

hence, e^t is another possible solution of (23.66), since

$$\frac{d^4 e^t}{dt^4} = e^t, \tag{23.78}$$

as well as, it is a solution of all the following ODEs:

$$\frac{dy(t)}{dt} = y(t);$$

$$\frac{d^2 y(t)}{dt^2} = y(t); \qquad\qquad (23.79)$$

$$\vdots = \vdots \qquad\qquad (23.80)$$

$$\frac{d^n y(t)}{dt^n} = y(t); \qquad\qquad (23.81)$$

$$\vdots = \vdots \qquad\qquad (23.82)$$

However, we also know that

$$\frac{d\,e^{-t}}{dt} = -e^{-t};$$

thus, we will also have:

$$\frac{d^2 e^{-t}}{dt^2} = e^{-t};$$

$$\frac{d^3 e^{-t}}{dt^3} = -e^{-t}; \qquad\qquad (23.83)$$

$$\frac{d^4 e^{-t}}{dt^4} = e^{-t}; \qquad\qquad (23.84)$$

$$\vdots = \vdots \qquad\qquad (23.85)$$

so that also e^{-t} is a solution of (23.66).

At moment, we have seen that $\sin(t)$, $\cos(t)$, e^t and e^{-t} are functions of t having the peculiar property to be equal to their respective fourth derivative, so that any of these functions is a possible solution of (23.66).

But this property is not the only common property of these functions: indeed, just citing the more evident ones, we see that all are continuous in t, and can be derived an infinite number of times. Moreover, for any of them we note that the relationship

$$\frac{d^{4k} y(t)}{dt^{4k}} = y(t)$$

is always verified for $k = 1, 2, 3, \ldots$.

We would have to search for the existence of other elementary functions equal to their fourth derivative, but they are not (later we will understand how one may obtain this info); thus, the elementary functions which can be a solution of our differential equations are the only ones, but none of them can be the *general solution*.

Equation (23.66) is a linear homogeneous differential equation: it is linear, since $y(t)$ and its derivatives are not raised at any power, and are not multiplied among them, and are also homogeneous because the nonzero term in the equation depends on the unknown $y(t)$. Indeed, on the basis of the *superposition principle*, we see that if an ODE is linear and homogeneous, then, any linear combination of the solutions is also a solution, and hence the general solution of (23.66) is

$$y(t) = A\sin(t) + B\cos(t) + Ce^t + De^{-t}, \qquad (23.86)$$

where A, B, C, D are four arbitrary real constants, for which we must assume that they are not all simultaneously zero, since, in this case, the differential equation would become $y = 0$, which is not a solution since it does not satisfy the (23.66) (and this means that the superposition principle may be stated also as saying that any linear combination of at least two solutions is a solution, too).

For (23.86) we may verify the superposition principle, since by successive derivations of $y(t)$ we get

$$y(t) = A\sin(t) + B\cos(t) + Ce^t + De^{-t}$$

$$\frac{dy(t)}{dt} = A\cos(t) - B\sin(t) + Ce^t - De^{-t}$$

$$\frac{d^2y(t)}{dt^2} = -A\sin(t) - B\cos(t) + Ce^t + De^{-t}$$

$$\frac{d^3y(t)}{dt^3} = -A\cos(t) + B\sin(t) + Ce^t - De^{-t}$$

$$\frac{d^4y(t)}{dt^4} = A\sin(t) + B\cos(t) + Ce^t + De^{-t}$$

$$= y(t), \qquad (23.87)$$

so the linear combination $y(t)$ is actually equal to its fourth derivative.

23.21 Systems of Linear Differential Equations

A system of two ODEs, of first order with constant coefficients, may be written as

$$\begin{cases} \dfrac{dy_1(t)}{dt} = a_{11}y_1(t) + a_{12}y_2(t) \\ \dfrac{dy_2(t)}{dt} = a_{21}y_1(t) + a_{22}y_2(t) \end{cases} \qquad (23.88)$$

that is, in matrix form, as

$$\begin{pmatrix} y_1'(t) \\ y_2'(t) \end{pmatrix} = \begin{pmatrix} a_{11} & a_{12} \\ a_{21} & a_{22} \end{pmatrix} \begin{pmatrix} y_1(t) \\ y_2(t) \end{pmatrix}$$

and in a more compact form as

$$\mathbf{y}' = \mathbf{A}\mathbf{y}.\qquad\qquad(23.89)$$

Any solution $y_1(t)$, $y_2(t)$ of the system (23.88) defines a curve, lying on the plane y_1, y_2, and called the *trajectory*, or the *orbit* of the system.

There are numerous applications of the system of ordinary equations, going from the Lotka-Volterra model of prey-predator dynamics (see it in a next section), until the dynamics of love affairs described by the Strogatz's Romeo and Juliet model:

$$\begin{cases}\dfrac{dR(t)}{dt} = \alpha R(t) + \beta J(t)\\[2mm]\dfrac{dJ(t)}{dt} = \gamma R(t) + \delta J(t)\end{cases},$$

in which, at a given time t, we define $R(t)$ the Romeo's love or hate for Juliet, and $J(t)$ is the Juliet's love or hate for Romeo, while α, β, γ, δ are real constant, which can be also negative, depending on the reciprocal mood of the two lovers.

Applications to medical problems are found, for example, in *farmacokinetics*, where the gastrointestinal tract concentration $y(t)$ and the blood concentration $x(t)$ of a drug administered at a rate $r(t)$ are described by the system:

$$\begin{cases}\dfrac{dy(t)}{dt} = -ay(t) + r(t)\\[2mm]\dfrac{dx(t)}{dt} = ay(t) + bx(t)\end{cases},$$

where a, b are real constants.

Perhaps, the most important application of the systems of linear equations is the solution of ordinary differential equations of higher order: indeed, any ordinary differential equation can be transformed in a system of first-order linear equations. Thus, it can be possible to reduce a problem of order n to a system of ordinary differential equations, that is, for example, by using this kind of transformations:

$$y'(t) = x(t)$$
$$y''(t) = x_1(t)$$
$$y'''(t) = x_2(t)$$
$$\vdots\quad=\quad\vdots$$
$$y^{(n)}(t) = x_{n-1}(t)$$

We can see the following example given by a simple second-order differential equation:

$$\frac{d^2y(t)}{dt^2} + \frac{dy(t)}{dt} + y(t) = 0$$

which we rewrite

$$y''(t) + y'(t) + y(t) = 0$$

then, putting $y'(t) = x_2$ and $y(t) = x_1$

$$x_2'(t) + x_2 + x_1 = 0$$

thus, since $x_2 = x_1'$

$$\begin{pmatrix} x_1'(t) \\ x_2'(t) \end{pmatrix} = \begin{pmatrix} x_2(t) \\ -x_2 - x_1 \end{pmatrix}$$

$$= \begin{pmatrix} 0 & 1 \\ -1 & -1 \end{pmatrix} \begin{pmatrix} x_1 \\ x_2 \end{pmatrix},$$

then our system is

$$\begin{pmatrix} 0 & 1 \\ -1 & -1 \end{pmatrix} \begin{pmatrix} x_1 \\ x_2 \end{pmatrix} = \begin{pmatrix} x_1' \\ x_2' \end{pmatrix}.$$

A bit more complicate equation could be

$$\frac{d^3y(t)}{dt^3} + \frac{d^2y(t)}{dt^2} - \frac{dy(t)}{dt} + y(t) = 0$$

which reads

$$x_3' + x_3 - x_2 + x_1 = 0$$

thus

$$\begin{pmatrix} x_1'(t) \\ x_2'(t) \\ x_3'(t) \end{pmatrix} = \begin{pmatrix} 0 & 1 & 0 \\ 0 & 0 & 1 \\ -1 & 1 & -1 \end{pmatrix} \begin{pmatrix} x_1 \\ x_2 \\ x_3 \end{pmatrix}.$$

Matrices are an excellent tool for solving a system of ordinary differential equations: the general form, as we have seen, is

$$\mathbf{y}'(t) = \mathbf{A}\mathbf{y}(t) + \mathbf{f}(t) \tag{23.90}$$

thus

$$\begin{pmatrix} y_1'(t) \\ y_2'(t) \\ \vdots \\ y_n'(t) \end{pmatrix} = \begin{pmatrix} a_{11} & a_{12} & \cdots & a_{1n} \\ a_{21} & a_{22} & \cdots & a_{2n} \\ \vdots & \vdots & \ddots & \vdots \\ a_{n1} & a_{n2} & \cdots & a_{nn} \end{pmatrix} \begin{pmatrix} y_1(t) \\ y_2(t) \\ \vdots \\ y_n(t) \end{pmatrix} + \begin{pmatrix} f_1(t) \\ f_2(t) \\ \vdots \\ f_n(t) \end{pmatrix},$$

if we impose $\mathbf{f}(t) = \mathbf{0}$, then Eqs. (23.90) reduce to

$$\mathbf{y}'(t) = \mathbf{A}\mathbf{y}(t),$$

whose solution are said the complementary solutions of (23.90).

Computing the characteristic equation of matrix $\mathbf{A}$

$$\det(\mathbf{A} - \lambda \mathbf{I})$$

we obtain a polynomial in λ with degree n; its solutions are the eigenvalues λ_i of $\mathbf{A}$, and for any eigenvalue we can determine an eigenvector $\mathbf{w}_i$ such that

$$(\mathbf{A} - \lambda_i \mathbf{I})\mathbf{w}_k = \mathbf{0}.$$

23.22 Prey-Predator Models

For the time being, we have evaluated situations in which we estimated the variation of a single population with unlimited growth (Malthusian model) and with growth limited by environmental pressure, or by the availability of land, or by the limitation of resources that can sustain the population (Verhulst model). While the Malthusian model reduces almost exclusively to a theoretical exercise in explaining the resolution of a simple first-order differential equation, the Verhulst model (and those derived from it) may have some practical applications in describing the growth of certain bacterial populations, while other models, such as Gompertz's model (and those derived from it), have more general and practical applicability, in that they may be suitable for describing the differentiation and growth of certain types of cancer.

Now, however, we begin to deal with the dynamics of populations that may interact with each other, in particular, situations in which mutual influence occurs, in the sense that variation in one population induces variation in the other; variation that may be immediate or delayed. One of the simplest interactions from which to derive a mathematical model is the dynamics of two populations, one of which is predator and the other is prey: this is a model based on differential equations worked out at different times and independently by Lotka and Volterra, from whose discoverers the model is named. It must be assumed that the two populations live in a closed environment and that the predated species may have sufficient food resources to avoid extinction problems due to this cause; instead, the dynamics of the predator species will be solely dependent on the dynamics of the prey species.

Of course, this is a very simplified situation and also quite unlikely. In fact, this model analyzes a situation with only one predator per predated species, which is not very common in nature: for example, rabbits in the wild can be preyed upon by foxes, lynxes, and eagles sharing the same hunting territory. Moreover, it is not considered the goddess of the food chain, since almost always a predated species is also a predator and one predator is also preyed upon by another predator closer to the top of the same food chain. The Lotka-Volterra model, even in its simplicity, is the basis for the development of more complex models involving many other aspects of the possible interaction between different species and between individuals of the same species.

For two coexisting and interacting species in the same environment, say Y, and X, which are quantified at time t by respectively $y(t)$ and $x(t)$, we could write the system:

$$\begin{cases} \dfrac{dy(t)}{dt} = y(t)f(x, y, t) \\ \dfrac{dx(t)}{dt} = x(t)g(x, y, t) \end{cases},$$

where $f(x, y, t)$ and $g(x, y, t)$ are two (at moment) unknown functions corresponding to instant growth rate for $y(t)$ and $x(t)$. Two coexisting species may have various types of interaction: from no interactions at all, e.g., when

$$f(x, y, t) \rightarrow f(y, t);$$

$$g(x, y, t) \rightarrow g(x, t),$$

to competition for the same food, to symbiosis, cooperation, parasitism (optional, transient, permanent, etc.), or predation of species Y toward species X. However, even more complicated situations may exist, such as when adult individuals of species X prey on young individuals of species Y, but are prey for adult individuals of Y, or even cannibalism situations in which Y may feed even on individuals of the same species, perhaps when the availability of prey is reduced.

In the above system, we set growth rates depending on time: this is a situation that happens when the interaction is seasonal, or governed by factors such the varying availability of food for the predated species (if the prey is a herbivore, grass availability may depend on the season).

Assuming that both f and g do not depend on t: for the two species we now write:

$$\begin{cases} \dfrac{dy(t)}{dt} = y(t)f(x, y) \\ \dfrac{dx(t)}{dt} = x(t)g(x, y) \end{cases},$$

where, in the case of noninteraction, we have

$$\frac{\partial f(x, y)}{\partial x} = 0,$$

$$\frac{\partial g(x, y)}{\partial y} = 0,$$

while for cooperating species

$$\frac{\partial f(x, y)}{\partial x} > 0,$$

$$\frac{\partial g(x, y)}{\partial y} > 0,$$

for food competition

$$\frac{\partial f(x, y)}{\partial x} < 0,$$

$$\frac{\partial g(x, y)}{\partial y} < 0,$$

and for predation, assuming Y is the predator

$$\frac{\partial f(x, y)}{\partial x} > 0,$$

$$\frac{\partial g(x, y)}{\partial y} < 0,$$

and the general, the evolution may be rewritten:

$$\begin{cases} \dfrac{dy(t)}{dt} = [c_y + a_y x(t) + b_y y(t)]y(t) \\ \dfrac{dx(t)}{dt} = [c_x + a_x x(t) + b_x y(t)]x(t) \end{cases},$$

in which we note that from the values assumed by the constants we may deduce that

$$a_y = 0, b_x = 0 \implies Y, X \text{ non interacting}$$

$$a_y > 0, b_x > 0 \implies Y, X \text{ cooperators}$$

$$a_y < 0, b_x < 0 \implies Y, X \text{ competitors}$$

$$a_y < 0, b_x > 0 \implies Y \text{ prey}, X \text{ predator}$$

$$a_y > 0, b_x < 0 \implies Y \text{ predator}, X \text{ prey}$$

The situation can be defined by the new system:

$$\begin{cases} \dfrac{dy(t)}{dt} = \gamma a x(t) y(t) - \mu y(t) \\ \dfrac{dx(t)}{dt} = r x(t) - a x(t) y(t) \end{cases} \tag{23.91}$$

The Lotka-Volterra model is given by the couple of differential equations describing the time evolution of the predator population $y(t)$ depending on the dynamics of the prey population $x(t)$.

Since we may expect that the number of prey killed by predators is $-ax(t)y(t)$ (where the product $x(t)y(t)$ represents the encounter between prey and predator), while the predator number increment in the time unit is $\gamma a x(t) y(t)$ (where γ is the number of predators born in the time unit for each killed prey in the same time unit), so that we write where a, r, μ are positive constants.

For first, we remark that the number $y(t)$ of predators depends only on the availability of prey, so that, in the absence of predators (thus if $y(t) = 0$), the prey population dynamics becomes:

$$\frac{dx(t)}{dt} = rx(t),$$

which means

$$x(t) = x_0 e^{rt};$$

thus, prey in the absence of predators will grow in an exponential fashion.

In turn, predators in the absence of prey, thus with $x(t) = 0$, will be governed by the equation:

$$\frac{dy(t)}{dt} = -\mu y(t)$$

so that

$$y(t) = y_0 e^{-\mu t}$$

and predators will face extinction, as expected.

The Lotka-Volterra system may have local solution in the form:

$$y(t) = y(0) \exp \left(\int_0^t (\gamma a x(\tau) - \mu) \, d\tau \right)$$

$$x(t) = x(0) \exp \left(\int_0^t (r - a y(\tau)) \, d\tau \right).$$

however, in any case, rewriting the Lotka-Volterra equations as

$$\begin{cases} \dfrac{dy(t)}{dt} = \gamma a x(t) y(t) - \mu y(t) \\ \dfrac{dx(t)}{dt} = r x(t) - a x(t) y(t) - b x^2(t) \end{cases}$$

with a factor $bx^2(t)$ depending on the density added to the differential equation of $x(t)$, we obtain the following results on the long run:

$$\frac{\mu}{\gamma a} \geq \frac{r}{b} \implies \begin{cases} x(t)|_{t \to +\infty} = \dfrac{r}{b} \\ y(t)|_{t \to +\infty} = 0 \end{cases}$$

$$\frac{\mu}{\gamma a} < \frac{r}{b} \implies \begin{cases} x(t)|_{t \to +\infty} = \dfrac{\mu}{\gamma a} \\ y(t)|_{t \to +\infty} = \dfrac{r - \dfrac{b\mu}{\gamma a}}{a} \end{cases}.$$

References

1. Kamke E. Differentialgleichungen. Vol. I, 10. Auflage. Wiesbaden: Springer Fachmedien; 1983.
2. Kamke E. Differentialgleichungen. Vol. II, 6. Auflage. Wiesbaden: Springer Fachmedien; 1979.
3. Dobrushkin VA. Applied differential equations. Boca Raton: CRC Press; 2015.
4. Farlow SJ. Partial differential equations for scientists and engineers. New York: Wiley; 1982.
5. Carvalho AM, Goncalves S. An analytical solution for the Kermack–McKendrick model. Physica A 2021; 2021:125659.
6. Mishra BK, Saini DK. SEIRS epidemic model with delay for transmission of malicious objects in computer network. Appl Math Comput. 2007; 118:1476–1482.
7. Mouaouine A, Boukhouima A, Hattaf K, Yousfi N. A fractional order SIR epidemic model with nonlinear incidence rate. Adv Differ Equations 2018; 2018:160. https://doi.org/10.1186/s13662-018-1613-z

Introduction to Partial Differential Equations 24

In general, a partial differential equation (PDE) of order n takes the form:

$$F\left(x_1, \ldots, x_m, w, \frac{\partial w(x_1, \ldots x_m)}{\partial x_1}, \ldots, \frac{\partial w(x_1, \ldots x_m)}{\partial x_m}, \frac{\partial^2 w(x_1, \ldots x_m)}{\partial x_1^2}, \ldots, \right.$$
$$\left. \ldots, \frac{\partial^n w(x_1, \ldots x_m)}{\partial x_1^n}, \frac{\partial^n w(x_1, \ldots, x_m)}{\partial x_1^{n-1} \partial x_2}, \ldots, \frac{\partial^n w(x_1, \ldots x_m)}{\partial x_m^n}. \right) = 0,$$

$w(x_1, \ldots x_m)$ being the unknown function.

A PDE contains some partial derivatives, so that the unknown function we are searching for is a function of two or more independent variables.

24.1 First-Order PDEs

We define the first-order partial differential equations (PDEs) as

$$F\left(x, y, w, \frac{\partial w(x, y)}{\partial x}, \frac{\partial w(x, y)}{\partial y}\right) = 0; \quad (x, y) \in \Omega,$$

where the space $C^1(\Omega)$ is the space where the function $w(x, y)$ has continuous partial derivatives of first order, so that Ω is whichever region in the plane (x, y) in which the continuity of partial derivatives is satisfied: the graph of the function $w(x, y)$ identifies a surface $z = w$ in the (x, y, z).

The three most relevant types of first-order PDEs are

- linear first-order PDEs

$$p(x, y)\frac{\partial w(x, y)}{\partial x} + q(x, y)\frac{\partial w(x, y)}{\partial y} + r(x, y)w(x, y) + s(x, y) = 0$$

© The Author(s), under exclusive license to Springer Nature Switzerland AG 2025
M. Nichelatti, *Mathematical Tools for Telemedicine*, TELe-Health,
https://doi.org/10.1007/978-3-031-81709-0_24

- quasilinear first-order PDEs

$$p(x, y, w)\frac{\partial w(x, y)}{\partial x} + q(x, y, w)\frac{\partial w(x, y)}{\partial y} + r(x, y, w)w(x, y) = 0$$

- homogeneous first-order PDEs

$$p(x, y)\frac{\partial w(x, y)}{\partial x} + q(x, y)\frac{\partial w(x, y)}{\partial y} = 0$$

where p, q, r, and s are some given functions.

24.2   Second-Order PDEs

A special attention must be paid to second-order PDEs with two independent variables, say, x and t, which can be represented in the general form:

$$A(x, t)\frac{\partial^2 w}{\partial x^2} + B(x, t)\frac{\partial^2 w}{\partial x \partial t} + C(x, t)\frac{\partial^2 w}{\partial t^2}$$

$$+D(x, t)\frac{\partial w}{\partial x} + E(x, t)\frac{\partial w}{\partial t} + F(x, t)w + G(x, t) = 0, \tag{24.1}$$

being $A(x, t)$, $B(x, t)$, $C(x, t)$, $D(x, t)$, $E(x, t)$, $F(x, t)$, and $G(x, t)$ some functions of x and t, which can also be constants. If we are dealing with a second-order PDE containing only constant terms, then (24.1) reads:

$$A\frac{\partial^2 w}{\partial x^2} + B\frac{\partial^2 w}{\partial x \partial t} + C\frac{\partial^2 w}{\partial t^2} + D\frac{\partial w}{\partial x} + E\frac{\partial w}{\partial t} + Fw + G = 0, \tag{24.2}$$

from which we can distinguish three types of equations:

(1) *elliptic equations* :   if $B^2 - 4AC < 0$;
(2) *parabolic equations* : if $B^2 - 4AC = 0$;
(3) *hyperbolic equations* : if $B^2 - 4AC > 0$.

It must be clear that this classification is valid also when $B^2(x, t) - 4A(x, t)C(x, t)$ is a function of x and t, thus if A, B, and C ain't all constants. However, one must bear in mind that if $B^2 - 4AC$ is a function of some independent variables, then a second-order PDE may potentially switch from one type to another on the basis of the domain (we will not discuss these special cases).

In general, elliptic equations, like

$$\frac{\partial^2 w(x, y)}{\partial x^2} + \frac{\partial^2 w(x, y)}{\partial y^2} = 0$$

deal with vibration and wave phenomena, while parabolic equations, like

$$\frac{\partial^2 w(x, y)}{\partial x^2} - \frac{\partial w(x, y)}{\partial t} = 0,$$

describe diffusion and flow phenomena, and hyperbolic equations, like

$$\frac{\partial^2 w(x, y)}{\partial x^2} - \frac{\partial^2 w(x, y)}{\partial t^2} = 0,$$

arise when studying wave phenomena, or also when working with steady-state phenomena.

An interesting case is the Tricomi equation, which reads

$$\frac{\partial^2 w(x, y)}{\partial x^2} + x\frac{\partial^2 w(x, y)}{\partial t^2} = 0,$$

where we can observe that the equation is elliptic if $x > 0$, parabolic if $x = 0$, and hyperbolic if $x < 0$.

24.3 Solitons and Biological Systems

Solitons are solutions in the form of similar self-reinforcing waves that appear for some partial differential equations, which are nonlinear and describe a variety of physical phenomena. Solitons are stable, and do not change amplitude or shape over time, so their behavior is very different from that of normal waves, which lose energy as they move. Solitons do not lose energy because their nonlinear characteristic counteracts scattering and allows propagation virtually without dissipation even over long distances (think tsunamis); they can collide with each other, but after the interaction they continue unchanged (barring any phase change) toward their original destination.

Solitons can occur in various modes, such as kinks and antikinks, which have an upward and downward step shape, or as positive or negative soliton waves (light solitons and dark solitons): either way, they tend to propagate steadily without apparent energy dissipation. They have been observed in many physical phenomena, as waves in water, as optical solitons, as plasma solitons, but also in some biological phenomena including DNA replication.

Solitons are stable solutions of some nonlinear wave equations: among the most important ones, we recall the *Kortweg-de Vries (KdV) equation*:

$$\frac{\partial u(x,t)}{\partial t} + u\frac{\partial u(x,t)}{\partial x} + \frac{\partial^3 u(x,t)}{\partial x^3} = 0,$$

and the *sine-Gordon (SG) equation*

$$\frac{\partial^2 u(x,t)}{\partial t^2} - \frac{\partial^2 u(x,t)}{\partial x^2} + \sin(u) = 0.$$

In the "soliton jargon," these equations read in a more simpler form as

$$u_t + uu_x + u_{xxx} = 0,$$

and

$$u_{tt} - u_{xx} + \sin(u) = 0,$$

respectively.

The KdV equation can be solved replacing $u(x,t)$ with the new function $v(x, c - t)$, so as to rewrite it as

$$-cv' + vv' + v''' = 0$$

and then, after a couple of integrations and some rearrangements, one obtains the solution in the form:

$$u(x,t) = 3c\,\text{sech}^2\left(\frac{\sqrt{c}(x - ct)}{2}\right)$$

which is a solitary wave of amplitude $A = 3c$ traveling at a speed c.

The SG equation can be solved, again, with the substitution of $u(x,t)$ with the function $v(x, c - t)$: in this case, equation becomes:

$$c^2 v'' - v'' + \sin(v) = (c^2 - 1)v' v'' + v' \sin(v) = 0,$$

and, again, after integrating and with some rearrangements, we obtain the solution:

$$u(x,t) = 4\arctan\left(\exp\left(\frac{ct - x}{\sqrt{1 - c^2}}\right)\right),$$

where c is still the velocity of wave propagation.

Solitons are very important in communication technology because they allow signals to be sent without scattering: it is therefore not surprising to verify that the transmission of nerve signals takes place via solitons. Indeed, the soliton constituting the nerve potential transmission is the solution of the partial differential equation:

$$\frac{\partial^2(\Delta\rho)}{\partial t^2} = \left(s^2 + (p + q\Delta\rho)\,\Delta\rho - \sigma\frac{\partial^2}{\partial x^2}\right)\frac{\partial^2(\Delta\rho)}{\partial x^2},$$

where $\Delta\rho$ is the variation of the membrane density determined by the action potential, s is the sound velocity along the nerve membrane, p and q are functions of the elasticity of the nerve membrane, and σ is a parameter taking into account the frequency of the sound velocity along the nerve membrane.

24.4   Fractional Differential Equations in Epidemics

In a previous chapter, we have seen that if $f(x)$ is differentiable at least n times, then we may define a differential operator D such that

$$D^n f(x) = f^{(n)}(x) = \frac{d^n f(x)}{dx^n},$$

with

$$Df(x) = f'(x) = \frac{df(x)}{dx},$$

and

$$D^n = D^m D^{n-m}; \quad n \geq m,$$

in which, $m, n \in \mathbb{N}$.

The fractional differential equations (FDEs) are a class of differential equations that involve fractional derivatives and integrals. Unlike traditional differential equations, which deal with integer-order derivatives (e.g., first, second, third derivatives), fractional differential equations involve derivatives of non-integer order (fractional derivatives), often expressed as fractional exponents. These equations have applications in various scientific and engineering fields, especially in modeling systems with complex, memory-dependent behaviors.

The general form of a FDE can be expressed as

$$D^\alpha u(t) = f(t, u(t))$$

where $f(t, u(t))$ is a function depending on t and on the unknown function $u(t)$. The fractional derivative operator D^α is defined according to the chosen fractional operator model (say, Riemann-Liouville, or Caputo, or others).

FDEs are used to model systems with complex dynamics, viscoelastic phenomena, systems with memory, until infection outbreak and spreading among populations, so their potential applicability ranges to practically all modelizable systems. However, the solution of a FDE is generally not easy at all, and often can be obtained only by means of numerical simulations.

As we saw, FDEs are widely applicable in the modeling of epidemic dynamics, providing a likely and realistic approach to the complex temporal evolution of an infectious disease, which depends on many factors like heterogeneity of the population immune response and possible anomalous behaviors in disease transmission. The option of the fractional order and FDE may then depend on the characteristics of the infection and infective agent and also on the available historical and current data, and on their reliability.

For example, a fractional SIR model has been proposed by Mouaouine et al. in the form:

$$\begin{cases} D^\alpha S(t) = \Lambda - \mu S(t) - \dfrac{\beta S(t)I(t)}{1 + \alpha_1 S(t) + \alpha_2 I(t) + \alpha_3 S(t)I(t)} \\ D^\alpha I(t) = -(1 + d + r)I(t) + \dfrac{\beta S(t)I(t)}{1 + \alpha_1 S(t) + \alpha_2 I(t) + \alpha_3 S(t)I(t)} \\ D^\alpha R(t) = rI(t) - \mu R(t) \end{cases},$$

reduced to

$$\begin{cases} D^\alpha S(t) = \Lambda - \mu S(t) - \dfrac{\beta S(t)I(t)}{1 + \alpha_1 S(t) + \alpha_2 I(t) + \alpha_3 S(t)I(t)} \\ D^\alpha I(t) = -(1 + d + r)I(t) + \dfrac{\beta S(t)I(t)}{1 + \alpha_1 S(t) + \alpha_2 I(t) + \alpha_3 S(t)I(t)} \end{cases}$$

since $R(t)$ does not appear in the first two equations. Obviously, $S(0) > 0$, and $I(0) > 0$.

The fractional derivative used in this model is the Caputo operator:

$$D^\alpha f(t) = \frac{1}{\Gamma(1 - \alpha)} \int_0^t \frac{1}{(t - x)^\alpha} f'(x) dx$$

defined over $0 < \alpha \le 1$, whereas Λ is the recruitment rate of the population at risk of the population, d is the death rate caused by the infection, μ is the death rate due to other causes, r is the recovery rate of the sick individual becoming healthy again, while in the functional response term

$$F(t) = \frac{\beta S(t)I(t)}{1 + \alpha_1 S(t) + \alpha_2 I(t) + \alpha_3 S(t)I(t)}$$

we find the infection rate β and the constants $\alpha_1, \alpha_2, \alpha_3 \geq 0$. The basic reproduction number of the model is

$$R_0 = \frac{\beta \Lambda}{(\mu + d + r)(\mu + \alpha_1 \lambda)}.$$

Note that in the possible case $\alpha_1 = \alpha = \alpha_3 = 0$, we would have

$$F(t) = \beta S(t) I(t)$$

so that the model would be reduced to

$$\begin{cases} D^\alpha S(t) = \Lambda - \mu S(t) - \beta S(t) I(t) \\ D^\alpha I(t) = \beta S(t) I(t) - (1 + d + r) I(t). \end{cases}$$

FDEs can account for spacetime heterogeneity in the population (nonlinear variations in individuals) and in the diffusion of the disease: this can be frequent in situations where population changes due to internal movements in the long run (immigration) and in the short period (commuting): in the latter case, potentially infected individuals, or those with the disease incubating, can carry the infection over medium to long distances facilitating the spread of the disease: this would also facilitate a fractal-like epidemic, since diffusion patterns would become self-similar on some different spatiotemporal scales.

24.5 An Example of Computer Virus Propagation in a Network

Some models have been proposed for the computer virus propagation: for example, according to Mishra and Saini, where the computer (node) population $N(t)$ at time t in a network may be expressed as

$$N(t) = S(t) + E(t) + I(t) + R(t),$$

being $S(t)$ the susceptibles, $E(t)$ the exposed, $I(t)$ the infected, and $R(t)$ the recovered nodes. The assumptions at the basis of these models are as follows: (1) any new node is susceptible; (2) the death rate ε due to virus attack is constant in any node; (3) the death rate μ not due to computer virus is constant in any node; (4) latent period ω is constant; (5) the temporary immune period τ is constant; (6) the waiting time in I, E, and R subpopulations is distributed in an exponential way; (7) when a node is not more infected, it acquires a temporary probabilistic immunity p, and can become infectious again with a probability $1 - p$.

From these assumptions, Mishra and Saini obtained an expression for $S(t)$, $E(t)$, $I(t)$, and $R(t)$ subpopulations as follows:

$$\frac{dS(t)}{dt} = bN(t) - \mu S(t) - \gamma \frac{S(t)I(t)}{N(t)} + \alpha I(t - \tau)e^{-\mu\tau},$$

$$E(t) = \int_{t-\omega}^{t} \gamma \frac{S(u)I(u)}{N(u)} e^{-\mu(t-u)} du,$$

$$\frac{dE(t)}{dt} = \gamma \frac{S(t)I(t)}{N(t)} - \gamma \frac{S(t-\tau)I(t-\tau)}{N(t-\tau)} e^{-\mu\omega} - \mu E(t)$$

$$\frac{dI(t)}{dt} = \gamma \frac{S(t-\omega)I(t-\omega)}{N(t-\omega)} e^{-\mu\omega} - (\mu + \varepsilon + \alpha)I(t),$$

$$R(t) = \int_{t-\tau}^{t} p\alpha I(u)e^{-\mu(t-u)} du,$$

$$\frac{dR(t)}{dt} = p\alpha I(t) - \alpha I(t - \tau)e^{-\mu\tau} - \mu R(t)$$

where α is the recovery rate and b the per capita birth rate, whereas γ is the number of contacts per unit time of a node times the probability of infection.

References

1. Drazin PG, Johnson RS. Solitons: an introduction. New York: Cambridge University Press; 1989.
2. Mishra BK, Saini DK. SEIRS epidemic model with delay for transmission of malicious objects in computer network. Appl Math Comput 2007;118:1476–82.
3. Mouaouine A, Boukhouima A, Hattaf K, Yousfi N. A fractional order SIR epidemic model with nonlinear incidence rate. Adv Differ Equ 2018:160. https://doi.org/10.1186/s13662-018-1613-z.

Some Mathematics for Neural Networks

25

Given the general architecture of a neural network (one input layer + at least one hiddel layer + one output layer) and given the information transmitted from the input layer, we may figure the transmission to the first hidden layer given by the matrix of weights which premultiplies the vectors of inputs as follows:

$$
\begin{pmatrix}
w_{11} & w_{12} & \cdots & w_{1n} \\
w_{21} & w_{22} & \cdots & w_{2n} \\
\vdots & \vdots & \ddots & \vdots \\
w_{m1} & w_{m2} & \cdots & w_{mn}
\end{pmatrix}
\begin{pmatrix}
x_1 \\ x_2 \\ \vdots \\ x_n
\end{pmatrix}
=
\begin{pmatrix}
y_1 \\ y_2 \\ \vdots \\ y_m
\end{pmatrix}
\longrightarrow
\begin{pmatrix}
f(y_1) \\ f(y_2) \\ \vdots \\ f(y_m)
\end{pmatrix},
$$

so we have n nodes in the input layer characterized by the x input data, which send the weighted signals to m nodes of the following layer, which produce m activating functions $f(y_k)$ [1, 2]. The output of the n-th layer is the input for the $(n + 1)$-th layer. We see that we are dealing just with a linear vector transformation, where we did not use the bias input so as not to burden the mathematical formalism.

25.1 Activation Functions

We already introduced the activation functions: we recall here the most known as follows:

$$A_{\text{lin}}(x) = \lambda x; \tag{25.1}$$

$$A_{\text{ramp}}(x) = \begin{cases} x & \text{if } x \geq 0 \\ 0 & \text{if } x < 0 \end{cases}; \tag{25.2}$$

$$A_{\text{log}}(x) = \frac{1}{1 + e^x}; \tag{25.3}$$

M. Nichelatti, *Mathematical Tools for Telemedicine*, TELe-Health,
https://doi.org/10.1007/978-3-031-81709-0_25

$$A_{\text{tanh}}(x) = \frac{e^x - e^{-x}}{e^x + e^{-x}};$$ (25.4)

$$A_{\text{step}}(x) = \begin{cases} 1 \text{ if } x \geq 0 \\ 0 \text{ if } x < 0 \end{cases}.$$ (25.5)

We see that activation functions may have profound effects on the $f(y_k)$ values: Eq. (25.1) is a simple linear transformation multiplying the output by a scalar λ, and leaving it unchanged in the case $\lambda = 1$, where in Eq. (25.2) we have a ramp, representing a linear behavior if $y \geq 0$, while the function is zero for negative y. In Eq. (25.3) we use a logistic activation function which represents a sigmoid curve ranging from 0 (when x approaches $-\infty$) to $+1$ (when x approaches $+\infty$), while in Eq. (25.4) we use a logistic activation function corresponding to a hyperbolic tangent, also representing a sigmoid curve, but ranging from -1 to $+1$. The last equation presented (25.5) is the Heaviside step, in which any value of $y \geq 0$ is flattened to one, and any value of $y < 0$ is flattened to zero.

25.2   Loss Function

During the training, we use the loss function L (also called the cost function) to measure how far is the network result from the target: for this purpose we can use many cost functions [1, 2], like the very simple sum of squared errors:

$$L = \sum_{k=1}^{n} (t_k - o_k)^2,$$

where t_k are the targets and o_k the outputs, or else the more complex cross-entropy:

$$L = -\sum_{k=1}^{n} t_k \log(h(o_k)) = -\sum_{k=1}^{n} t_k \log \frac{e^{o_k}}{\sum_{j=1}^{n} e^{o_j}},$$

where $h(o_k)$ is the softmax activation function. It is immediate to verify that if all outputs match the target, the L is zero, whereas, if all the outputs differ from the targets, then L tends to infinity.

The loss function must be minimized to minimize the difference between output and target: the most used technique is the *gradient descent*, consisting in obtaining the derivative of L with respect to the weights w, and then to go ahead in the direction in which L decreases, such that, for any layer jump from n to $n + 1$, one has:

$$w_{n+1} = w_n - \rho \frac{\partial L}{\partial w_n},$$

where ρ is the learning rate, so the weights w are gradually corrected and adjusted, until the output is reasonably close to the expected target.

25.3 Backpropagation: The Chain Rule in Neural Networks

Assume we are dealing with a very simple network; assume also that we want to know the specific effect exerted by a weight w on the generic loss function L. It will generally be a composed function of the weight, such that, for example,

$$L = p(q(r(s(t(w)))))$$

so that

$$\frac{\partial L}{\partial w} = \frac{\partial L}{\partial p} \frac{\partial p}{\partial q} \frac{\partial q}{\partial r} \frac{\partial r}{\partial s} \frac{\partial s}{\partial t} \frac{\partial t}{\partial w}.$$

In practice, we can compute and save the gradient at any step along the layers, and calculate $\frac{\partial L}{\partial w}$ at any node, which will be used when going back along the layers: the technique is called *backpropagation*.

At this point, we can also take the loss function L, to see how the given weight $w_{n-1,n}$ between the hidden nodes $n-1$ and n influences the error: hence, for a single path, if the total error is Z, we get:

$$\frac{\partial L}{\partial w_{n_{l-1},n_l}} = \frac{\partial n_l}{\partial w_{n_{l-1},n_l}} \frac{\partial L}{\partial Z} \left(\frac{\partial L}{\partial n_j} \prod_{k=l}^{j-1} \frac{\partial n_{k+1}}{\partial n_k} \right),$$

whereas, for a set of different paths n_l toward the output, we have:

$$\frac{\partial L}{\partial w_{n_{l-1},n_l}} = \frac{\partial n_l}{\partial w_{n_{l-1},n_l}} \frac{\partial L}{\partial Z} \left(\sum_{n_l} \frac{\partial L}{\partial n_j} \prod_{k=l}^{j-1} \frac{\partial n_{k+1}}{\partial n_k} \right).$$

References

1. Deisenroth MP, Faisal AA, Ong CS. Mathematics for machine learning. Cambridge: Cambridge University Press; 2020.
2. Jiang H. Machine learning fundamentals. Cambridge: Cambridge University Press; 2021.

The manufacturer's authorised representative in the EU is Springer
Nature Customer Service Centre GmbH, Europaplatz 3, 69115 Heidelberg,
Germany. If you have any concerns regarding our products, please
contact ProductSafety@springernature.com

Printed and bound by CPI Group (UK) Ltd, Croydon, CR0 4YY
29/04/2026
02099535-0002